# Applied AI and Computational Intelligence in Diagnostics and Decision-Making


Danish Ather
*Amity University, Tashkent, Uzbekistan*

Ng Khai Mun
*Kuala Lumpur University of Science and Technology (KLUST), Malaysia*

Sachin Jain
*Ajay Kumar Garg Engineering College, Ghaziabad, India*

Vishal Jain
*Kuala Lumpur University of Science and Technology (KLUST), Malaysia & Vivekananda Institute of Professional Studies, New Delhi, India*

Vinay Kukreja
*Chitkara University Institute of Engineering and Technology, Chitkara University, India*



IGI Global
Scientific Publishing
Publishing Tomorrow's Research Today

Vice President of Editorial Melissa Wagner
Director of Acquisitions Mikaela Felty
Director of Book Development Jocelynn Hessler
Production Manager Mike Brehm
Cover Design Jose Rosado

Published in the United States of America by
IGI Global Scientific Publishing
701 East Chocolate Avenue
Hershey, PA, 17033, USA
Tel: 717-533-8845 | Fax: 717-533-7115
Website: https://www.igi-global.com E-mail: cust@igi-global.com



Library of Congress Cataloging-in-Publication Data

Names: Ather, Danish editor | Ng, Khai Mun, 1984- editor | Jain, Sachin, 1986- editor | Jain, Vishal, 1983- editor | Kukreja, Vinay editor
Title: Applied AI computational intelligence in diagnostics and decision-making / edited by Danish Ather, Khai Mun Ng, Sachin Jain, Vishal Jain, Vinay Kukreja.
Description: Hershey, PA : IGI Global Scientific Publishing, [2026] | Includes bibliographical references and index. | Summary: "This book aims to provide a clear understanding of how AI models learn from interactions and continuously improve decision-making"-- Provided by publisher.
Identifiers: LCCN 2025019851 (print) | LCCN 2025019852 (ebook) | ISBN 9798337333113 hardcover | ISBN 9798337333120 paperback | ISBN 9798337333137 ebook
Subjects: LCSH: Medicine--Decision making--Data processing | Reinforcement learning | Medical care--Decision making | Medical informatics
Classification: LCC R859.7.D42 H37 2026 (print) | LCC R859.7.D42 (ebook)
LC record available at https://lccn.loc.gov/2025019851
LC ebook record available at https://lccn.loc.gov/2025019852

British Cataloguing in Publication Data
A Cataloguing in Publication record for this book is available from the British Library.

# Table of Contents

**Preface**.......................................................................................................... xvi

**Chapter 1**
AI and Computational Intelligence in Healthcare: An Introductory Guide........... 1
*Sanchali Kapoor, SAITM, India*
*Reeta Parmar, SAITM, India*
*Neetu Sharma, Galgotias University, India*
*Puneet Garg, KIET Group of Institutions, India*
*Narinder Jit Singh, INTI International University, Malaysia*

**Chapter 2**
Introduction to AI and Computational Intelligence in Healthcare ...................... 27
*G. Sivakarthi, Anna University, India & Velammal College of Engineering and Technology, India*
*A. Vinora, Velammal College of Engineering and Technology, India*
*Nancy Deborah R., Velammal College of Engineering and Technology, India*
*M. Soundarya, Velammal College of Engineering and Technology, India*

**Chapter 3**
AI-Powered Healthcare Solutions: Bridging the Medical Gap in Underserved Communities Worldwide ........................................................................... 57
*Leelawati Pokhrel, SAITM, India*
*Mohd Arsalan, SAITM, India*
*Priyanka Rani, GITAM University, India*
*Puneet Garg, KIET Group of Institutions, India*
*Placido Rogerio Pinheiro, University of Fortaleza, Brazil*

**Chapter 4**
Machine Learning and Computational Intelligence for Smart Healthcare: Advancing Diagnosis and Treatment ........ 87
*Siva Subramanian R., SRM Institute of Science and Technology, India*
*R. Asha, Sathyabama Institute of Science and Technology, India*
*J. Sangeetha, S.A. Engineering College, India*
*A. Adaikkammai, RMD Engineering College, India*
*T. Thilagam, Vel Tech Rangarajan Dr. Sagunthala R&D Institute of Science and Technology, India*
*P. Aparna, RMK College of Engineering and Technology, India*

**Chapter 5**
Advancing Healthcare With Predictive Analytics for Disease Diagnosis and Risk Assessment ........ 111
*Siva Subramanian R., SRM Institute of Science and Technology, India*
*Subhash Chandra N., CVR College of Engineering, India*
*S. Vijayaselvarani, Veltech Tech Multi Tech Dr. Rangarajan Dr. Sakunthala Engineering College, India*
*Anand Babu R., Panimalar Engineering College, India*
*Anto Gracious L. A., R.M.K. College of Engineering and Technology, India*
*K. Jeyakarthika, Ramco Institute of Technology, India*
*D. Raja, Thiagarajar College of Engineering, India*

**Chapter 6**
Harnessing Predictive Analytics for Disease Diagnosis and Risk Assessment: Transforming Preventive Healthcare With AI ........ 133
*Mukul Sharma, Swami Vivekanand Subharti University, Meerut, India*
*Shashiraj Teotia, Swami Vivekanand Subharti University, Meerut, India*
*Vivek Aggarwal, Ajay Kumar Garg Engineering College, Ghaziabad, India*
*Vikas Sharma, SRM Institute of Science and Technology, Delhi, India*
*Tarun Kumar Vashishth, IIMT University, Meerut, India*
*Barkha Samania, SRM Institute of Science and Technology, Delhi, India*

**Chapter 7**
Collaborative Health Intelligence: Federated Learning as the Foundation of Future Medical Care ........ 163
*Mohammad Nasar, Mazoon College, Oman*
*Mohammad Abu Kausar, University of Nizwa, Oman*
*Nasser Al Musalhi, Mazoon College, Oman*

**Chapter 8**
Medical Imaging and Radiology: AI-Powered Diagnostics ............................. 191
*Swathi V. N. V. L. S., CVR College of Engineering, India*
*S. Sugapriya, Velammal Engineering College, India*
*Suraj Garg, Chandigarh Group of Colleges, Jhanjeri, India*
*Amruta Mahalle, Datta Meghe Institution of Management Studies, India*
*Atharva Umakant Yewale, Datta Meghe Institute of Management Studies, India*
*P. Selvakumar, Department of Science and Humanities, Nehru Institute of Technology, Coimbatore, India*
*Manjunath T. C., Rajarajeswari College of Engineering, India*

**Chapter 9**
AI-Driven Clinical Decision Support Systems Enhancing Decision-Making in Modern Healthcare ........................................................................... 219
*Vikas Sharma, SRM Institute of Science and Technology, Delhi, India*
*Tarun Kumar Vashishth, IIMT Univeristy, Meerut, India*
*Renu Kumar, IIMT Engineering College, Meerut, India*
*Sanjukta Vidyant, Shobhit University, Meerut, India*
*Asheesh Pandey, ABES Engineering College, Ghaziabad, India*
*Barkha Samania, SRM Institute of Science and Technology, Delhi, India*

**Chapter 10**
AI-Enhanced Clinical Decision-Making Through a Collaborative Approach .. 249
*Ravikumar R. N., Marwadi University, Rajkot, India*
*S. Aarthi, Marwadi University, Rajkot, India*
*Bekhzod Ruzimbaev Saparbaevich, Mamun University, Khiva, Uzbekistan*
*Satheesh Kumar A., Nandha Engineering College, Erode, India*
*Muhabbat Jumaniyozova, Urgench State University, Urgench, Uzbekistan*
*Shakhnoza Toshova, Termez University of Economics and Service, Termez, Uzbekistan*

**Chapter 11**
Reinforcement Learning for Adaptive Healthcare: Deep Q-Networks in Clinical Decision Optimization........................................................................ 281
*Mohammad Arafah, University of Petra, Jordan*
*Ahmad Aladawi, Loughborough University, UK*

**Chapter 12**
Optimizing Personalized Treatment Decisions Using Deep Q-Networks in Reinforcement Learning ........ 315
*Arpita Nayak, KIIT School of Liberal Studies, KIIT University, India*
*Ipseeta Satpathy, KSOM, KIIT University, India*
*Vishal Jain, School of Engineering & Technology, Vivekananda Institute of Professional Studies, New Delhi, India*

**Chapter 13**
Learning to Heal: Deep Q-Networks as the Future of AI-Driven Healthcare ... 337
*Sapandeep Kaur Dhillon, Guru Nanak Dev University, Amritsar, India*
*Ikvinderpal Singh, Trai Shatabdi Guru Gobind Khalsa College, Amritsar, India*
*Parminder Kaur, Guru Nanak Dev University, Amritsar, India*

**Chapter 14**
Drug Discovery and Optimization With AI ........ 379
*Dipesh Uike, Dr. Ambedkar Institute of Management, Studies, and Research, India*
*S. Sugapriya, Velammal Engineering College, India*
*Manpreet Kaur, Chandigarh Group of Colleges, Jhanjeri, India*
*Amruta Mahalle, Datta Meghe Institution of Management Studies, India*
*Neha Dhule, Datta Meghe Institute of Management Studies, India*
*P. Selvakumar, Department of Science and Humanities, Nehru Institute of Technology, Coimbatore, India*
*Manjunath T. C., Rajarajeswari College of Engineering, India*

**Chapter 15**
Future Trends in AI and Smart Healthcare ........ 405
*Amandeep Kaur, Chandigarh Group of Colleges Jhanjeri, Mohali, India*
*Ramandeep Sandhu, Lovely Professional University, Phagwara, India*
*Gaganpreet Kaur, Chandigarh Group of Colleges Jhanjeri, Mohali, India*
*Deepika Ghai, Lovely Professional University, Phagwara, India*

**Compilation of References** ........ 437

**About the Contributors** ........ 481

**Index** ........ 495

# Detailed Table of Contents

**Preface** ........................................................................................................ xvi

**Chapter 1**
AI and Computational Intelligence in Healthcare: An Introductory Guide........... 1
*Sanchali Kapoor, SAITM, India*
*Reeta Parmar, SAITM, India*
*Neetu Sharma, Galgotias University, India*
*Puneet Garg, KIET Group of Institutions, India*
*Narinder Jit Singh, INTI International University, Malaysia*

The transformation of healthcare through artificial intelligence (AI) and computational intelligence creates new approaches for healthcare diagnosis, treatment, patient monitoring, administrative processes etc. This chapter covers how these technologies support clinical decision-making and workflow improvement in healthcare, tackling the issues such as data privacy and bias as well as requirements for ethical frameworks for enhanced patient outcomes. Specific, real-world case studies crystallize use of AI for outcomes ranging from early disease detection to the remote patient care. Finally, the significance of inter-disciplinary cooperation between clinicians, data scientists and policymakers is key in order for us to develop responsible AI systems. With healthcare fully on the digital innovation bandwagon, learning the code of AI/CI enables us to play an important role in the fabric of future of medicine. The following introduction is a short guide for researchers, practitioners and students interested in the transformative impact of intelligent technologies on healthcare today.

**Chapter 2**
Introduction to AI and Computational Intelligence in Healthcare ...................... 27
*G. Sivakarthi, Anna University, India & Velammal College of Engineering and Technology, India*
*A. Vinora, Velammal College of Engineering and Technology, India*
*Nancy Deborah R., Velammal College of Engineering and Technology, India*
*M. Soundarya, Velammal College of Engineering and Technology, India*

Artificial Intelligence (AI) and Computational Intelligence are transforming healthcare, enabling intelligent decision-making, predictive analytics, and personalized treatment strategies. The integration of Deep Q-Networks (DQNs) and reinforcement learning has introduced powerful techniques for optimizing complex medical environments. It provides an in-depth exploration of how AI models, particularly reinforcement learning-based approaches, enhance clinical decision-making, disease prediction, and hospital resource management. By leveraging computational intelligence, The transformative impact of AI in medicine is undeniable, and its continued evolution will shape the future of healthcare in profound ways. This provides the necessary insights to navigate this rapidly changing landscape, empowering readers to embrace AI-driven innovations and contribute to the advancement of intelligent healthcare systems.

**Chapter 3**
AI-Powered Healthcare Solutions: Bridging the Medical Gap in Underserved Communities Worldwide ........ 57
*Leelawati Pokhrel, SAITM, India*
*Mohd Arsalan, SAITM, India*
*Priyanka Rani, GITAM University, India*
*Puneet Garg, KIET Group of Institutions, India*
*Placido Rogerio Pinheiro, University of Fortaleza, Brazil*

This chapter examines the transformative ability of artificial intelligence when it comes to dealing with global health challenges with a specific attention to developing countries. However, the implementation of AI in developing countries is facing unique challenges, including moral ideas around infrastructure limits, data shortages, regulatory structure and rights and inclusion. Through the extensive analysis of case studies, new technologies and political structure, this book examines both opportunities and obstacles that are effective in global health contexts. It provides a roadmap for researchers, decision makers, health professionals and technology developers to ensure that these innovations meet local needs, respect cultural references and promote the health care system. AI contributes to the on-going discourse on the role of technology in achieving sustainable development and universal health coverage by investigating the intersection of global health and development.

**Chapter 4**
Machine Learning and Computational Intelligence for Smart Healthcare: Advancing Diagnosis and Treatment ........ 87
*Siva Subramanian R., SRM Institute of Science and Technology, India*
*R. Asha, Sathyabama Institute of Science and Technology, India*
*J. Sangeetha, S.A. Engineering College, India*
*A. Adaikkammai, RMD Engineering College, India*
*T. Thilagam, Vel Tech Rangarajan Dr. Sagunthala R&D Institute of Science and Technology, India*
*P. Aparna, RMK College of Engineering and Technology, India*

Machine Learning (ML) and Computational Intelligence (CI) are revolutionizing the healthcare sector by enhancing diagnostic accuracy, personalizing treatments, and optimizing healthcare delivery. This chapter explores the applications, challenges, and emerging trends of ML and CI in smart healthcare, focusing on areas such as medical imaging, disease prediction, personalized medicine, and treatment recommendations. Key challenges such as data quality, algorithmic bias, and model interpretability are discussed, alongside emerging technologies like federated learning, explainable AI, and digital twins. The integration of ML and CI with clinical workflows promises to improve patient outcomes, reduce costs, and foster a more personalized approach to healthcare. The future of smart healthcare lies in developing transparent, collaborative, and scalable AI systems that enhance human expertise while preserving patient privacy and safety.

**Chapter 5**
Advancing Healthcare With Predictive Analytics for Disease Diagnosis and Risk Assessment ........................................................................................ 111
*Siva Subramanian R., SRM Institute of Science and Technology, India*
*Subhash Chandra N., CVR College of Engineering, India*
*S. Vijayaselvarani, Veltech Tech Multi Tech Dr. Rangarajan Dr. Sakunthala Engineering College, India*
*Anand Babu R., Panimalar Engineering College, India*
*Anto Gracious L. A., R.M.K. College of Engineering and Technology, India*
*K. Jeyakarthika, Ramco Institute of Technology, India*
*D. Raja, Thiagarajar College of Engineering, India*

Predictive analytics has emerged as a transformative tool in healthcare, enabling early disease diagnosis, risk assessment, and personalized treatment. This chapter examines the application of machine learning and statistical models in clinical settings, highlighting their impact on disease prediction and prevention. Key data sources such as electronic health records (EHRs), medical imaging, genomics, and wearable devices are explored, alongside methods including deep learning, ensemble techniques, and statistical models. The chapter also addresses challenges such as data quality, bias, and privacy concerns, while discussing emerging trends like federated learning, real-time analytics, and integration with wearable devices.

**Chapter 6**
Harnessing Predictive Analytics for Disease Diagnosis and Risk Assessment: Transforming Preventive Healthcare With AI ................................................ 133
*Mukul Sharma, Swami Vivekanand Subharti University, Meerut, India*
*Shashiraj Teotia, Swami Vivekanand Subharti University, Meerut, India*
*Vivek Aggarwal, Ajay Kumar Garg Engineering College, Ghaziabad, India*
*Vikas Sharma, SRM Institute of Science and Technology, Delhi, India*
*Tarun Kumar Vashishth, IIMT University, Meerut, India*
*Barkha Samania, SRM Institute of Science and Technology, Delhi, India*

In healthcare, applying AI alongside predictive analytics is transforming disease diagnosis, risk assessment, and treatment management. This chapter addresses the multidisciplinary impact of algorithm and data model sophistication on early detection, outcome forecasting, and patient identification stratified by risk. Health predictive analytics offers numerous possibilities by deconstructing vast and intricate datasets like electronic health records, genomic information, and data from wearables into actionable, anticipatory, tailored Healthcare-focused on proactive personal preventive intervention. Predictive models like logistic regression, decision trees, and ensemble and deep learning are covered, along with their use in chronic disease management, cancer risk forecasting, and cardiovascular risk assessment. The chapter also analyses critical data concerns such as accuracy, explainability, bias and fairness, usability, and integration into clinical workflows.

**Chapter 7**
Collaborative Health Intelligence: Federated Learning as the Foundation of Future Medical Care ................................................................................ 163
*Mohammad Nasar, Mazoon College, Oman*
*Mohammad Abu Kausar, University of Nizwa, Oman*
*Nasser Al Musalhi, Mazoon College, Oman*

Cryptographic federated learning (FL) transforms healthcare with privacy-preserving AI using decentralized data. This chapter explains FL, highlighting case studies: breast cancer detection up 15% (80% to 92%) across 10 hospitals, COVID-19 mortality prediction up 12% (75% to 84%), and 80% accurate acute kidney injury risk prediction. FL shines in imaging (92% tumor detection), personalized care (20% fewer hospital visits), rare disease diagnosis (22% higher accuracy), and informatics (10% better EHR models). Homomorphic encryption cuts breach risks by 80%. Challenges like 10% accuracy loss from data heterogeneity, 65% patient unawareness, and GDPR compliance are tackled with weighted algorithms and clear consent. FL envisions global surveillance, integrating 1 billion wearable records and 10 petabytes of imaging data by 2030, saving $3.5 billion and improving 15 million outcomes across 1,500 institutions. For researchers, clinicians, technologists, and policymakers, it clarifies FL, assesses achievements and challenges, and promotes innovation for secure, equitable healthcare.

**Chapter 8**
Medical Imaging and Radiology: AI-Powered Diagnostics .............................. 191
*Swathi V. N. V. L. S., CVR College of Engineering, India*
*S. Sugapriya, Velammal Engineering College, India*
*Suraj Garg, Chandigarh Group of Colleges, Jhanjeri, India*
*Amruta Mahalle, Datta Meghe Institution of Management Studies, India*
*Atharva Umakant Yewale, Datta Meghe Institute of Management Studies, India*
*P. Selvakumar, Department of Science and Humanities, Nehru Institute of Technology, Coimbatore, India*
*Manjunath T. C., Rajarajeswari College of Engineering, India*

Medical imaging has become a cornerstone of human body without the need for invasive procedures. This non-invasive capability allows for early detection, precise diagnosis, and personalized worldwide. medical imaging in diagnostics, its wide range of applications, the numerous benefits it future potential of this technology. of imaging modalities, each designed to offer unique insights into the human body. Early X-ray technology, while groundbreaking at the time, was limited in its ability to provide detailed images of soft tissues. As a result, subsequent innovations (PET) have dramatically expanded the capabilities of medical imaging, allowing healthcare professionals to visualize bones, soft tissues, organs, blood vessels, and even cellular and molecular structures in unprecedented detail.The advent of digital imaging, which replaced film-based techniques, has further enhanced diagnostic accuracy, allowing for faster image acquisition, enhanced image clarity, and easier storage and sharing of medical images.

**Chapter 9**
AI-Driven Clinical Decision Support Systems Enhancing Decision-Making in Modern Healthcare ............................................................................ 219
*Vikas Sharma, SRM Institute of Science and Technology, Delhi, India*
*Tarun Kumar Vashishth, IIMT Univeristy, Meerut, India*
*Renu Kumar, IIMT Engineering College, Meerut, India*
*Sanjukta Vidyant, Shobhit University, Meerut, India*
*Asheesh Pandey, ABES Engineering College, Ghaziabad, India*
*Barkha Samania, SRM Institute of Science and Technology, Delhi, India*

The incorporation of AI into clinical CDSS enables real-time insights which can be acted upon, thus improving the quality of care provided to the patients. The architecture as well as the features and development methods of CDSS focusing on machine learning and natural language processing as well as other predictive analytics capabilities are analysed. It discusses relevant cases that allow performing medical diagnosis and prescription of medicines so as to mitigate automation-enabled medical negligence and malpractice. Also, it addresses concerns with integration of AI into clinical workflows such as data silos, clinician gatekeeping, social contexts, and legal contexts. With the use of case studies, this chapter illustrates the effect of AI tools on CDSS by showing the improvement in the heightened healthcare opportunities that are readily available after the use of AI, as well as the provision of individualized treatment meant for specific unique patients due to the flexible nature offered by AI.

**Chapter 10**
AI-Enhanced Clinical Decision-Making Through a Collaborative Approach .. 249
*Ravikumar R. N., Marwadi University, Rajkot, India*
*S. Aarthi, Marwadi University, Rajkot, India*
*Bekhzod Ruzimbaev Saparbaevich, Mamun University, Khiva, Uzbekistan*
*Satheesh Kumar A., Nandha Engineering College, Erode, India*
*Muhabbat Jumaniyozova, Urgench State University, Urgench, Uzbekistan*
*Shakhnoza Toshova, Termez University of Economics and Service, Termez, Uzbekistan*

AI integration in healthcare transforms medical decision-making and treatment processes, enhancing patient care and advancing research. Deep Q-Networks (DQNs) with reinforcement learning help healthcare professionals analyze data for personalized treatment plans. AI automation boosts diagnostic accuracy and operational efficiency through collaboration between humans and machines. This chapter focuses on AI-powered clinical decision support systems that assist in diagnosing complex diseases and developing treatment strategies. Real-time analysis of medical imaging and health records enables early detection of cancers, cardiovascular disorders, and neurological disorders. Reinforcement learning also streamlines hospital resource use and cuts costs. Despite progress, ethical oversight is essential to address privacy, algorithmic bias, and ensure transparency. This study explores human-AI synergy in clinical settings, pointing out the importance of trustworthy, ethically guided AI that complements human intuition for improved patient outcomes.

**Chapter 11**
Reinforcement Learning for Adaptive Healthcare: Deep Q-Networks in Clinical Decision Optimization............................................................................ 281
*Mohammad Arafah, University of Petra, Jordan*
*Ahmad Aladawi, Loughborough University, UK*

The chapter explores the conditioning of Deep Q Networks (DQNs) and computational intelligence for changing the healthcare decision making. We study the role of reinforcement learning for sequential optimization of clinical decisions in different kinds of healthcare domains. Innovations regarding application of DQNs in complex medical environments as well as the theoretical foundations of DQNs are presented. This paper shows how these technologies transform clinical decision supporting systems, predictive analytics, disease diagnosis, personalized treatment optimization as well as IoT-enabled patient monitoring. Demonstrating wide spread implementation in settings of chronic disease management, critical care and diagnostic pathways results in very substantial improvements of clinical outcomes over traditional approaches.

**Chapter 12**
Optimizing Personalized Treatment Decisions Using Deep Q-Networks in Reinforcement Learning ........................................................................... 315
*Arpita Nayak, KIIT School of Liberal Studies, KIIT University, India*
*Ipseeta Satpathy, KSOM, KIIT University, India*
*Vishal Jain, School of Engineering & Technology, Vivekananda Institute of Professional Studies, New Delhi, India*

Healthcare treatments have found new paths through personalized strategy development made possible by Deep Q-Networks (DQNs) working together with computational intelligence and data-driven adaptive choices. Medical diagnosis receives support from DQNs through their analysis of extensive patient data combinations including reports together with test results and imaging data to establish diagnostic trends which boost diagnostic accuracy while functioning. The prescription process of drugs becomes more effective using DQNs because they deploy simulation techniques to identify the best drug treatment combinations by processing both genetic data and patient-specific medical status. DQNs generate adjustable treatment strategies by processing live patient feedback that optimizes the management of long-term health problems especially when treating diabetes or cancer. The full capabilities of this technology require resolving present privacy issues and interpretability barriers and workflow implementation requirements to achieve the potential outcomes.

**Chapter 13**
Learning to Heal: Deep Q-Networks as the Future of AI-Driven Healthcare ... 337
*Sapandeep Kaur Dhillon, Guru Nanak Dev University, Amritsar, India*
*Ikvinderpal Singh, Trai Shatabdi Guru Gobind Khalsa College, Amritsar, India*
*Parminder Kaur, Guru Nanak Dev University, Amritsar, India*

Deep Q-Networks (DQNs) in smart healthcare enable artificial intelligence to rapidly alter medical decisions and learn from mistakes. DQNs build smart healthcare agents by leveraging reinforcement learning rather than rules. Dynamic learning advances diagnosis, treatment, and hospital operations. DQNs enable artificial intelligence systems to assess activities by using rewards and punishments, thereby optimizing their strategies. They draw on deep learning and Q-learning. Robotic-assisted procedures and ICUs save lives through educated judgments. DQNs identify diseases, develop drugs and tailored therapies. AI bots use patient data to tailor treatment. Problems abound. Think about morality, openness in decision-making, and data security. Explainable artificial intelligence in human-AI decision systems increases dependability and utility. As wearable's and telemedicine interfaces offer smart, responsive healthcare, DQNs also do. Human knowledge remains enormous. The DQNs should help physicians. Beyond data analysis, systems help enhance patient care.

**Chapter 14**
Drug Discovery and Optimization With AI ....................................................... 379
*Dipesh Uike, Dr. Ambedkar Institute of Management, Studies, and Research, India*
*S. Sugapriya, Velammal Engineering College, India*
*Manpreet Kaur, Chandigarh Group of Colleges, Jhanjeri, India*
*Amruta Mahalle, Datta Meghe Institution of Management Studies, India*
*Neha Dhule, Datta Meghe Institute of Management Studies, India*
*P. Selvakumar, Department of Science and Humanities, Nehru Institute of Technology, Coimbatore, India*
*Manjunath T. C., Rajarajeswari College of Engineering, India*

Across many scientific disciplines, and application is in modern development long, costly over a can cost billions of dollars. predictive analytics, are now playing pivotal roles in revolutionizing this process by making. The drug discovery process typically includes generating hypotheses about drug interactions. Using vast datasets derived from genomics, proteomics, chemical libraries, and biomedical literature, AI algorithms can process and analyze complex biological information in a fraction of the time it would take using conventional methods. response to emerging diseases, where speed is critical—as demonstrated during the COVID-19 pandemic.omics data to reveal previously unknown associations between biological markers and diseases. interpret thousands of scientific articles, extracting valuable insights about genes, proteins, and potential disease mechanisms. By integrating this information with experimental data, error experimentation. predictive ability helps researchers filter out unsuitable compounds early, reducing the risk of late-stage failures.

**Chapter 15**
Future Trends in AI and Smart Healthcare ....................................................... 405
*Amandeep Kaur, Chandigarh Group of Colleges Jhanjeri, Mohali, India*
*Ramandeep Sandhu, Lovely Professional University, Phagwara, India*
*Gaganpreet Kaur, Chandigarh Group of Colleges Jhanjeri, Mohali, India*
*Deepika Ghai, Lovely Professional University, Phagwara, India*

The healthcare industry will experience revolutionary medical practices through Artificial Intelligence (AI) integration up to 2030. This chapter analyzes future tendencies in AI coupled with smart healthcare through a discussion about advanced technologies helping medical staff with prediction capabilities, tailored treatment solutions, and immediate clinical choices. Through Systematic Literature Review (SLR) methodology, this chapter sets out major investigation paths that highlight federated learning as a data protection and Explainable AI (XAI) method for decision processes and digital twin modeling for precise healthcare delivery. This chapter identifies AI-powered diagnostic technologies, along with robotic surgery systems and wearable health monitoring. Remote patient care services can be improved through the combination of Internet of Medical Things (IoMT) technology with 5G-enabled smart healthcare infrastructure. The chapter also presents the essential framework needed to deploy AI in healthcare and achieve ethical standards and security requirements for healthcare data.

**Compilation of References** ................................................................................ 437

**About the Contributors** ....................................................................................... 481

**Index** ..................................................................................................................... 495

# Preface

The integration of Artificial Intelligence (AI) and Computational Intelligence (CI) into healthcare has ushered in a new era of medical innovation, one that combines data-driven decision-making with advanced diagnostic and treatment capabilities. This volume, *Applied AI and Computational Intelligence in Diagnostics and Decision-Making*, brings together a wide range of perspectives, applications, and methodologies that highlight the transformative role of intelligent technologies in healthcare.

From predictive analytics and machine learning to federated learning and reinforcement learning, the chapters explore how computational intelligence not only improves diagnosis and treatment but also reshapes the delivery of medical care across diverse global contexts. The discussions include both technical developments and ethical considerations, underscoring the need for responsible, transparent, and inclusive AI systems. Readers are offered a balance of foundational knowledge and forward-looking insights, making this collection relevant to researchers, practitioners, policymakers, and students alike.

The following chapters provide a comprehensive journey through the state-of-the-art applications of AI in healthcare:

## CHAPTER OVERVIEW

- **Chapter 1** introduces the transformative role of AI and computational intelligence in healthcare, emphasizing diagnostic innovation, patient monitoring, ethical concerns, and interdisciplinary collaboration.
- **Chapter 2** explores reinforcement learning and Deep Q-Networks as tools for predictive analytics, personalized treatment, and optimized healthcare resource management.

- **Chapter 3** highlights the application of AI in underserved and developing communities, examining opportunities, barriers, and pathways to equitable and sustainable healthcare access.
- **Chapter 4** investigates the role of machine learning and computational intelligence in advancing smart healthcare, focusing on medical imaging, personalized medicine, explainable AI, and digital twin technologies.
- **Chapter 5** presents predictive analytics as a powerful tool for early disease detection and risk assessment, examining data from sources such as electronic health records, genomics, and wearable devices.
- **Chapter 6** expands on predictive analytics by addressing the role of AI in preventive healthcare, chronic disease management, and personalized interventions, while also discussing concerns of accuracy, fairness, and clinical integration.
- **Chapter 7** introduces federated learning as a privacy-preserving approach to collaborative healthcare intelligence, showcasing its potential through case studies and future projections.
- **Chapter 8** provides a deep look at AI-powered medical imaging and radiology, tracing the evolution of imaging technologies and their role in accurate, non-invasive diagnostics.
- **Chapter 9** examines AI-driven clinical decision support systems, focusing on their design, integration into workflows, and ability to enhance real-time decision-making.
- **Chapter 10** emphasizes collaborative AI-human decision-making, showing how reinforcement learning and automation improve diagnostic precision and treatment planning while raising ethical questions.
- **Chapter 11** delves into reinforcement learning and Deep Q-Networks as adaptive tools for clinical decision optimization across chronic disease management, critical care, and diagnostics.
- **Chapter 12** explores how personalized treatment decisions can be optimized through reinforcement learning, particularly in contexts such as cancer and diabetes management.
- **Chapter 13** envisions the broader role of Deep Q-Networks as future agents of AI-driven healthcare, highlighting dynamic learning, robotic-assisted procedures, telemedicine, and explainable AI.
- **Chapter 14** shifts focus to drug discovery, illustrating how AI accelerates hypothesis generation, compound screening, and data integration to reduce costs and improve innovation in pharmaceutical development.
- **Chapter 15** concludes by examining emerging trends in AI and smart healthcare, including federated learning, explainable AI, digital twins, robotic systems, and IoMT-enabled personalized care.

This volume collectively demonstrates how AI and computational intelligence are reshaping healthcare into a more intelligent, precise, and accessible system. It underscores the importance of developing technologies that balance innovation with ethics, ensuring that healthcare advances remain patient-centered, equitable, and sustainable. By bridging technical detail with real-world application, the chapters provide a roadmap for the ongoing evolution of intelligent healthcare systems that will define the next decade of medical practice.

**Danish Ather**
*Amity University, Tashkent, Uzbekistan*

**Khai Mun Ng**
*Kuala Lumpur University of Science and Technology (KLUST), Malaysia*

**Sachin Jain**
*Ajay Kumar Garg Engineering College, Ghaziabad, India*

**Vishal Jain**
*Kuala Lumpur University of Science and Technology (KLUST), Malaysia & Vivekananda Institute of Professional Studies, New Delhi, India*

**Vinay Kukreja**
*Chitkara University Institute of Engineering and Technology, Chitkara University, India*

Chapter 1

# AI and Computational Intelligence in Healthcare:
## An Introductory Guide

**Sanchali Kapoor**
https://orcid.org/0009-0002-7392-9622
*SAITM, India*

**Reeta Parmar**
https://orcid.org/0009-0003-7189-1226
*SAITM, India*

**Neetu Sharma**
*Galgotias University, India*

**Puneet Garg**
https://orcid.org/0000-0002-4635-546X
*KIET Group of Institutions, India*

**Narinder Jit Singh**
*INTI International University, Malaysia*

## ABSTRACT

*The transformation of healthcare through artificial intelligence (AI) and computational intelligence creates new approaches for healthcare diagnosis, treatment, patient monitoring, administrative processes etc. This chapter covers how these technologies support clinical decision-making and workflow improvement in healthcare, tackling the issues such as data privacy and bias as well as requirements for ethical frame-*

DOI: 10.4018/979-8-3373-3311-3.ch001

*works for enhanced patient outcomes. Specific, real-world case studies crystallize use of AI for outcomes ranging from early disease detection to the remote patient care. Finally, the significance of inter-disciplinary cooperation between clinicians, data scientists and policymakers is key in order for us to develop responsible AI systems. With healthcare fully on the digital innovation bandwagon, learning the code of AI/CI enables us to play an important role in the fabric of future of medicine. The following introduction is a short guide for researchers, practitioners and students interested in the transformative impact of intelligent technologies on healthcare today.*

## 1. OVERVIEW OF ARTIFICIAL INTELLIGENCE IN HEALTHCARE

*AI for Healthcare Artificial Intelligence (AI) refers to the use of advanced technologies to mimic human intelligence for tasks like diagnosis, treatment recommendations from data monitoring etc. AI systems are built to quickly process large amounts of data, detect trends and help healthcare professionals in making quicker, more precise evidence-based decisions (Prabha et. al., 2023).*

There are quite a few AI technologies that are currently disrupting healthcare in meaningful ways. Machine learning models that identify disease risks, individualize therapy choices, and optimize clinical decision-making Artificial Intelligence (AI) Natural Language Processing (NLP) helps to understand and structure the unstructured clinical notes, research papers, and patient reports so that only valuable information is available. This is achieved through Computer Vision algorithms which can read medical images, like X-rays, MRIs and CT scans to detect abnormalities with great accuracy. Robotics assists surgeries, and even the rehabilitation phase or patient care in general with more precision while reducing human errors (Engelbreht, 2007).

One of the most advantages is to reduce human mistakes and augment diagnosis with AI being one of the greatest integration. With large dataset AI systems, also capable of learning certain minute patterns that may slip past human vision. This creates the opportunity for early disease detection, including cancer or diabetic retinopathy which in turn can meaningfully improve outcomes with treatment. Furthermore, AI being at the core of predictive analytics predicts health deteriorations before they occur leading to interventions in advance.

AI even helps in automating administrative work such as patient record storage, appointment scheduling, billing and medical coding that gives the health care professional time to see more patients (Malik, Pathania & Rathaur, 2019). Virtual health assistants and AI chatbots are assisting to route patient inquiries, taking care of monitoring patients with chronic diseases or reminding them to take their meds, providing support off the hospital setting too. AI is also extremely important in closing the gaps of healthcare, especially for the underserved and rural areas with a higher absence of access to specialist care. AIpowered remote diagnostic tools can virtually connect patients with the specialists for timely and relevant healthcare delivery.

Digital transformation is continuing with ferocity to the various sub sectors in the healthcare domain and AI stands firmly on top of this frenzy. It is redefining the future of medicine by enabling improved patient outcomes, improved efficiency & access to health services for everyone and for affordable cost. Yet to be realized, full of the promise of AI in healthcare are we only through careful realization, and ethical considerations for how technology developers may also need to work more closely together with its future practitioners.

## 2. FOUNDATIONS OF COMPUTATIONAL INTELLIGENCE

Computational Intelligence (CI) is a branch of AI which focuses on the adaptive mechanisms which is devoted to intelligent behaviour in adaptive and unstructured environment. CI, versus traditional AI that typically requires hand-crafted rules and logic, are data-driven learning systems able to self-adapt and self-correct over time as well suit autonomous behaviour under uncertainty suited for health applications (Verma, Paul & Johri 2020).

The **core techniques** of Computational Intelligence include:

i. Artificial Neural Networks (ANNs):

Artificial Neural Networks (ANNs) - Modelled after the structure and function of human brain, artificial neural networks are used to solve complex problems by interconnected processing nodes or neurons (Manocha et. al., 2021) ANNs are typically used for a wide range of purposes in the healthcare domain like disease classification (cancer detection from biopsy) medical image interpretation(MRI, CT scan reading) and predictive modelling (disease deterioration prediction or risk of readmission to hospital for the patient). ANNs are such robust tools of diagnostics augmentation and decision support capabilities.

ii. Fuzzy Logic Systems:

Fuzzy logic is the area of reasoning that are not crisp or exact, instead fitting human reasoning when it is between absolute "yes/no" and values which can be somewhere between like: "high," or "somewhat", or negated forms like "very low". Fuzzy logic systems are especially efficient in fields of health care where fuzziness and uncertainty prevail (Huang, Kangas & Rasco, 2007). They are, for use in symptom assessment on the basis of vague patient inputs (pain levels), as well as building intelligent decision support systems, and simulating general medical diseases that are highly non-diagnostic and full of grey areas. This malleability allows for more subtle and tailored clinical assessments.

iii. Evolutionary Computing:

Evolutionary algorithms (such as Genetic Algorithm - GAs and Particle Swarm Optimization - PSO) which are inspired by processes in nature (Verma, Paul & Johri 2020) are suitable to solve a variety of complex optimization problems. Significant role in augmenting decision making and operational efficiency (Agatonovic-Kustrin& Beresford, 2000) Due to the fact these are the algorithms, Healthcare most relevantly contribute in; they are widely used for personalized treatment plans, determining optimal time of drug dosing based on individual patients and thus reducing side-effects while maximizing effectiveness or allocation of scarce resources within hospitals. In practice, the solutions proposed by these techniques contribute to more adaptive and intelligent healthcare solutions (Gürsel, 2016) through the simulation of evolving heuristics to solve problems.

## 3. EVOLUTION OF AI AND CI IN MEDICAL SCIENCE

From conceptual experimentations to indispensable instruments in contemporary healthcare systems Artificial Intelligence (AI) and Computational Intelligence (CI) (Tupe & Kulkarni, 2015) have come of age in the field of medical science. The path they take mirrors some of the great technological advances that have transformed medicine, practice and delivered illnesses.

*Figure 1. The Evolution of AI and CI in Medical Science*

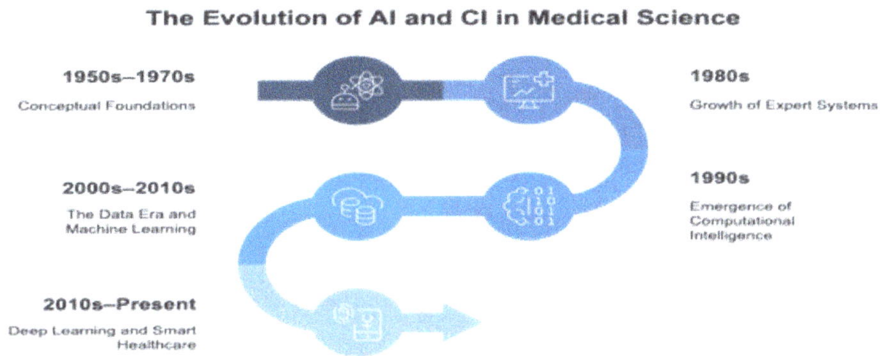


i. Conceptual Foundations (1950s–1970s):

Machines modelled after human intelligence started in the 1950s. The philosophical foundation of AI was originally set by Alan Turing through his famous question "Can machines think? Some of the initial AI efforts in Medicine include expert systems like MYCIN (originally developed in the 70s) for organ infecting bacterial infections. Rule-based logic in healthcare was shown to have potential, albeit by rule-heavy systems limited by computing power (Avanzo et. al. 2024).

ii. Growth of Expert Systems (1980s):

Expert Systems (1980s: if-then rules to mimic clinical reasoning (Behare et. al., 2025), these systems were employed in tasks as diagnosis and drug interaction checks but were not equipped for data learning. This was a necessary step towards the arrival of decision support tools in hospitals, nevertheless.

iii. Emergence of Computational Intelligence (1990s):

Computational Intelligence (neural networks, fuzzy logic and genetic algorithms) have enabled more flexible and adaptive models to solve complex medical problems during 1990s. So, these kinds of techniques enable systems to improve by learning from examples, deal with semi-qualitative inputs and tune treatments along to afford time dependent applications of AI (Chaddad et. al., 2023).

iv. The Data Era and Machine Learning (2000s–2010s):

Machine learning came into the picture with the proliferation of digital health records and substantial computing advancements. A set of algorithms were created to identify trends in patient data, post-outcome prediction and driven decision support for personalized treatment. Medical imaging analysis, patient risk stratification and population health management have scaled up to be the major areas of applications(Davenport & Kalakota, 2019).

v. Deep Learning and Smart Healthcare (2010s–Present):

Over the last few years, deep learning (a form of neural network with deep structure) significantly increased the medical imaging capabilities, speech recognition and genomics prospects. AI can now surpass or at the very least match human experts in the detection of diseases, such that AI outperforms (Shahsavarani et. al., 2015) cancer or diabetic retinopathy from scans. CI meanwhile, still keeps on peeling the skin off drug discovery and hospital operations as well as home-based patient monitoring with CI.

vi. Integration and Real-World Impact:

AI and CI are no longer confined in the research labs; they are getting ingrained in EHRs, robotic surgeries, telemedicine platforms, and wearable devices or analytics apps. Those technologies are enabling a move from reactive to predictive care with characteristics of personalized medicine and in time decision support (Muhiyaddin et. al., 2020).

## 4. TYPES OF AI TECHNIQUES USED IN HEALTHCARE

*Figure 2. AI Techniques in Healthcare*

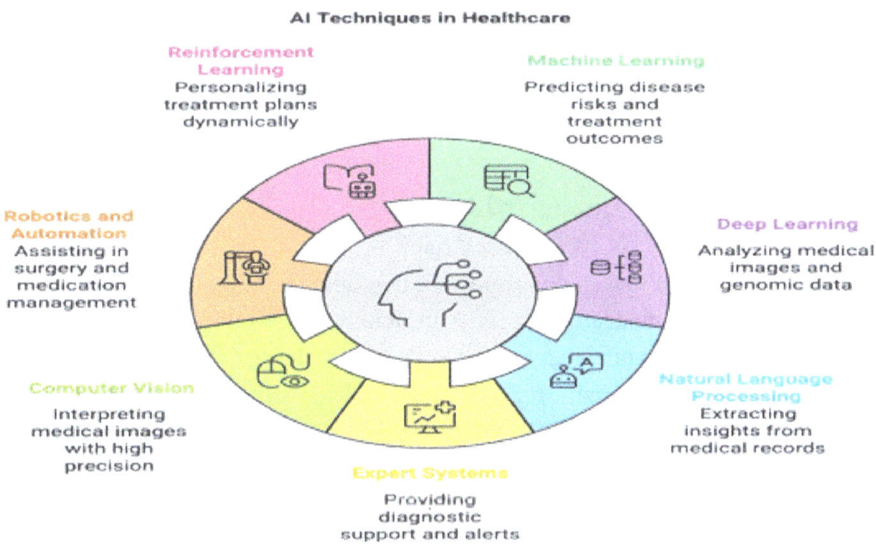


Artificial Intelligence (AI) in Healthcare: Different techniques that try to mimic the cognitive functions by human's e.g. learning, reasoning and decision-making in healthcare. These methods help in differentiate how machines can process intricate medical data, streamline clinical workflows and enhance patient caring methods. (Beeler, Bates & Hug, 2014).In Healthcare, Majority of AI techniques are of the following below as main as used:

i. Machine Learning (ML)

Machine Learning has been one of the prevalent AI methods that widely implemented in healthcare sector. This is the training of algorithms on historical clinical data to detect patterns and predict things without any explicit programming for certain tasks (Zhou et. at. 2022). ML helps in predicting disease risks like for example the probability of heart disease or diabetes in patients. It is used for calculating treatment response by data extracted from medical history; and early detection of prevalent conditions so treatment can be started pre-emptively.

ii. Deep Learning (DL)

Deep Learning (subset of Machine Learning) uses multi-layer neural networks to solve high dimensional and complex problems. It has a multi-layered architecture that learns the structure of human brain thus it can detect very subtle pictures in data. Deep learning works particularly well for medical image analysis in health care i.e. detecting tumors or lesions from MRI/CT scans. It also is of importance for processing textual and spoken language (transcription of medical conversations or) still very broadly used in genomic experiments/ drug discovery efforts to shorten research (Hudaa et. al., 2019).

iii. Natural Language Processing (NLP)

Natural Language Processing empowers machines to comprehend, analyse and deliver responses to human language. NLP in Healthcare: To analyse the unstructured data from Electronic Health Records (EHR) s we are doing NLP (Roy et. al., 2021) and deriving relevant information for clinical decision support. It speeds up access to all the medical literature as well it also NLP underpins intelligent voice assistants that address clinicians and patients by listening for voice commands or questions.

iv. Expert Systems

Expert systems are AI programs that attempt to mimic human medical expert decision-making, making a set of heuristic rules. These systems might not be trained on data like ML models but they have their place in many clinical applications. They are used in alerting drug interactions, suggesting diagnosis and guiding according to clinical guidance. They are very transparent and given their reliability, (Makanjee, Hoffmann& Bergh, 2015) especially well for regulated area.

v. Computer Vision

Computer vision enables AI systems to understand and process visual information. It is mainly used in radiology of healthcare for example reading and recognizing X-rays, MRI scans or CT images with high degree of accuracy (Behare et. al., 2025). It also serves an important purpose in pathology wherein it assists to photograph tissue samples for abnormalities. In dermatology also, computer vision algorithms are used to detect and classify skin conditions and sometimes outperform human dermatologists in accuracy.

vi. Robotics and Automation

AI robotics and automation, in particular are beginning to be used more and more for both clinical as well as operational activities within health care settings. Surgical systems like the Da Vinci Surgical System, robotic-assisted surgery make it possible for surgeons to perform complex procedures with increased precision. It too makes use of automation in medication management systems for proper dispensing. Moreover robotic technologies have been applied for the rehabilitation of the patients and helping those elderly or disabled people in quality life (Rahim, Afroz & Akinola, 2025).

vii. Reinforcement Learning

Reinforcement Learning (RL) is the approach for AI, where it learns the actions of optimal behaviours by doing and fixing via rewards/penalties from its actions. RL is making a splash in healthcare, allowing systems to continuously adapt algorithms in real-time once the oncologist gets a mind change about treatment plans. Similarly, it is also being investigated with adaptive drug dosing in chronic therapy and rescheduling of healthcare resources such as ICU beds or surgical teams (Lin et. al., 2017).

## 5. CLINICAL DECISION SUPPORT SYSTEMS (CDSS)

Clinical Decision Support Systems (CDSS) are AI based tools that assist the clinicians at the time of decision-making, with timely and evidence-based insights in healthcare delivery. These systems review numerous data sets in the field of medical (eg, patients history lab values, imaging and clinical guidelines) helping healthcare professionals reach proper diagnosis and develop treatment plans that are effective to their patients.

CDSS use The CDSSs can be embedded with Electronic Health Records (EHRs) and use sophisticated algorithms to understand contextual patient information. From flagging drug interactions, to differential diagnoses or flagged test results they can suggest starting points for individualized treatment pathways. Rule base (the system may provide recommendations based on pre-defined clinical rules) and others which are machine learning based, to get better and learn over time.

CDSS reduces the potential for human error and improves patient safety by facilitating informed decision-supports informed by evidence; enhances diagnostic accuracy and expedites the efficiency of clinical workflows. That is particularly important in challenging cases where so many diagnostic categories or medications simultaneously need to be considered. CDSSs which are becoming more natural, predictive and provide real-time context aware support in a number of medical specialties with the advancements of AI.

## 6. ROLE OF NATURAL LANGUAGE PROCESSING (NLP) IN HEALTHCARE

Natural Language Processing (AI and an important subfield of) re-invents healthcare by allowing machines to understand, interpret & produce human languages. The importance of NLP at this point in time cannot be overstated within an industry where vast store of life-critical information (clinical notes, discharge summaries, pathology reports and narrative from patient) lays in strangled text data which needs further structured analysis or clinical insights

A major domain of NLP in health science is EHR data manipulation to extract the essential medical facts. Text and textual data are generated in such a quantity during care of patient that it becomes difficult for healthcare providers to process his or her textual data. NLP tools can take this information and quickly classify it to bring to the top the most vital details like history, current conditions, treatment + medications(s) registered for follow-up. NLP automates data extraction that allows clinicians to make quicker decisions in a more informed fashion, thus improving care quality and decreasing errors.

NLP also rationalises administrative workflows in the domain of Healthcare. NLP makes it easier for NLP systems performing automated coding, billing (long and boring tasks for healthcare professionals) In this regard these tools have the ability to read physician notes correctly and place the right codes for streamlined compliance and lower overhead. It not only saves time, but also reduces errors and hefty financial penalties.

One of the significant fields in which NLP is applied is clinical decision support systems (CDSS). NLP algorithms that run in real time on patient records would help to detect rising risks, such as a soon to be missed diagnosis or upcoming drug-drug interactions adverse events from the guidelines. If for example the medication that a patient is currently taking in his/her list collides with the medication that he/she were just prescribed NLP systems will flag this and alert the provider resulting with safer and efficient patient care.

Furthermore in the field of patient engagement NLP is impacting at a big way. Conversational AI, in which virtual health assistants and chatbots use NLP to speak with patients in a natural, almost humanlike conversation form. These tools can help answer health questions, schedule appointments, prescribe medication, send reminders for prescriptions and check on chronic conditions. Delivered outside the clinical setting, NLP driven tools bring information and support to patients at times of their convenience to empower them to be more engaged.

NLP in medical research; allowing researchers to hunt though these crazy sea of scientific paper. NLP allows researchers to quickly aggregate evidence and trends through the analysis of thousands of research articles, clinical trial reports and case studies triggering new hypotheses. This speeds up rate of medical advances and ensures better evidence in practice. In general, NLP facilitates the communication between human language and machine intelligence in healthcare. It facilitates systems to consume and interpret natural language with greater efficiency, streamline care delivery, drive improved patient outcomes throw personalized health. Healthcare will see a larger role of NLP with its digital transformation, even in future more accurate and efficient but more innovation to be brought in the medical field (Lin et. al., 2017).

## 7. MEDICAL IMAGING AND DIAGNOSTIC SUPPORT

Artificial Intelligence and Computational Intelligence is changing healthcare, the most experience impact may be observed in the area of medical imaging / diagnostic support. They improve the accuracy, speed and performance rates of image interpretation and disease diagnosis to almost same as or better than expert human using such technologies.

i. Role of AI/CI in Radiology:

Radiology with technique of Imaging X-rays, MRI, and CT scans ultrasounds. AI models, and notably deep learning algorithms are fed to understand these images and spot abnormalities from them.

- **Tumor Detection**:AI can spot brain, lung, breast or other tumor types by finding very small patterns not visible to the human eye.
- **Fracture and Lesion Identification**: With thousands of annotated images per class, systems can detect fractures, haemorrhages and other lesions with high precision on.
- **Chest X-ray Interpretation**:By scanning and analysing chest X-rays, AI tools can screen for conditions such as pneumonia, TB, COVID-19 very quickly.

ii. Diagnostic Support in Pathology:

In pathology, AI assists in examining tissue samples and blood slides.

- **Digital Pathology**:Whole slide imaging (WSI) digitizes pathology slides which are subsequently read by AI algorithms in order to find cells with cancer potential or anything weird.
- **Cell Counting and Classification**:AI helps in the automation of laborious cells counting, cell-type identification and screening of blood smears or biopsy samples for anomalies (Amarasingham et. al.. 2014).

iii. Early Disease Detection:

AI and CI systems are particularly useful in **predicting diseases at an early stage**, even before symptoms appear.

- **Diabetic Retinopathy Screening**:AI systems analyse retinal scans for the indication of diabetic retinopathy so that early intervention and vision saving are possible.
- **Alzheimer's and Neurological Conditions**:Brain imaging and machine learning models are helping to pick up the ever early signs of neuron generation on a new level.
- **Cardiovascular Risk Prediction**: AI analyses echocardiograms or angiograms Images for heart imaging data to diagnose diagnosis and risk stratification.

iv. Integration with Clinical Workflows:

- **Decision Support:** AI imaging tools produce reports, raise alerts on abnormal findings and guide the consultation for further imaging/molecular testing to radiologists/Physicians.
- **Real-Time Analysis:** Some systems able to deliver near real-time analysis of medical imaging during procedures, thereby improving workflow in critical care environments (Ho et. al., 2020).

## 8. PREDICTIVE ANALYTICS AND PATIENT RISK ASSESSMENT

AI and predictive healthcare analysis the predictive analytics in health care utilizes AI algorithms to making broad inferences from mass amounts of patient data to make predictions on future health occurrences. This facilitates, the healthcare providers to move from reactive care delivery to proactive and preventive care thus proactively detecting people who have a high risk of deteriorating. Understanding Predictive Analytics in Healthcare.

Predictive analytics in healthcare is using historical and real-time data (e.g. medical records, lab results, vital signs and lifestyle patterns) through artificial intelligence like machine learning techniques to predict future health events. This works, to detect patterns and trends in the data of patients making it possible for disease progression forecasting, readmission or adverse consequences from medical care estimation. It can also prescribe evidence-based care strategies that may be what will prevent ill-health and promote health proactivity, tailoring care to the individual patient.

i. Patient Risk Assessment with AI Models

The wide-ranging patient variables use in AI models helps to derive risk scores estimation so as to inform clinical decisions at the point of care with greater credibility and accuracy. For chronic disease, it allows the application of AI for predicting chances of things perking into diabetes, hypotension, heart disease based on patient behaviours (readmissions), medication adherence and clinical metrics. On the other hand, these models predict readmission for 30 days inpatients so as to target high-risk patients and allow early follow-ups or even alternative care strategies. In an intensive care unit, AI can track (almost) real-time physiological data such as heart rate and oxygen levels to alert when the patient is deteriorating. AI is utilized in the prediction of prognosis for cancer, by predicting tumor growth, treatment response and survival using images, biopsies and genetic testing data (Mhlanga, 2025).

ii. Tools and Techniques Used

Many tools and practices work, together to implement predictive analytics in healthcare. We train the machine learning models (e.g., Random forests, Decision Trees and Neural Networks on health state labelled datasets to discover latent patterns and risk-metric. Natural Language Processing (NLP) is the other big technique, which untaps clinical value from unstructured sources (doctor notes and EMR narratives) Raw Data The data Integration Platforms too are very important; they combine data coming from multiple channels such as wearable devices, lab reports, genetics profiles releases. Portals, over a unified picture of the client's health provide patient inputs from disparate integrations such as wearable devices lab, reports genetic profiles.

iii. Benefits of Predictive Analytics

Predictive analytics has major advantages that take healthcare delivery to a whole new level. A big advantage is creating care plans that are individually relevant to each patient based on their unique risk profile. It also promotes early interventions, which help to prevent more serious health concerns and unnecessary hospital admissions. Also, on the other side predictive models help in more optimal resource utilization by predicting the needs of a hospital like staffing requirements, bed availability and equipment. This is important in the long run as preventive strategies reduce emergency admissions, lengths of stay and costs.

iv. Real-World Applications

Predictive analytics is already starting to make an impact in the real-world clinical settings. Sepsis early warning systems use predictive models in the identification of the condition before it is too late, allowing for timely and potentially life-saving treatment. Programs for mental health tracking monitor behaviour and mood patterns to predict the emergence of disorders such as depression or suicidal behaviour. At a larger level, population health management programs utilize predictive analytics for community-level health risk assessment allowing governments/ insurers to launch targeted health initiatives and improve public health outcomes (Malik & Solaiman, 2024).

## 9. PERSONALIZED AND PRECISION MEDICINE

Precision and personalized medicine is a paradigm shift in healthcare where the treatment, prevention strategies are individualized to every unique aspect of patient. It is the result of a shift from "one size fits all" using computational intelligence (CI), artificial intelligence (AI) that analyses very large genetically-clinical-lifestyle datasets and allow more precise effective targeted care.

i. Role of Computational Intelligence in Personalization

Using complex datasets computational intelligence approaches (machine learning, deep learning, genetic algorithms and such) extract patterns & relationships that are often beyond human comprehension. These models can be used to combine genomic sequences, biomarker profiles, environmental exposures and electronic health records (EHR) for explaining how a given patient will respond to a disease, and by consequence how they can be treated.

ii. Genetic and Molecular Data Analysis

Precision medicine, one of the core pillars involves genetic data usage. CI systems could be trained to study DNA sequencing data for detection mutations, gene expressions and biomarkers linked to diseases like cancer, rare genetic disorders or cardiovascular conditions. Tracing these genetic markers, clinicians are able to choose drugs or therapies more likely to be effective based on the patient's genetic profile reducing trial and error for that patient group.

iii. Tailored Treatment Plans

Using AI insights, the doctors could build personalized treatment plans for the patient considering not only her genetic data but also her age (gender), medical history, lifestyle and even relocation (Cartolovni, Tomicic & Mosler, 2022). Precision medicine in cancer, for example, determines which patients will respond to immunotherapy or targeted therapy based on their tumor profiles.

iv. Disease Prevention and Early Detection

Beyond care, computational models predict the risk for developing diseases at an individual level. With genetic susceptibilities and early biomarkers examined, healthcare providers could take prevention-oriented actions such as advising lifestyle modifications, recommend early screening programs and producing better health results with reduced healthcare expenditures.

v. Drug Development and Clinical Trials

AI also accelerates drug discovery by utilising genetic data to find what may become drug targets, as well as predicting how individuals would respond to various compounds in silico. Moreover, precision-based clinical trials leverage CI to make sure that only patients genetically likely to respond to the test drug enter the trial thereby increasing trial success (Schonberger, 2019).

## 10. AI IN HOSPITAL AND HEALTHCARE MANAGEMENT

Artificial Intelligence (AI) is not only changing the face of patient care and diagnostics but also in hospital and healthcare management. Through the automation of operations, AI drives best-in-class resource utilization & service delivery, which drives operational excellence and improved patient experiencefor staff and patients alike.

i. Improving Administrative Efficiency

Hospitals process large amounts of administrative work every day, everything from patient registration & insurance processing, to billing and discharge summary. These are usually routine and time-consuming but AI processes automate them to avoid human errors and time saving. Streamlines workflows so that the staff is available more time to handle patient work and CS.

- **Automated Scheduling:** One of thissuch area where AI has added huge value. Provides scheduling of appointments using historical data to identify no-shows, therefore increasing availability for doctors & staff and reduces last minute drudgery. That enables better time management and lesser wastage of time.
- **Medical Billing and Coding:**Yet another essential task that AI makes simple. With the help of AI, you can give diagnosis and procedures to claim codes at the point in time reducing claim denials and also increase insurance approval time (faster through a claims process). This leads less financial error and improves revenue cycle efficiency (Upadhyay et. al., 2023).
- **Document Management:**AI Natural Language Processing (NLP) tools make this easier. These tools are able to pull critical information from disjointed clinical documents, convert hand written notes into digital and bring to structured records. This enhances data fetching, compliance and accuracy of documentation.

ii. Optimizing Resource Allocation

Efficient resource management is fundamental for high-quality patient care as well as operational cost minimization in hospitals. Human resource, medical equipment and the facilities are used in the optimum manner with the help of AI systems that process data in real-time to these systems.

AI optimization staffing: uses AI to predict patient flow patterns and places healthcare personnel on the floor Staffing optimization-AI will be trained to predict patient inflow rates; when there has an ideal number of healthcare personnel available or at peak hours/seasonal demand, AI can easily direct nurses/doctors to where there are understaffed/overstaffed spots.

Another part Equipment Utilization is critical too. By using predictive analytics for example equipment demand, best high value machines such as MRI and CT scanners are employed to the max. That minimizes downtimes and thus the amount of patients waiting for care.

By AI, the inventory management is also optimized whereby it is being able to identify how much of medical supplies and medicines are being used on real time basis. AI can accurately predict the supply of things so as not to run out or stock up as we cannot, and ensure stock availability of critical goods to be always there.

iii. Enhancing Patient Flow and Experience

The navigational path that patients take from first coming into the hospital through to discharge affects two parties: that of the patient and the efficiency in which a facility operates. AI that identifies possible delays and plays a role in resource management to unblock the workflow happens in patient flow.

AI-enabled bed management which keeps a real time eye on bed occupancy, significantly improve the Bed Management AI-powered systems regulate bed function An algorithm takes into account discharge timings and aids in admissions right, is particularly useful when in emergencies or patient surge.

AI powered AI tools triage severity of patients' Emergency Room (ER) Triage is supported this provides better outcome for the critical patients as it reduces waiting times and saves people's life.

One other area where AI is good for the patient experience is Personalized Communication. Questions that are commonly asked appointments or meds reminders through virtual assistants/chatbots and guiding patients along the administrative process to make their hospital experience feel more natural and interactive.

iv. Decision Support for Hospital Management

AI as a decision making tool for hospital administrators and C suites allows them to run the hospital by helping analyse terabytes of operational clinical data to provide strategic insights.

AI Performance Dashboards show critical metrics such as patient satisfaction, average days in hospital, readmission rates, and financial performance to management. Dashboards provide the telemetry to track progress and spot potential problem areas where leaders can do fine-tuning in real-time.

Another key capability is Operational Forecasting. With AI, you can forecast the future patient inflow by analysing seasonal data, admission histories and external health factors (i.e., disease X broke out now affecting Y population). This anticipatory insight enables hospitals to set up ahead of time initiate staffing and inventory agreements, scheduling patterns etc.

# 11. ETHICAL, LEGAL, AND SOCIAL IMPLICATIONS OF AI IN HEALTHCARE

As Artificial Intelligence (AI) steps further into the foreground of the healthcare canvas, it underlies both major advantages as well as significant ethical, legal and social issues. AI technologies need to be tackled on these challenges in order to ensure that they are safe, fair, and patient/healthcare provider trustworthiness.

i. Data Privacy and Security

AI for Healthcare requires access to huge amounts of patient data which is very sensitive, like histories, genetic enhancements and diagnostic results. Privacy and security of this data is an important part as ethical concern. Inadequate Handling or Breach could lead to disclosure of sensitive personal health information, eroding patient trust and legal protections. Compliant with data privacy laws such as HIPAA (U.S.) or GDPR (in Europe) for the information to be kept secure, the following requirements on data encryption, secure storage and restricted access are warranted.

ii. Algorithmic Bias and Fairness

AI systems train on historical data, they can also be biased due to race, gender age or socioeconomic status. If ignored, these biases are likely to get encoded in AI algorithms and result in biased answers poorer treatment recommendations or misdiagnoses for particular population. The ethical implementation of AI involves developers using diverse and inclusive datasets, running continuous audits for algorithmic bias in order to identify and correct bias, so that AI tools may serve as unbiased care for all patients (Mhlanga, 2025).

iii. Informed Consent and Transparency

Patients have a right to knowledge when AI is playing a part in the decision making process of medicine and what exactly does the AI do. Consent must inform not only of the treatment itself but also what AI tools are to be used. That is in order to educate patients about what AI is, how it works, what data is used for and what the risks or biases may be – in simple terms. Lastly, the need for algorithmic transparency explainable and interpretable by clinicians in the decision-making process will continue to drive trust within AI systems.

iv. Regulatory Compliance and Accountability

AI Health Applications must adhere to medical device regulations and be certified to be used. In several countries regulatory bodies (like FDA of U.S. or EMA for Europe) are formulating guidelines on AI based tools. They typically govern over the basics of safety, correctness and reliability as well as ethical use. Additionally, the issue of accountability comes in what is the developer or the healthcare provider or even an institution liable for when an AI diagnosis/treatment plan causes harm? Strict legal frameworks must be in place to establish liability and drive ethical deployment.

v. Social Acceptance and Human Oversight

AI must augment, not substitute for human Healthcare professionals. Human-in-the-loop is the concept that medical experts should always get final say in most important decisions. AI social accept is keeping a balance between technology progress and soft of human empathy The need for training healthcare professionals, as well as the public on AI (what is it, how does it work on their field and what are its limits) to foster awareness and responsible uptake.

## 12. FUTURE DIRECTIONS AND RESEARCH OPPORTUNITIES

Integration of Artificial Intelligence (AI) & Computational Intelligence (CI) in Healthcare is still evolving and there are plenty of sci-fi scenarios waiting to happen. Though current applications have been invaluable so far, the future hold even greater transformations as well as new research challenges and issues from an ethical standpoint. Section summarizes trends within their infancy, difficulties facing the development and potential breakthrough areas [6].

i. Emerging Trends in AI/CI in Healthcare

The biggest trend in AI gets with real-time AI-driven decision-making. AI is being embedded into tools that analyse patient data in near-time (or real-time), with wearable's and remote monitoring advanced offering AI constructs ready for continuous health monitoring, and automated response in case critical health events occur.

A new trend is the emergence of multi-modal AI systems that bring data from diverse sources genomics, imaging, electronic health records (EHRs), patient reported outcomes etc. together to form a more complete picture of patient health. Such systems can enhance diagnostic accuracy and allow for more tailored treatment guidelines.

Federated learning and privacy-preserving AI are attracting growing interest stand to. Via these techniques, the models can learn from data distributed in healthcare data without actually moving the sensitive patient data and meet privacy needs also facilitates hospitals and research institutions collaboration in broader spectrums (Malik & Solaiman, 2024).

ii. Key Research Opportunities

Explainable AI (XAI) has an enormous potential in the field of AI, developed so that clinicians and patients can understand the reason for decision of these systems. The more AI solutions get woven into the tissue of clinical decision support, the greater the need for authority and interpretability.

AI in Drug Discovery and Vaccine development is another bright spot too. Using AI to predict the efficacy of compounds and simulate molecular interactions, the time and money needed to develop new treatments can be reduced by decades (Beniwal et. al., 2021).

Research on precision medicine is equally rich, especially when the utilization of AI in genetic and molecular profiling gets used for personalizing healthcare. More research is required to better predict disease, treatment response, and health outcomes.

iii. Challenges Ahead

There are however many challenges to overcome before that potential can be reached. Key one is some high-quality and well-defined healthcare data. Generalization and the ability to generalize on different populations is hindered by the variety or discrepancies inherent within healthcare systems and institutions (Sharma, Gupta & Garg, 2022), such as AI.

A second challenge is the problem of governance ethics. As AI will make even more autonomous decisions, it becomes necessary to take a principled stance on legal and ethical issues of accountability and consent as well as fairness.

We also require interdisciplinary partnership among healthcare workers, data scientists, ethicists and policymakers to guarantee that AI applications will be technically solid as well socially sustainable, and legally practical.

iv. Potential Breakthroughs

Breakthroughs are in store for the future of AI robotic surgery, where robots, guided by AI will be performing intricate procedures with unprecedented levels of accuracy. Likewise, virtual health assistants might become all-the-way interactive platforms that handle relatively routine care management, prescription monitoring and mental health crisis-suspected-care support.

AI-based mental health diagnostics is the second transformative area in which small changes in speech, facial expression and behaviour (analysed from video and voice inputs) may lead to early detection/intervention for mental health disorders (Ramasamy et. al., 2024).

AI with brain-computer interfaces (BCIs) combined could bring an upheaval in treatments for neurological diseases, thereby providing novel forms of therapies and control/communication of artificial substitute for disabled (patient).

## 13. GLOBAL IMPACT OF AI INNOVATIONS ON HEALTHCARE ACCESSIBILITY

Artificial Intelligence (AI) is transforming healthcare in making services accessible, particularly in such parts of the world where traditional healthcare infrastructure is non-existent. By providing scalable solutions that were infeasible to deliver at scale before using AI to drive innovation, the ground breaking healthcare innovations made possible by AI are bridging critical gaps for many populations.

One of those major AI influence on health accessible is the diffusion of remote care. Patients in rural or underserved communities now have the ability to see healthcare providers via telemedicine platforms enabled by AI, eliminating the need for a patient to go miles. AI algorithms help triage patient clinical needs, prescribe treatments and even flags frontline for emergent conditions (Makanjee, Hoffmann & Bergh, 2015). AI chatbots and diagnostic tools provide virtual consultations that allow for faster penetration as well as the reach of a larger patient base.

AI is also normalizing medical diagnostics with the masses. Techno such as computer vision allow for the imaging of medical images (X-rays MR, CT) less expensive and sometimes even at the same high accuracy as human specialists do. AI and health apps can help health care workers that are not specialists with screenings for diabetic retinopathy TB or cervical cancer in community settings also portable diagnostic devices. The ability to detect early greatly enhances the outcome of treatment and decreases disease burden (Singh et al., 2024).

AI in regions with a lack of trained health workers can help them by automating routine activities like patient record keeping, clinical documentation and medication. Through AI-based decision support systems the workforce sets a patient environment where, even in those places where the required specialist knowledge is scarce; the care (or provision) of the patient is evidence informed.

AI is also important for public health. Disease surveillance for the early detection of disease outbreaks and its forecasting are done with the help of predictive analytics models to resources efficient allocation. AI systems aided governments and healthcare organizations in tracking infection trends during health crises such as the one due to COVID-19 outbreak, managing capacity for hospitals globally as well coordinating vaccination efforts (Malik et al., 2020).

While these are promising developments, it should be noted about data privacy and security, algorithmic biases and the cost of technology. To truly make AI more accessible globally, solutions must be tuned to local contexts, thoughtfully grapple with ethics and make sure it is the most marginalized groups who do not get left behind.

## SUMMARY

Artificial Intelligence (AI) and Computational Intelligence (CI) integration in healthcare: A disruptive revolution towards medical service delivery, diagnosis & management. In this chapter, the basics of AI and CI, their growth, development & examples of applications are discussed in context to the healthcare field. Artificial Intelligence (AI) is the development of smart machines led to the performance of tasks in the way a human does. Computational Intelligence (a branch of AI) includes neural networks, fuzzy systems and evolutionary algorithms that can work with vague uncertain imprecise data, hence they are extensively used on healthcare.

The history of AI is based on rule-based expert systems in the 1970s (e.g., MYCIN), which has evolved into data driven adaptive systems driven by machine learning/deep learning/natural language processing. The techniques cover the medical applications from disease prediction and medical imaging to diagnosis through personalized treatment planning and robotic surgeries. With the help of AI enabled modern tools (Clinical Decision Support System CDSS), for example, clinicians can follow data driven indications during the assessment and treatment of patients that improve both quality of diagnosis/treatment as well reduce medical errors.

The chapter further lists the AI techniques applied in healthcare such as machine learning for sufferer risk prediction, NLP models to text-based clinical notes and vision based medical image analysis. AI and CI are likely to get further developments in future; which brings hope especially for precision medication, preventive care & the efficient Healthcare management. But there are ethical, legal and privacy issues that need to be tackled for responsible and open adoption. AI & CI, on the other hand are the way forward to smarter safer healthcare systems that will make both patient and doctors/healthcare providers healthier.

## REFERENCES


Agatonovic-Kustrin, S., & Beresford, R. (2000). Basic concepts of artificial neural network (ANN) modeling and its application in pharmaceutical research. *Journal of Pharmaceutical and Biomedical Analysis*, *22*(5), 717–727.

Amarasingham, R., Patzer, R. E., Huesch, M., Nguyen, N. Q., & Xie, B. (2014). Implementing electronic health care predictive analytics: Considerations and challenges. *Health Affairs*, *33*(7), 1148–1154.

Avanzo, M., Stancanello, J., Pirrone, G., Drigo, A., & Retico, A. (2024). The evolution of artificial intelligence in medical imaging: From computer science to machine and deep learning. *Cancers (Basel)*, *16*(21), 3702.

Beeler, P. E., Bates, D. W., & Hug, B. L. (2014). Clinical decision support systems. *Swiss Medical Weekly*, *144*, w14073.

Behare, N., Keerthi, V. M., Vasmatkar, A., Waghulkar, S., Behare, S. N., Mohture, A., & Sharma, S. (2025). AI, CI, and Society 5.0: A Historical Overview. *Open AI and Computational Intelligence for Society*, *5*(0), 1–26.

Beniwal, S., Saini, U., Garg, P., & Joon, R. K. (2021). Improving performance during camera surveillance by integration of edge detection in IoT system. [IJEHMC]. *International Journal of E-Health and Medical Communications*, *12*(5), 84–96.

Chaddad, A., Peng, J., Xu, J., & Bouridane, A. (2023). Survey of explainable AI techniques in healthcare. *Sensors (Basel)*, *23*(2), 634.

Davenport, T., & Kalakota, R. (2019). The potential for artificial intelligence in healthcare. *Future Healthcare Journal*, *6*(2), 94–98.

1. Gürsel, G. (2016). Healthcare, uncertainty, and fuzzy logic. *Digital Medicine*, *2*(3), 101–112.

Ho, D., Quake, S. R., McCabe, E. R., Chng, W. J., Chow, E. K., Ding, X., & Zarrinpar, A. (2020). Enabling technologies for personalized and precision medicine. *Trends in Biotechnology*, *38*(5), 497–518.

Huang, Y., Kangas, L. J., & Rasco, B. A. (2007). Applications of artificial neural networks (ANNs) in food science. *Critical Reviews in Food Science and Nutrition*, *47*(2), 113–126.

Hudaa, S., Setiyadi, D. B. P., Lydia, E. L., Shankar, K., Nguyen, P. T., Hashim, W., & Maseleno, A. (2019). Natural language processing utilization in healthcare. *International Journal of Engineering and Advanced Technology*, *8*(6), 1117–1120.

Lin, Y. K., Chen, H., Brown, R. A., Li, S. H., & Yang, H. J. (2017). Healthcare predictive analytics for risk profiling in chronic care. *Management Information Systems Quarterly, 41*(2), 473–496.

Makanjee, C. R., Hoffmann, W. A., & Bergh, A. M. (2015). Healthcare provider and patient perspectives on diagnostic imaging investigations. *African Journal of Primary Health Care & Family Medicine*, *7*(1), 1–10.

Malik, A., &Solaiman, B. (2024). AI in hospital administration and management: Ethical and legal implications. *Research handbook on health, AI and the Law*, 20-40.

Malik, M., Singh, Y., Garg, P., & Gupta, S. (2020). Deep Learning in Healthcare system. *International Journal of Grid and Distributed Computing, 13*(2), 469–468.

Malik, P., Pathania, M., & Rathaur, V. K. (2019). Overview of artificial intelligence in medicine. *Journal of Family Medicine and Primary Care, 8*(7), 2328–2331.

Manocha, A. K., Jain, S., Singh, M., & Paul, S. (Eds.). (2021). *Computational Intelligence in Healthcare*. Springer.

Mhlanga, D. (2025). AI in Hospital Administration: Revolutionizing Healthcare.

Muhiyaddin, R., Abd-Alrazaq, A. A., Househ, M., Alam, T., & Shah, Z. (2020). The impact of clinical decision support systems (CDSS) on physicians: a scoping review. *The Importance ofHealth Informatics in Public Health during a Pandemic*, 470-473.

Prabha, C., Singh, J., Agarwal, S., Verma, A., & Sharma, N. (2023). Introduction to computational intelligence in healthcare: Applications, challenges, and management. In *Computational Intelligence in Healthcare* (pp. 1–15). CRC Press.

Rahim, M. J., Afroz, A., & Akinola, O. (2025). Predictive Analytics in Healthcare: Big Data, Better Decisions. *International Journal of Scientific Research and Modern Technology*, *4*(1), 1–21.

Ramasamy, L. K., Khan, F., Joghee, S., Dempere, J., & Garg, P. (2024, March). Forecast of Students' Mental Health Combining an Artificial Intelligence Technique and Fuzzy Inference System. In *2024 International Conference on Automation and Computation (AUTOCOM)* (pp. 85-90). IEEE.

Roy, K., Debdas, S., Kundu, S., Chouhan, S., Mohanty, S., & Biswas, B. (2021). Application of natural language processing in healthcare. *Computational Intelligence and Healthcare Informatics*, 393-407.

Schönberger, D. (2019). Artificial intelligence in healthcare: A critical analysis of the legal and ethical implications. *International Journal of Law and Information Technology*, *27*(2), 171–203.

Shahsavarani, A. M., Azad MarzAbadi, E., HakimiKalkhoran, M., Jafari, S., &Qaranli, S. (2015). Clinical decision support systems (CDSSs): State of the art review of literature. *International Journal of Medical Reviews*, *2*(4), 299–308.

Sharma, R. Gupta, S. and Garg, P., "Model for Predicting Cardiac Health using Deep Learning Classifier," (2022) Fifth International Conference on Computational Intelligence and Communication Technologies (CCICT), pp. 25-30, doi: DOI: 10.1109/CCiCT56684.2022.00017

Singh, M., Garg, P., Srivastava, S., & Saggu, A. K. (2024, April). Revolutionizing Arrhythmia Classification: Unleashing the Power of Machine Learning and Data Amplification for Precision Healthcare. In *2024 Sixth International Conference on Computational Intelligence and Communication Technologies (CCICT)* (pp. 516-522). IEEE.

Tupe, S., & Kulkarni, N. P. (2015). eca: Evolutionary Computing Algorithm for E-Healthcare Information System. *iPGCON-2015*, 24-25.

Upadhyay, D., Garg, P., Aldossary, S. M., Shafi, J., & Kumar, S. (2023). A Linear Quadratic Regression-Based Synchronised Health Monitoring System (SHMS) for IoT Applications. *Electronics (Basel)*, *12*(2), 309.

Verma, J. K., Paul, S., & Johri, P. (Eds.). (2020). *Computational Intelligence and Its Applications in Healthcare*. Academic Press.

Zhou, B., Yang, G., Shi, Z., & Ma, S. (2022). Natural language processing for smart healthcare. *IEEE Reviews in Biomedical Engineering*, *17*, 4–18.

Chapter 2
# Introduction to AI and Computational Intelligence in Healthcare

**G. Sivakarthi**
https://orcid.org/0009-0009-3434-418X
*Anna University, India & Velammal College of Engineering and Technology, India*

**A. Vinora**
https://orcid.org/0009-0006-2049-3457
*Velammal College of Engineering and Technology, India*

**Nancy Deborah R.**
https://orcid.org/0009-0004-9186-3318
*Velammal College of Engineering and Technology, India*

**M. Soundarya**
*Velammal College of Engineering and Technology, India*

## ABSTRACT

*Artificial Intelligence (AI) and Computational Intelligence are transforming healthcare, enabling intelligent decision-making, predictive analytics, and personalized treatment strategies. The integration of Deep Q-Networks (DQNs) and reinforcement learning has introduced powerful techniques for optimizing complex medical environments. It provides an in-depth exploration of how AI models, particularly reinforcement learning-based approaches, enhance clinical decision-making, disease prediction, and hospital resource management. By leveraging computational intelligence, The transformative impact of AI in medicine is undeniable, and its continued evolution will shape the future of healthcare in profound ways. This provides the*

DOI: 10.4018/979-8-3373-3311-3.ch002

*necessary insights to navigate this rapidly changing landscape, empowering readers to embrace AI-driven innovations and contribute to the advancement of intelligent healthcare systems.*

## 1. INTRODUCTION

The fusion of artificial intelligence (AI) and computational intelligence (CI) with health systems is revolutionizing the field of medical science, clinical decision support, and patient treatment. As healthcare information increases in complexity due to electronic health records, wearable sensors, medical imaging, and genomics, the necessity for intelligent systems to enable data interpretation, pattern recognition, outcome prediction, and decision optimization becomes unavoidable. AI in general means that computers can emulate human intelligent behavior like learning, problem-solving, and reasoning and has traveled a long distance in health care. From expert systems based on rules to sophisticated deep algorithms, AI today drives diagnosis engines, virtual medical assistants, robotic surgery, and predictive analytics platforms. In contrast, computational intelligence techniques such as neural networks, fuzzy logic, genetic algorithms, and swarm intelligence is providing nature-inspired, adaptive solutions to non-linear, high-dimensional healthcare challenges where conventional mathematical modeling cannot assert control (Gupta et al., 2023). Their worth is not just in the automation but in how they can bring out human capability, minimize error, and be tailored to suit individual needs. Machine learning software, for example, is able to predict the progression of disease in patients who are chronically ill from historical trends and patterns (Al-Jarrah et al., 2015). Deep learning software, a category of AI software, has been astounding medical image diagnostics with the ability to beat radiologists in most cases to spot tiny defects. Meanwhile, CI software such as fuzzy logic is in the best position to deal with vagueness in medical diagnosis, where crisp classification is not desirable (Forczek & Rudzki, 2018). These technologies enable better understanding of patient state and aid clinicians in making timely, evidence-based decisions. Deep Q-Networks (DQNs), a family of deep reinforcement learning techniques, are a new breakthrough in AI technology for dynamic and sequential decision-making challenges. DQNs are capable of learning optimal treatment policies by engaging with simulated or actual patient data environments and receiving feedback from clinical outcomes. This model-free learning approach enables AI agents to acquire policies that are not necessarily intuitive for human experts, thus improving the effectiveness of personalized treatment regimens. For example, in intensive care units (ICUs), DQNs have been utilized to decide on the best intervention sequence for sepsis patients with high survival rates and minimal unnecessary interventions (Li et al., 2020). The combination of CI and AI in medicine also allows one to construct hybrid models that combine the strengths of several methodologies. Neural-fuzzy systems, for example, blend the learning capability of neural networks with the interpretability of fuzzy logic such that high performance and interpretability in decision-making are possible a first step to clinical acceptance. Evolutionary algorithms, a borrowing from biological evolution, are applied to evolve model parameters or identify relevant features from big healthcare data. The combination of CI and AI in medicine also enables the development of hybrid models that exploit the strengths of several approaches. Neural-fuzzy systems, for example, combine the learning capability of neural networks with fuzzy logic explainability so that high performance and explainability can both be attained in decision-making a first requirement for clinical acceptability. Evolutionary algorithms, a borrowing from the process of biological evolution, are utilized to evolve model parameters or pick relevant features out of vast health data, making the model more generalizable and decreasing its dimension (Choi et al., 2016). This chapter provides an overview of the fundamental concepts of AI and CI, their origins, key elements, and some medical applications. We also explore how deep Q-networks, being a new paradigm of reinforcement learning, are changing the intelligent healthcare future of decisions. As background, readers get an appreciation of the transformative power of computational intelligence and how it is constructing a new future of data-driven, patient-centered healthcare (Forczek & Rudzki, 2018).

## 1.2. Importance Of Technology In Modern Healthcare

The 21st century has seen the never-before convergence of healthcare and technology, transforming the diagnosis, treatment, and disease management. Advanced healthcare challenges arising from new emerging chronic diseases, aging populations, and pandemics must be countered by solutions that are smart, scalable, and responsive (Battineni et al., 2020). Technology, particularly AI and CI, has now become a basis in the fight against the same, bringing healthcare providers to the technology level that offers maximum precision, efficiency, and personalization to patients. Contemporary healthcare is now practiced in an information-rich world. Electronic health records (EHRs), imaging, genomic sequencing, wearable sensors, and telemedicine platforms produce enormous amounts of information. But that data is typically lost by virtue of being too much, vague, and fuzzy. CI and AI technologies bridge this lacuna. In real-world clinical healthcare environments, for example, in optimizing the timing of drug administration or adjusting ventilators in intensive care, DQNs can replicate most treatment pathways and decide on the best methods based on patient outcomes. In contrast to fixed decision support systems, DQNs learn dynamically from the environment and improve over time and are of special value in adaptive and customized healthcare interventions. The advantages of technology implementation are experienced in practically every aspect of healthcare. Machine learning algorithms are the stars of predictive analytics for patient risk stratification, readmission prediction, and disease progression prediction. For instance, recurrent neural networks (RNNs) and time-series analysis can longitudinally monitor patient vitals and prompt early sepsis notification (Choi et al., 2016). Using patient-specific information, including genetic information, lifestyle, and clinical history, AI platforms can generate treatment plans tailored to the patient. The tools of computational intelligence, like genetic algorithms, are best suited to solve multi-objective problems in this scenario like efficacy, cost, and side effect balance while choosing drug treatment (Manocha et al., 2022). To this end, CI approaches such as neuro-fuzzy systems are viable compromises between transparency and precision. Furthermore, health is a high-risk venture in which human lives are at stake, and therefore strict validation and regulatory control must be adhered to before employing AI or CI systems in clinical practice (Gupta et al., 2023). Generalizability across various populations and healthcare venues continues to be a pressing issue among researchers and practitioners alike. However, the path of technological progress in healthcare is evident. Moving from reactive to proactive care, facilitated by predictive modeling and intelligent monitoring, is a paradigm shift in the provision of healthcare. AI and CI are not healthcare automation technologies they are engines of innovation, driving smarter, more connected, and more responsive healthcare. The utility of technology in healthcare today rests on the promise that it has to disrupt in bettering outcomes, improving access, reducing cost, and individualizing care. As technologies continue to advance, such as deep Q-networks and hybrid computational intelligence systems, they will increasingly dominate the future of intelligent healthcare decision-making. The journey to intelligent healthcare is just beginning, and its cornerstone is our capacity to harness the full potential of AI and CI in a responsible, inclusive, and ethical manner (Haddiya & Ramdani, 2024).

## 1.3. Role Of Intelligent Systems In Decision-Making

Smart systems today are an established component of current healthcare, predominantly in how the clinical and administrative decisions are made. Due to the explosion in medical information as well as a growing degree of patient care sophistication, health providers are beckoning AI and CI systems to augment faster, more accurate, and patient-focused decision-making processes. These intelligent systems, including machine learning, deep learning, fuzzy logic, evolutionary computing, and hybrid models, represent a paradigm shift away from rule-based, conventional methods to adaptive, data-driven methods with real-time, evidence-based decision support (Goodfellow, Bengio, & Courville, 2016). The potential of intelligent systems is in their capability to interpret vast amounts of heterogeneous healthcare data anything from structured EHR data to unstructured clinical notes and high-dimensional imaging files. Through identifying concealed patterns, associations, and trends in this data, shrewd systems help physicians to make diagnoses, forecast the course of illnesses, choose the best treatments, and allocate resources ideally. Of all these technologies, DQNs, one among the reinforcement learning models, are highly effective tools in dynamic and sequential decision-making scenarios (Anagnostou et al., 2003). In clinical practice in the real world, decisions have to be made often in uncertain situations, with limitations of time, and in differential responses from patients. Classic statistical models or deterministic-biased decision trees will generally not be able to capture the subtleties of such complexity. Intelligent systems, however, learn from experience and continually refine their method based on results. A DQN can, for example, encode a sequence of treatment of a patient by learning based on clinical incidents, rewards (e.g., better health parameters), and penalties (e.g., side effects). This renders them highly appropriate for treatment protocol optimization, particularly for chronic disease or intensive care administration, where order of action determines long-term results (Financial Times, 2025). The system can be optimized in terms of policies by time using DQNs to enhance treatment choice and patient-specific decision-making. Intelligent systems are not only increasingly affecting clinical decision-making but are also increasingly having an impact on operational and administrative decision-making at hospitals. Machine learning predictive analytics can forecast patient admissions, manage staffing shifts, and optimize supply chain management. The algorithms are based on hospital trends of resource consumption, seasonality of illness, and demographics to give insight to inform policy and save operating expenses. Evolutionary algorithms, being a subclass of CI, are generally used in such applications to solve multi-objective and constraint problems (Khan et al., 2020). Ethical and interpretability issues are of the highest priority when using intelligent systems for decision-making. Clinicians should have confidence and comprehend the basis of AI recommendations so that they can incorporate them into their routines confidently. Methods such as explainable AI (XAI) and fuzzy logic-inferred interpretable models bridge this gap by promoting transparency and accountability of the decision-making process. Neuro-fuzzy systems, for instance, offer a combination of the learnability of neural networks with the interpretability of fuzzy systems, providing a performance-trust balance. Even though promising, intelligent systems are not perfect. Non-quality of data, biased algorithms, lack of standardization, and interfacing issues with existing systems could affect the efficiency of such systems. Human-AI collaboration is now, therefore, the area of concern where human decisions are augmented through intelligent systems and not substituted. This collaborative framework allows end decisions to be made with clinical expertise alongside data-informed decisions and thereby ensures improved accountability and outcomes. In the times to come, the smart system's role in health care decision-making will continue to grow even further with improvement in deep reinforcement learning, transfer learning, and federated learning (Hossain et al., 2019). These technologies will enable more generalizable and scalable AI models to be learned from distributed sources of data without sacrificing patient confidentiality. Federated learning, for instance, can facilitate hospitals' ability to train intelligent models cooperatively without sharing data, the way towards inclusive and equitable decision-support solutions. Intelligent system implementation in healthcare decision-making is a revolution in medicine. Through the application of AI and CI technologies hybrid models and Deep Q-Networks, specifically the doctors are able to make smarter, faster, and more personalized choices. With better clinical outcomes and resource utilization, these systems have the potential for a future of proactive, patient-centered, and informed healthcare achieved through continuous learning. With every passage of time and technological and research advancement, the intelligent augmentation of human judgment in medicine will continue to be a powerful driving force for the development of next-generation medical systems (Haddiya & Ramdani, 2024).

## 1.4. Overview Of Artificial Intelligence And Computational Intelligence In Health Care

Artificial intelligence is a cutting-edge branch of computer science that involves the creation of machines that are capable of executing tasks requiring human intellect. Such tasks involve learning, reasoning, solving problems, perceiving, and understanding language. Technically, AI attempts to replicate or extend human intellectual processes by creating intelligent systems and algorithms that are able to process massive information, detect patterns, and make independent choices (Bohr & Memarzadeh, 2020). AI has, in the past, transitioned from symbolic reasoning and rule-based systems to more complex methods like machine learning, deep learning, and reinforcement learning. Such a transition, in medicine, has come at a very steep cost, where AI systems are now capable of helping with diagnosis, predicting disease onset, providing customized treatment, and handling administrative duties. Machine learning, being one of the forms of AI, enables systems to enhance performance over time without explicit programming. It is especially helpful in healthcare scenarios where AI is learned from patient history to identify anomalies, predict potential health risks, and assist in clinical decision-making (Goodfellow, Bengio, & Courville, 2016).

Deep learning, in which artificial neural networks are composed of several layers, has also enhanced AI, particularly in processing unstructured data such as medical images, speech, and text. Algorithms of RNN and CNN have been extremely accurate in identifying pictures and processing sequence data, respectively (Hossain et al., 2019). Deep Q-Networks (DQNs), a learning algorithm for reinforcement, have found new paths to healthcare through intelligent agents' potential to learn optimum treatment policies in more detail upon interacting with systems that change in real time recently. Agents are provided with feedback for their actions in the form of penalties or rewards, thus allowing them to refine their strategies over time. The adaptability and learning nature of DQNs position them best in healthcare's high-level decision-making problems like ICU therapy or managing chronic diseases (Battineni et al., 2020). Artificial intelligence in healthcare moves from drug discovery, robots, and virtual health assistants into the realm of areas beyond diagnosis and decision-making. As the AI becomes more embedded in the healthcare system, though, there are data privacy, algorithmic fairness, transparency, and ethical concerns. Solving these will be essential to realizing the vast potential of AI while ensuring trust and its integration into practice. As a basis for smart healthcare, AI is both a promise and a challenge to reimagine human well-being through smart, data-driven solutions (Ashrafian et al., 2015).

## 1.5. Definition And Historical Evolution Of AI

Artificial intelligence refers to the engineering and science of creating computer programs or machines to perform tasks that are usually associated with human intelligence. They include reasoning, learning, making decisions, interpreting natural language, and vision (Jiang et al., 2017). At its basic level, AI seeks to mimic human intelligence and, to some extent, excel at it as far as efficiency and precision are concerned. AI can be called narrow AI, for a specific purpose like image recognition or translation, and general AI, which would have the potential to do anything mentally that an individual would. AI's capacity to replicate human mental processes like reasoning, decision-making, and vision perception makes it a highly valuable tool in medicine. For example, AI systems can help in disease diagnosis, treatment planning, medical image interpretation, and patient outcome prediction. These are central to enhancing efficiency, accuracy, and quality of care within healthcare (Haddiya & Ramdani, 2024). AI embraces a number of subdomains, such as machine learning, natural language processing, robotics, computer vision, and knowledge representation. Deep learning, a subset of ML concerned with multi-layer neural networks and reinforcement learning trained agents learning through trial, error, and feedback, subsequently emerged as children of their utility to tackle difficult problems, particularly in medicine, finance, and autonomous systems. Specifically, Deep Q-Networks, where deep learning is integrated with Q-learning (one of the sub-disciplines of reinforcement learning), now pervasively live in decision settings with temporally changing preferences or intervally altering decisions made by covering multiple times, e.g., planning to treat a patient (LeCun et al., 2015).

### 1.5.1. Historical Evolution Of AI

In the past, artificial intelligence has experienced a series of concepts unfolding, technological innovations, and revolutionary applications across various sectors, one being healthcare. The history of AI begins as far back as the 1940s and 1950s, when Alan Turing articulated the fundamental concepts of machine intelligence, and in 1956, at the Dartmouth Conference, referred to the term "artificial intelligence." Early enthusiasm led to rule-based systems such as the Logic Theorist and General Problem Solver, but computer capabilities and knowledge representation limitations gave rise to the first "AI winter" of the 1970s in response to disillusionment (Kumar & Sharma, 2023). Expert systems such as MYCIN rekindled it in the 1980s, employing programmed medical rules in decision-making. As promising as they were, the systems turned out to be expensive and inflexible to maintain, bringing about another AI winter in the late 1980s. The 1990s saw the shift towards machine learning because of greater data and computational resources. Most importantly, IBM's Deep Blue beat world chess champion Garry Kasparov in 1997, increasing the strategic thinking ability of AI. The 2000s were replete with revolutionary innovation in statistical learning and neural networks that set the stage for deep learning to dominate the 2010s. Computational achievements on the basis of theories within CNNs and triumphs within such architectures as AlexNet to identify images also fueled implementations in the AI within mainstream applications for medical imaging, diagnosis, and genomics. Evolution of reinforcement learning, Deep Q-Networks by DeepMind, further spread the application of AI in sequential decision-making a field at the core of complicated healthcare environments such as care management of chronic diseases, treatment decision-making, and optimization of the ICU. AI is at the very forefront of clever healthcare systems with real-time decision support, forecasting, and patient-focused intervention capability (Jiang et al., 2017). Blending AI with computational intelligence methods fuzzy logic, evolutionary computation, and hybrid models is making it more effective at dealing with uncertainty, reacting to intricate patterns in data, and providing clear, actionable insight. As AI continues to advance, focus increasingly turns to ethics frameworks, explainability, and responsible use, especially in high-consequence domains like healthcare. The shift from rule-based reasoning towards self-learning systems represents a paradigm change in how machines are able to augment human intelligence opening up immense possibilities to revolutionize the delivery of healthcare through intelligent, data-driven, and patient-centric solutions (Bohr & Memarzadeh, 2020).

## 1.5.2. Types Of Artificial Intelligence

Artificial intelligence has been categorized into three broad types on the basis of its ability: narrow AI, general AI, and super AI. These classifications assist in determining the ability and scope of AI systems, particularly in high-risk and dynamic sectors like medicine, where decision-making, flexibility, and safety are of utmost concern. Figure.1.5.2 shows the types of Artificial Intelligence.

*Figure 1. Types Of Artificial Intelligence*

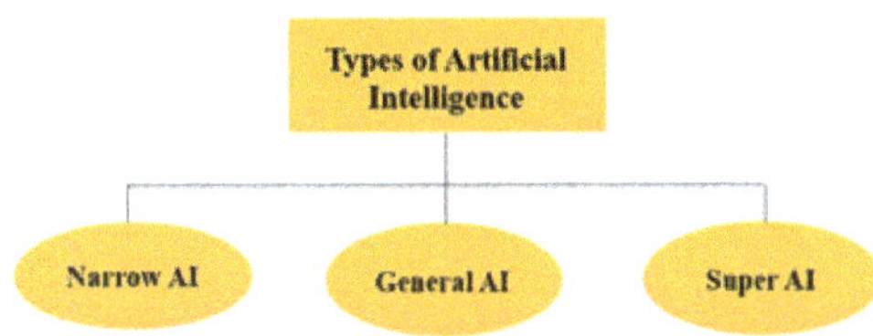


1. Narrow AI (ANI - Artificial Narrow Intelligence)

Weak AI, or narrow AI, are those AI systems trained and programmed to do a specific task or set of tasks. The systems operate on predetermined parameters and are unable to broaden their domains further. All current uses of AI are under this umbrella, such as face recognition systems, voice assistants Siri and Alexa, spam mail detection, and medical diagnosis software that utilizes AI (Reuters, 2024). Narrow AI has an important function in the health industry. Computer vision systems can use X-rays and MRIs to identify anomalies, whereas other systems can be used for patient deterioration prediction in intensive care units from real-time monitoring data. DQNs, a type of reinforcement learning, are also used in narrow applications like identifying the optimal dose of medication or proposing personalized treatment regimens for chronic illnesses. While narrow AI systems are highly efficient in their designated tasks, they lack self-awareness and the ability to transfer knowledge between different activities (Shen, 2024).

2. General AI (AGI - Artificial General Intelligence)

General AI is a type of AI that has the capacity to comprehend, learn, and utilize intelligence across various tasks much like human intelligence. AGI systems, unlike narrow AI, can execute any intellectual task that the human person can do.

They can develop the capacity to adjust to novel situations, think in novel contexts, and transfer the ability gained in one context to another. AGI is still a theory and something that researchers and scientists are in progress towards. In medicine, general AI would be having intelligent agents capable of reading complicated medical histories, diagnosing, forecasting outcomes, proposing treatments, and even empathizing with patients all with some extent of nuance and general reasoning like an extremely skilled human doctor. Although advances in deep learning and reinforcement learning have moved us closer to this utopia, real AGI remains to be accomplished (Reuters, 2024).

3. Super AI (ASI - Artificial Superintelligence)

Super AI is a theoretical plane on which not only humanly superior machines reign over human intelligence in all aspects of reasoning, deciding, feeling sympathy, and imagining, but also develop in an existence independent of their creators. Super AI would surpass the top human minds in all dimensions of imagination, sciences, general wisdom, and social skills.

In healthcare, super AI would result in revolutionary transformation, i.e., healing disease, controlling world health systems, and even making human life longer through research and interventions. But advanced AI poses deep security and ethical issues. Control, unpredictability, and human values alignment are most critically on the agenda currently. Therefore, the creation of super AI must be pursued with utmost prudence and under robust ethical guidelines and global collaboration.

Each level of AI is a level of intelligence and autonomy. We are firmly in the era of narrow AI today and progressing towards general AI with the help of algorithms like DQNs that learn to produce the best policies in changing environments. Realization of these categories not only facilitates an understanding of the trajectory of AI technology but also enables stakeholders in healthcare to harness its potential in a strategic manner for enhanced, safer, and more personalized decision-making (Al-Jarrah et al., 2015).

### 1.5.3. Core Technologies Behind In AI Healthcare

Artificial Intelligence healthcare is underpinned by an array of technologies that allow machines to perceive, learn, reason, and act in order to augment or simulate human intelligence. These technologies are the backbone of smart healthcare systems and enable them to handle vast amounts of data, recognize patterns, and facilitate clinical decision-making with unprecedented accuracy. Among these, machine learning, deep learning, natural language processing and expert systems are key enablers in transforming the provision of healthcare (Chen et al., 2017). Figure.1.5.3 shows the Technologies in AI Healthcare.

*Figure 2. Core Technologies Of Artificial Intelligence In Healthcare Systems*

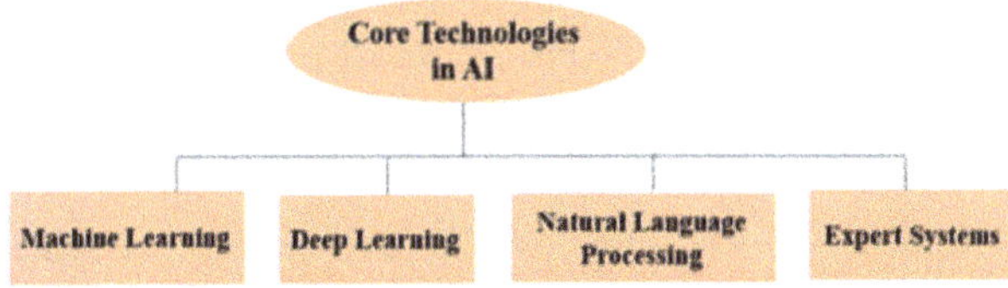


1. Machine Learning in healthcare

Machine Learning being one of the fundamental subsets of Artificial Intelligence, computerizes the learning of the computer to learn patterns within data and make data-driven decisions with minimal human involvement. Machine Learning (ML) fundamentally redefines clinical work habits in the healthcare domain using predictive analytics, risk stratification, and accurate diagnostics (Beam & Kohane, 2018).

Machine Learning algorithms like decision trees, support vector machines (SVM), and k-nearest neighbors (KNN) are extensively applied for:

Detection of abnormalities in radiological and pathological images (e.g., detection of growing tumors).
Trend disease onset or development (e.g., diabetes or cancer).
Classify patients into different risk groups for tailored care plans.

One of the greatest strengths of ML in medicine is that it can become better over time as it becomes exposed to more and more data.

For instance, an ML model trained on electronic health records (EHRs) can predict hospital readmission, side effects of drugs, or decline in chronic patients. These predictions can pre-emptively alert clinicians, enhancing intervention schedules and patient protection. As medicine continues to become increasingly data-intensive, the capability of ML to facilitate real-time, smart, and personalized decision-making is growing (Beam & Kohane, 2018).

2. Deep Learning for healthcare

Deep Learning while a more sophisticated version of ML, uses multilayer artificial neural networks to represent complex patterns in high-dimensional data. DL has transformed imaging in medicine such as medical imaging, genomics, drug discovery, and personalized medicine (Amato et al., 2013).

Gargantuan applications of CNNs are used in pathology and radiology for detecting abnormalities like tumor, fracture, or blood cell abnormality in images.
Recurrent Neural Networks are used to investigate sequential data, including ECG signals and online ICU patient monitoring data.DL also makes reinforcement learning approaches possible, particularly DQNs which apply deep learning to Q-learning so that intelligent systems can learn maximum policies in difficult, dynamic health environments.
For example: In treatment optimization, DQNs can learn to select progressively the optimal therapy plan for long-term diseases. They could enable resource planning and real-time decision-making in ICU care through the prediction of patient trajectories. DL has come to be regarded as the gravity point of future smart healthcare systems by enabling the possibility of real-time, high-stakes decision-making (LeCun et al., 2015).

3. Natural Language Processing (NLP) in Clinical Practice

Natural Language Processing (NLP) enables computers to read, understand, and respond to human language. This feature is particularly useful in medicine, where more than 80% of clinical information is unstructured trapped in physician comments, discharge summaries, radiology reports, and research studies. Uses of NLP in medicine are:

Clinical text mining for extracting symptom, diagnosis, and treatment information from free-text comments.
Real-time transcription of doctor-patient dialogue directly into EHRs.
Literature summarization and retrieval for evidence-based medicine.
Sentiment analysis of patient feedback forms and online reviews.
BERT and GPT-adopted state-of-the-art NLP models have started to make conversational AI a reality for healthcare.

Virtual health assistants, symptom guides, and smart chatbots on these platforms can converse with patients, respond to queries, and lead them through pre-diagnosis steps all in natural language. This enhances access and continuity of care, particularly in telemedicine and remote environments.

4. Expert Systems for Healthcare Decision Support

Expert Systems are computer programs that simulate the problem-solving ability of an expert human. They employ an inference engine and a knowledge base of medical rules and facts to produce clinical decision support. Early instances such as MYCIN illustrated how medical expertise could be programmed to aid physicians in diagnosing infectious diseases and suggesting antibiotics (Dey et al., 2018). Although current AI promotes data-driven methods such as ML and DL, rule-based expert systems are still useful in certain healthcare settings:

Emergency triage, where formal logic is required for quick decision-making,
Orphan diseases, where data are limited but specialist consensus is clearly defined,
Medical compliance systems, where transparency and explainability of decisions are required for legal and ethical responsibility.

In modern deployments, hybrid architectures combining expert systems and neural networks (i.e., neuro-symbolic AI) are being developed. These models offer precision as well as transparency, so that clinical decision-making is not only effective but also explainable an imperative in controlled health environments (Kaul et al., 2020).

## 1.6. Integrating Core Technologies For Smart Healthcare

With the progress in the digital medicine environment, the use of central technologies such as Artificial Intelligence, Computational Intelligence, Deep Q-Networks, Machine Learning, Deep Learning, Natural Language Processing and expert systems is essential in the design of intelligent, adaptive healthcare systems (Chen et al., 2017). The technologies offer unmatched data analysis, pattern recognition, predictive model capacity, and real-time decision-making. Their union represents a paradigm shift toward the provision of health care from reactive to proactive, patient-focused, and evidence-based systems that empower clinicians and patients as well. The integration of AI and CI in intelligent healthcare also enhances interoperability across various healthcare subsystems. High-level decision support systems can gather and analyze data from disparate sources genomic databases, body sensors, imaging devices, and patient self-reports into a cohesive image. The combined data architecture offers real-time analysis and rapid response capability, thereby allowing healthcare professionals to make faster and better decisions (Financial Times, 2025). But an additional important benefit of such convergence is the convenience of precision medicine. Treatment plans can be improved with DQNs to learn to adapt depending on treatment response from the patient. Because they continue to learn from treatment response, DQNs continuously refine strategies to optimize maximum efficacy while minimizing side effect. For cancer chemotherapy, reinforcement learning can be used to customize chemotherapy regimens depending on tumor response and tolerance of the patient. Home care and telemedicine services will be significantly enhanced by incorporating such simple technologies. AI systems will be able to track patients' vital signs in real-time, identify abnormalities, and alert the healthcare team of impending emergencies. NLP algorithms enable natural language conversational agents and virtual health assistants to talk naturally to patients, walking them through symptom tracking, medication reminders, and well-being tracking. This not only increases the accessibility of healthcare service among rural and underprivileged populations but also takes the burden off of the hospital infrastructures. Although it is valuable, deployment of support CI and AI technologies also proves to be challenging. Standards of data interoperability and data privacy have to be maintained, particularly during processing of cross-platform data exchange. The "black-box" model nature of some deep learning models also calls for novel explainability frameworks and clinician trust. Nevertheless, progress in interpretable AI and transparent CI systems is being made very fast with a view to crafting these technologies to wider clinical adoption and faithfulness.

Training health professionals in the understanding and implementation of these technologies will be crucial to the successful rollout of the same. Interdisciplinary education fusing medical science and data science along with machine learning will be critical to the development of the next generation of scientists and clinicians (Khan et al., 2020). Deployment of core technologies in health care in the future will also gain further traction with improvements in computing power, cloud computing, and state support for digital health innovation. As DQNs and hybrid CI models get more mature, they will further augment the functioning of health care systems and make them more responsive, context-aware, and patient-specific. The shared underlying AI and CI technologies about the adaptive learning aspect of Deep Q-Networks are the bases of a healthier, more cost-effective, and more equitable system of healthcare. This revolutionary approach not only increases clinical performance but also enables the broader vision of universal health coverage through smart, data-driven options. As we become aware of such innovations in intelligent healthcare systems, we prepare ourselves for a future where quality care becomes affordable, accessible, and customized to the unique needs of each individual patient (Shen, 2024).

## 1.7. An Insight Into Computational Intelligence In Smart Healthcare Decision-Making

Computational intelligence is one of the pillars of next-generation intelligent healthcare systems that possess adaptive, robust, and intelligent problem-solving paradigms drawing inspiration from nature and natural phenomena (Chen et al., 2017). CI stands superior to conventional artificial intelligence that usually relies on logic programs since CI performs better in complex, uncertain environments where data can be noisy, incomplete, or nonlinear the very nature of real-world healthcare environments. In the age of digital revolution, CI offers the computing capability and flexibility required to enable DQNs and other AI models to make real-time, patient-specific, and context-dependent decisions. CI combines various biologically inspired subfields such as ANNs, fuzzy logic systems, evolutionary algorithms, swarm intelligence, and hybrid systems. These approaches become even more central to healthcare applications such as personalized medicine, ICU management, real-time clinical decision support, and predictive analytics application domains where deep reinforcement learning techniques such as DQNs excel when combined in intelligent, adaptive learning paradigms.

WHAT IS COMPUTATIONAL INTELLIGENCE?

Computational intelligence is a nature-inspired AI subdiscipline focusing on the abilities of learning, self-adaptation, and problem-solving without pre-defined sets of rules. CI systems capitalize on the dynamics of evolution, cognition, and swarms to create intelligent agents that can make decisions under uncertainty perfect for the dynamic, high-stakes healthcare landscape. When combined with deep Q-networks, CI offers extra resilience to reinforcement learning capabilities by allowing agents to optimize long-term health care decisions through trial-and-error learning alongside cautious adaptation (Gupta et al., 2023).

WHY CI MATTERS IN HEALTHCARE

The significance of CI in contemporary healthcare arises from its capacity to:

Heterogenous, high-dimensional, and missing patient data.
Non-linear medical diagnostic and treatment progression patterns.
Long-horizon decision-making, a key component of chronic disease management and ICU monitoring.
Interoperate with agents that conduct reinforcement learning, i.e., DQNs, to produce autonomous, explainable, and optimized care paths.

## 1.7.1. Core Components Of CI Techniques In Healthcare

Computational Intelligence techniques, human and nature-based, usher in epoch-making times in intelligent healthcare. CI techniques enhance Deep Q-Networks to make data-driven, efficient, and adaptive decisions possible in advanced clinical environments. The new CI techniques are ANNs, fuzzy systems, evolutionary computing, swarm intelligence, and hybrid techniques and how they enable intelligent healthcare systems. Figure.1.7.1 shows the technologies of Computational Intelligence in Medical Healthcare.

*Figure 3. Core Components Of Computational Intelligence In Healthcare Systems*

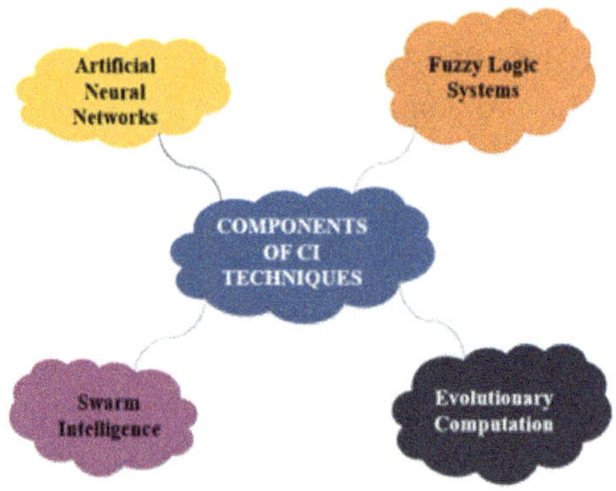


1. Artificial Neural Networks (ANNs)

ANNs model brain function and are central to finding complicated, non-linear patterns within clinical information. ANNs are foundation deep learning models that are used commonly in DQNs to learn state-action mappings in dynamical health settings like emergency response systems or adaptive treatment strategies. ANNs find outliers in ECG signals, predict patient deterioration, and aid diagnostic imagery in intelligent healthcare (Amato et al., 2013).

2. Fuzzy Logic Systems

Fuzzy logic yields truth values so that computers can calculate fuzzy or uncertain patient data such as "mild pain" or "intermittent fever." Fuzzy rules may screen policy choices in risk or uncertainty values in DQN-enhanced healthcare systems. Fuzzy-based CDSS introduce complexity to triage choices and help to direct interventions among limited resources.

3. Evolutionary Computation

After natural selection, evolutionary algorithms (for example, Genetic Algorithms) find solutions in large problem spaces, i.e., multi-objective radiotherapy treatment planning, medical scheduling of resources or tuning of AI model hyperparameters.

Combined with DQNs, evolutionary strategies can be used to evolve action selection policies, finding solutions to reinforcement learning agents where large state-action spaces exist, i.e., hospital bed allocation or modeling of chronic disease pathways (Ashrafian et al., 2015).

4. Swarm Intelligence

Swarm intelligence propels the tendency of problem-solving based on ant group and bird collective animal movement. Swarm algorithms like Ant Colony Optimization (ACO) and Particle Swarm Optimization (PSO) are utilized to perform telemedicine routing, medical image segmentation, and workflow optimization during surgeries with ease. Swarm methods with the use of DQNs have the ability to accelerate multi-agent reinforcement learning convergence rates in systems like distributed healthcare networks or smart ICU.

5. Hybrid Systems

Hybrid CI systems combine two or more CI methods to achieve better performance and flexibility. Fuzzy neural networks are utilized for single diagnosis, or neuro-evolutionary algorithms can be applied to train policy networks in DQNs. In medicine, the hybrid methods can provide context-sensitive, personalized, and scalable solutions, particularly where heterogeneous sources of data and decision variables have to be combined in real time.

### 1.7.2. The Role Of CI In Facilitating Deep Q-Networks

Deep Q-Networks, the blending of deep learning and Q-learning, depend on CI frameworks to process different input information, learn from new scenarios, and improve healthcare decisions with the passage of time. CI methods i.e., ANNs and fuzzy systems are feasible to be utilized as either the function approximator or reward modulator for DQNs and improve their performance in sparse-reward environments or high-dimensional sensory inputs.

For instance, in intelligent management of chronic diseases, a DQN can use fuzzy logic for decomposing subjective symptom reporting and ANNs to simulate the progression of a disease, optimized with evolutionary algorithms after patient feedback loops. In the fast-evolving world of contemporary medicine today, computational intelligence is more of a central idea rather than an adjunct technology (Lee et al., 2024). By facilitating systems to learn, evolve, and make decisions under uncertainty, CI makes possible reinforcement learning frameworks such as Deep Q-Networks to provide intelligent, adaptive, and optimized healthcare services.

As healthcare shifts towards patterns of personalized, predictive, and precision-medicine-based care, the integration of CI and DQNs will be central to bringing out the best in intelligent healthcare decision-making.

## 1.8. Difference Between AI And CI

Table 1 gives an overview of key features, strategies, and functions of artificial intelligence and computational intelligence and a brief comparison of the latter. While CI employs statistically derived adaptive processes appropriate for fuzzy, complicated scenarios such as medicine, AI employs effort and logical rules to simulate human intelligence.

*Table 1. Comparison of AI and CI*

| Artificial Intelligence (AI) | Computational Intelligence (CI) |
|---|---|
| General term for creating systems that mimic human intelligence. | CI is a branch of AI that is concerned with nature-inspired learning, adaptation, and problem-solving. |
| Generally, logic-oriented, employs rule-based, symbolic reasoning systems. | Nature-inspired, frequently data-driven, adaptive, and heuristic in character. |
| Expert systems, decision trees, classical machine learning, NLP, etc. | Neural networks, fuzzy logic, evolutionary algorithms, swarm intelligence, hybrids. |
| Optimized to work with well-structured, complete data and well-defined rules. | Thrives in uncertain, noisy, incomplete, and imprecise environments such as healthcare. |
| Very limited flexibility unless consciously reprogrammed. | High adaptability systems learn and get better over time based on data and feedback. |
| Rule-based AI is most likely to be transparent; ML-based AI is likely to be a black box. | CI methods such as fuzzy logic provide very high interpretability; neural networks may be black boxes. |
| An expert system for disease diagnosis from recognized symptoms. | A fuzzy neural network for patient triage in an emergency department under uncertainty. |
| Traditional AI is not necessarily compatible with deep reinforcement learning in an easy manner. | CI methods are typically integrated into DQNs for improved decision-making in sophisticated health care environments. |
| Clinical guidelines, chatbot triage, rule-based decision support. | ICU management, chronic disease simulation, treatment optimization under uncertainty. |

### 1.8.1. Need For AI And CI In Healthcare

The fusion of artificial intelligence and computational intelligence in healthcare systems enables paradigms for medical decision-making to be redesigned, patients' outcomes optimized, and operationally optimized effectiveness. Speaking of complexity growing in healthcare as well as growing information volume, there isn't any process in clinical decision-making that won't be able to manage the kind of complexity and volume of information. AI and CI, especially when provided by algorithms such as Deep Q-Networks, provide dynamic, smart, and scalable solutions that overcome such limitations. Figure.1.8.1 shows the essential need for healthcare systems in AI and CI.

*Figure 4. Need for AI and CI in Healthcare Systems*

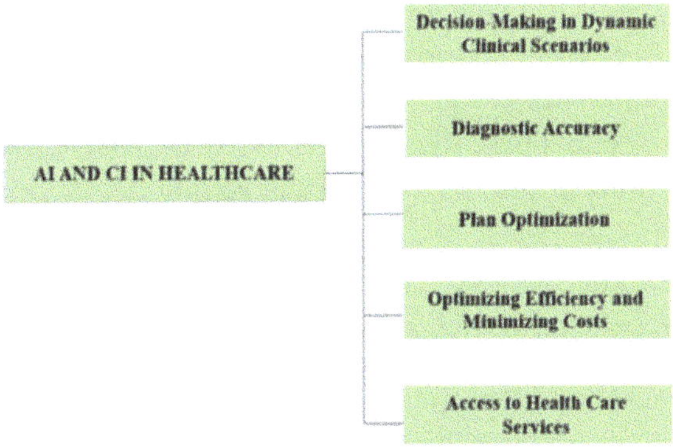


1. Enabling Improved Decision-Making in Dynamic Clinical Scenarios

Clinical decision-making involves several variables that are dependent on each other, like patient history, diagnostic information, and results of treatment. AI and CI platforms such as DQNs are especially helpful in dynamic situations because they can learn, change, and provide real-time, data-driven recommendations.

**Example:** A DQN algorithm can be trained from EHRs and even mirror treatment protocols, using previous performance as a learning foundation and adapting decision-making approaches over time. It leads to patients' care plans that minimize trial and error in the treatment protocols.

2. Enhanced Diagnostic Accuracy

Quality care relies upon accurate diagnosis, but traditional techniques of diagnosis are slow and subject to human error. AI techniques such as convolutional neural networks (CNNs) are far more effective in medical image analysis, recognizing patterns and abnormalities with incredible sensitivity.

Example:

The use of CNNs is on the rise for radiology, with the ability to identify early indications of lung cancer from CT scans faster and more accurately than experienced radiologists.

CI Perspective: Fuzzy logic processing assists in translating imprecise symptom sentences, like “moderate pain” or “irregular heartbeat,” to allow for more realistic and subtle tests (University of Pittsburgh & Leidos, 2025).

3. Personalized Treatment Plan Optimization

AI and CI also play a vital role in personalized medicine by optimizing treatment plans with respect to patient profiles. DQNs assist in personalizing the plans by learning optimal actions in sequential treatment settings.

Example

In oncology treatment, DQNs may be trained to suggest chemotherapy doses adaptively based on patients' responses over time with an optimal balance of effectiveness and side effect (Bibault et al., 2016).

4. Optimizing Efficiency and Minimizing Costs

Administrative overhead is one of the principal burdens of the healthcare system. Through AI and CI, patient triage, scheduling, billing, and claims processing can theoretically be automated, and other resources utilized for actual patient treatment. Natural Language Processing technology streamlines clinical documentation through transcription and summarization of physician-patient consultations, lowering administrative burden by as much as 40%.

5. Enhancing Access to Health Care Services

Artificial intelligence technologies enhance access to medical knowledge via telemedicine, mobile health, and smart diagnostic devices, particularly among underserved or rural communities.

Example:

An AI-driven mobile app can aid rural community health workers in first patient interviews and triage, connecting patients to experts via virtual consultations.

## 1.8.2 Benefits And Challenges Of AI & CI In Traditional Healthcare Systems

Benefits of AI & CI In Healthcare Systems

The merge of artificial intelligence and computational intelligence with the application of medicine practice is revolutionizing the health care sector. Both technologies provide improved diagnostic, treatment planning, and functional efficiency utilities to the doctors. Both of them, together with data-driven, exhibit a possible benefit of delivering more accurate, specific, and economic treatment.

1. Improved Diagnostic Accuracy

Artificial intelligence techniques like convolutional neural networks (CNNs) have transformed medical imaging, reaching or even beating the performance of medical experts at identifying diseases like cancer, pneumonia, and diabetic retinopathy. CI techniques, particularly fuzzy logic systems, are useful because they enable vague and subjective input data e.g., patients' own described symptoms making diagnostic support available even in unclear clinical situations (Kaul et al., 2020).

2. Personalized Treatment Planning

With the emphasis shifting to precision medicine, AI and CI technologies enable the development of personalized treatment protocols. Deep Q-Networks, learning through interacting and giving feedback, are especially helpful in improving treatment protocols over time based on multiple variables such as genetic predisposition, lifestyle, and disease history, generating better patient-specific results.

3. Augmented Decision Support

Artificial Intelligence and Cognitive Insight-based Clinical Decision Support Systems (CDSS) assist clinicians in filtering through enormous amounts of heterogeneous data to produce insights not necessarily based on traditional analysis. The systems are invaluable in time-sensitive environments such as emergency rooms or intensive care units, where real-time, evidence-based guidance is critical.

4. Operational Efficiency and Cost Reduction

The use of AI in the automation of the routine administrative task's appointment scheduling, medical coding, and insurance claim processing liberates clinical staff from these tasks so that they spend more time caring for patients. NLP also proves useful by transforming unstructured clinical documentation into structured data for Electronic Health Records enhancing workflow and minimizing administrative burden.

5. Accessibility and Remote Healthcare Delivery

Where there are not as many health facilities or during pandemics, AI platforms enable remote diagnosis, consultation of patients, and monitoring. Telemedicine platforms, virtual assistants, and chatbots enable the delivery of care in such a way that even poorer or rural communities receive medical care in a timely manner.

The application of CI and AI, particularly when coupled with Deep Q-Networks, has incredible potential to re-engineer the delivery and results of healthcare but will only work if there is an integrated solution. Simultaneously addressing technical, ethical, operational, and educational challenges will lead to a smarter, equitable, and more sustainable future of healthcare.

Challenges of AI & CI In Healthcare Systems

Though AI and CI possess transformational potential, their integration with current models of healthcare presents a range of challenges to be confronted cautiously to allow ethical, secure, and effective adoption

1. Data Privacy and Security

Security must be robust in health information security. Convergence of AI and CI solutions must be in accordance with data protection laws such as HIPAA and GDPR. Breach of security can lower the public's trust and lead to huge regulatory penalties.

2. Legacy System Integration

Healthcare departments typically possess old platforms and software that are not compatible with the existing platforms of AI. It is difficult to integrate new platforms into the existing systems and requires a lot of technical time and expense.

3. Interpretability and Trust

AI systems, especially deep learning models, are opaque in their decision-making. This “black box” nature is a hindrance to clinical uptake since doctors require interpretable outputs to be able to trust and verify AI recommendations.

4. Bias and Fairness

AI systems trained from representative data sets may have systemic or societal biases. These may cause unequal treatment or recommendation for a diagnosis and diagnosis failure, particularly in the underrepresented populations. Ethical monitoring and an inclusive sample data should be integrated to avoid such possibilities.

5. Overly High Costs and Technical Skills Gap

The application of AI and CI solutions also requires a great deal of capital and human resources. Most health institutions, particularly those in the low- and middle-income countries, experience resource constraints that inhibit their capacity to adopt and maintain such tools. Educating administrators and clinicians on how to utilize these devices is also greatly needed but once more nearly forgotten.

## 1.9. Real-World Healthcare Scenarios Using AI And CI

Artificial intelligence and computational intelligence are transforming the healthcare industry in terms of improved decision-making and patient health. From algorithms like Deep Q-Networks, AI- and CI-based systems are transforming healthcare into efficient, predictive, and personalized care. In this section, it elaborates on some real-life instances where AI and CI are being utilized for intelligent healthcare decision-making.

✓ **Customized Treatment Plans**

AI and CI methods of Deep Q-Networks (DQN) can be employed such that specific patients having chronic conditions such as cancer and diabetes get customized treatment plans ready. Using AI, the patient's best possible treatment plan can be established based on his or her genes, habits, and past history; real-time adjustment of the doses of drugs; and recommendations for lifestyle modifications for enhancing outcomes (University of Pittsburgh & Leidos, 2025).

✓ **Early Disease Detection**

AI and CI systems are used in applications such as early cancer detection by scanning medical images (e.g., CT, MRI) and patient histories for patterns that would show the development of disease before the appearance of symptoms. DQNs may be utilized to guide decision-making in the direction of optimizing detection of anomalies, achieving the highest diagnosis accuracy, and aiding clinicians in prioritizing patients at the highest risk for follow-up examination (University of Pittsburgh & Leidos, 2025).

✓ **Real-Time Decision Support and Monitoring**

In the case of postoperative or critically ill patients, artificial intelligence-based real-time monitoring systems can measure vital signs and other physiological data. CI algorithms are capable of analyzing streams of continuous data and forecasting impending complications such as sepsis or cardiac failure and alerting clinicians in a position to make informed, timely decisions that improve recovery times as well as the patient's survival rates.

✓ **Effective Utilization of Health Resources**

AI and CI methods like reinforcement learning can be employed in managing hospitals and clinics in a manner where the utilization of resources, manpower, bed occupancy, and health equipment can be optimized. For instance, Deep Q-Networks can be applied to predict patient arrival, schedule shifts of personnel, and assign resources optimally so that waiting time is minimized as well as healthcare service delivery in general. For instance, in intelligent management of chronic diseases, a DQN can use fuzzy logic for decomposing subjective symptom reporting and ANNs to simulate the progression of a disease, optimized with evolutionary algorithms after patient feedback loops. In the fast-evolving world of contemporary medicine today, computational intelligence is more of a central idea rather than an adjunct technology. By facilitating systems to learn, evolve, and make decisions under uncertainty, CI makes possible reinforcement learning frameworks such as Deep Q-Networks to provide intelligent, adaptive, and optimized healthcare services. As healthcare shifts towards patterns of personalized, predictive, and precision-medicine-based care, the integration of CI and DQNs will be central to bringing out the best in intelligent healthcare decision-making.

## 1.10. Deep Q-Networks: (An Overview Of Reinforcement Learning And Its Importance In Clinical Decision-Making)

Reinforcement learning is a machine learning discipline that teaches an agent to make a series of decisions by interacting with its environment with the aim of maximizing a cumulative reward. Unlike supervised learning, where the model is learned based on labeled data, RL employs the feedback that the agent receives from the environment rewards or penalties to drive the learning process. In medical contexts, RL applies itself to optimizing medical decisions by duplicating the sequential, dynamic, and compound quality of medical interventions. It seeks to establish AI systems in learning effective actions, such as therapeutic regimens, through error and trial over an extended period of time and make decisions based on better choice experience through the incorporation of previous experience. Reinforcement learning is the agent, who interacts with the environment, and the reward function, which indicates the agent's goals. For example, in medicine, the environment would be a patient's state, and the agent would be a treatment recommendation algorithm. The agent receives feedback from the environment as a positive (recovery) or negative (side effect) outcome and improves subsequent actions to attempt to maximize long-term rewards. Deep Q-Networks integrate RL and deep learning to solve complex, high-dimensional worlds. DQNs employ deep neural networks to estimate the Q-function, an integral part of the RL algorithm. The Q-function estimates the sum of all the expected rewards for taking any action in the present state in order to control future actions of the agent (Esteva et al., 2017). While conventional RL methods possess a discrete action space, DQNs extend this strength to continuous action spaces, which are common in medicine, with examples being continuous values such as drug dosing or treatment regimen. The principal components of the DQN architecture are a deep neural network utilized to approximate the Q-function and an experience replay buffer utilized to cache past interactions in order to eliminate correlations between consecutive training examples (Fogel, 2018). The neural network accepts the current state (e.g., patient data) as input and returns Q-values for potential actions (e.g., treatment). With the usage of reinforcement learning, DQNs enable AI systems to learn, evolve, and optimize based on actual patient data, which results in improved decision-making and optimum treatment of the patient. This dynamic decision-making, data-driven capability puts DQNs at the forefront of smart healthcare systems of the future, allowing healthcare professionals to make smart decisions to optimize patient care.

## 1.11. Emerging Pattern And The Future Path To Intelligent And Personalized Medicine In AI And CI

With the evolution of the AI and computational intelligence domain, a range of emerging trends is transforming the healthcare paradigm, requiring more sophisticated, adaptive, and customized healthcare solutions. Federated learning, explainable AI, and AIoT (Artificial Intelligence of Things) are leading the transformation and providing innovations in patient care, decision support, and individualized treatment planning (Dey et al., 2018). Federated learning, which is a machine learning method in a decentralized manner, is most crucial in the case of healthcare, as patient information is extremely sensitive and privacy is absolutely critical. Federated learning makes it possible to train AI models on multiple devices or institutions without moving sensitive information to a centralized server. Rather than communicating all data to one another, the model gets trained locally in a device or hospital network and only shares model updates. As such, personal health information does not get communicated, maintains compliance with privacy regulations (such as GDPR and HIPAA), yet still allows rich machine learning models to be built. Wearable technology, intelligent sensors, and networked medical devices now continuously track patients' vital signs, mobility, and environmental information, creating vast amounts of data (Forczek & Rudzki, 2018). AIoT systems are able to record and interpret such information in real-time, allowing for ongoing monitoring of health and more prompt interventions when necessary. For example, intelligent devices that monitor blood glucose levels will send alerts if a patient's levels are critically high or low, prompting immediate response. This IoA combination not just facilitates remote monitoring but also predictive analytics, helping doctors to predict future complications beforehand. If health systems employ AIoT, physicians can achieve more precise, real-time data pertaining to patients' well-being and thus become competent in faster, accurate decision-making. These new trends are propelling healthcare toward a smarter, personalized future. CI and AI are helping healthcare systems to transcend one-size-fits-all care to more individualized, customized care. With analytics driven by AI, clinicians can sift through a patient's personal medical history, genetic makeup, lifestyle, and surroundings to develop highly personalized treatment plans. For example, AI machines can foretell how a patient will react to a given drug based on their genetic structure and thereby fine-tune treatment schedules and eliminate side effects. Also, AI-driven diagnostic applications can offer individualized recommendations for prevention, and the patients can better their lives by preventing the onset of chronic disease (Kumar & Sharma, 2023). As AI and CI evolve further, their influence on healthcare will intensify, shaping healthcare systems into intelligent, more responsive, and more efficient systems for addressing the varied needs of patients (Lee et al., 2024). The advent of federated learning, explainable AI, and AIoT is just the starting point of a patient-centric healthcare revolution. With these technologies, healthcare can be anticipatory, with information-driven choices facilitated by entire, real-time information and learning AI systems that continuously evolve and improve, resulting in improved health for patients and populations.

## 1.12. CONCLUSION

Reflecting on the advancements and potential of artificial intelligence and computational intelligence in healthcare, we find that these technologies are revolutionizing the healthcare system and the process of medical decision-making. In this chapter, we have seen how AI, specifically Deep Q-Networks and some CI methods, are revolutionizing clinical decision-making by delivering real-time, data-informed insights endorsing personalized care, optimized treatment plans, and patient outcomes. Not only do these technologies optimize current healthcare procedures, but they are also enabling smarter, better, and more patient-focused healthcare systems to be realized. One of the highlights of the conversation was incorporating deep Q-networks into clinical decision support. Leverage the implied reinforcement learning axioms, and DQNs can learn by experimentation how to enhance decision algorithms from massive patient data sets to make more responsive and accurate recommendations. This is particularly so in scenarios such as personalized medicine, where treatments need to be created based on individualized profiles of medical history, health, and genetic profiles.

DQNs allow the system to provide the most suitable interventions based on this dynamic information, resulting in improved outcomes as well as minimizing the risks for negative reactions. This forward-looking healthcare trend holds the potential to significantly relieve pressure from healthcare systems and enhance long-term patient outcomes. A major area for future work is the increased use of AI-based decision support systems across all levels of healthcare. These systems will present clinicians with AI-based information that aids in diagnosis, treatment planning, and patient management. By lessening the cognitive load that is put on healthcare professionals, these systems will minimize the chances of human error and take action on the latest information available. The coupling of CI and AI with healthcare operations will bring about increased human-AI collaboration in coordinating human capabilities with AI systems. Moreover, rather than replacing the medical professionals, AI will also be employed as a tool to enhance their knowledge base so that they can provide higher-order functions in patient care that require human discrimination and empathetic skills. The future is one of clinicians collaborating with AI in delivering more compassionate, improved, and more efficient care. All in all, the path to smarter and more targeted medicine has traveled far with the relentless advancement of AI and CI as primary drivers. The merging of technologies such as DQNs, Federated Learning, XAI, and AIoT is dictating the trajectory for patient-centric, adaptive, and responsive health systems. The future holds much promise, and the potential to revolutionize the face of healthcare delivery, enhance patient outcomes, and transform the process of medical decision-making is limitless. In the future years, the partnership between AI systems, doctors, and patients will shape the intelligent healthcare of the future.

## REFERENCES


Al-Jarrah, O. Y., Yoo, P. D., Muhaidat, S., Karagiannidis, G. K., & Taha, K. (2015). Efficient machine learning for big data: A review. *Big Data Research*, *2*(3), 87–93. DOI: 10.1016/j.bdr.2015.04.001

Amato, F., López, A., Peña-Méndez, E. M., Vaňhara, P., Hampl, A., & Havel, J. (2013). Artificial neural networks in medical diagnosis. *Journal of Applied Biomedicine*, *11*(2), 47–58. DOI: 10.2478/v10136-012-0031-x

Anagnostou, T., Remzi, M., Lykourinas, M., & Djavan, B. (2003). Artificial neural networks for decision-making in urologic oncology. *European Urology*, *43*(6), 596–603. DOI: 10.1016/S0302-2838(03)00165-5 PMID: 12767358

Ashrafian, H., Darzi, A., & Athanasiou, T. (2015). A review of clinical applications of artificial neural networks. *The Journal of Surgical Research*, *192*(1), 164–170. DOI: 10.1016/j.jss.2014.06.022

Battineni, G., Sagaro, G. G., Chinatalapudi, N., Amenta, F., & Tayebati, S. K. (2020). Applications of machine learning predictive models in the chronic disease diagnosis. *Journal of Personalized Medicine*, *10*(2), 21. DOI: 10.3390/jpm10020021 PMID: 32244292

Beam, A. L., & Kohane, I. S. (2018). Big data and machine learning in health care. *Journal of the American Medical Association*, *319*(13), 1317–1318. DOI: 10.1001/jama.2017.18391 PMID: 29532063

Bibault, J. E., Giraud, P., & Burgun, A. (2016). Big data and machine learning in radiation oncology: State of the art and future prospects. *Cancer Letters*, *382*(1), 110–117. DOI: 10.1016/j.canlet.2016.07.036 PMID: 27241666

Bohr, A., & Memarzadeh, K. (2020). The rise of artificial intelligence in healthcare applications. In Bohr, A., & Memarzadeh, K. (Eds.), *Artificial Intelligence in Healthcare* (pp. 25–60). Academic Press., DOI: 10.1016/B978-0-12-818438-7.00002-2

Chen, M., Ma, Y., Li, Y., Wu, D., Zhang, Y., & Youn, C. H. (2017). Wearable 2.0: Enabling human-cloud integration in next generation healthcare systems. *IEEE Communications Magazine*, *55*(1), 54–61. DOI: 10.1109/MCOM.2017.1600278CM

Choi, E., Schuetz, A., Stewart, W. F., & Sun, J. (2016). Using recurrent neural network models for early detection of heart failure onset. *Journal of the American Medical Informatics Association: JAMIA*, *24*(2), 361–370. DOI: 10.1093/jamia/ocw112 PMID: 27521897

Dey, N., Ashour, A. S., & Balas, V. E. (2018). *Smart medical data sensing and IoT systems design in healthcare*. Springer., DOI: 10.1007/978-3-319-73960-1

Esteva, A., Kuprel, B., Novoa, R. A., Ko, J., Swetter, S. M., Blau, H. M., & Thrun, S. (2017). Dermatologist-level classification of skin cancer with deep neural networks. *Nature*, *542*(7639), 115–118. DOI: 10.1038/nature21056 PMID: 28117445

Financial Times. (2025, January 15). How we can use AI to create a better society. Financial Times. https://www.ft.com/content/33ed8ad0-f8ad-42ed-983a-54d5b9eb2d27

Fogel, D. B. (2018). Factors associated with clinical trials that fail and opportunities for improving the likelihood of success: A review. *Contemporary Clinical Trials Communications*, *11*, 156–164. DOI: 10.1016/j.conctc.2018.08.001 PMID: 30112460

Forczek, E., & Rudzki, E. (2018). Artificial intelligence in healthcare: Opportunities and risks. *European Journal of Medical Research*, *23*(1), 1–5. DOI: 10.1186/s40001-018-0341-0 PMID: 29304843

Goodfellow, I., Bengio, Y., & Courville, A. (2016). *Deep learning*. MIT Press.

Gupta, M., Ahmed, S., Kumar, R., & Altrjman, C. (Eds.). (2023). *Computational intelligence in healthcare: Applications, challenges, and management*. CRC Press., https://www.routledge.com/Computational-Intelligence-in-Healthcare-Applications-Challenges-and/Gupta-Ahmed-Kumar-Altrjman/p/book/9781032304939

Haddiya, I., & Ramdani, S. (2024). Artificial intelligence in healthcare: A focus on the best practices. ITM Web of Conferences, 69, 02010. https://doi.org/DOI: 10.1051/itmconf/20246902010

Hossain, M. S., Muhammad, G., & Alhamid, M. F. (2019). Automatic fruit classification using hybrid deep learning model. *IEEE Access : Practical Innovations, Open Solutions*, *7*, 116146–116158. DOI: 10.1109/ACCESS.2019.2933562

Jiang, F., Jiang, Y., Zhi, H., Dong, Y., Li, H., Ma, S., & Wang, Y. (2017). Artificial intelligence in healthcare: Past, present and future. *Stroke and Vascular Neurology*, *2*(4), 230–243. DOI: 10.1136/svn-2017-000101 PMID: 29507784

Kaul, A., Ali, S., & Gupta, D. (2020). Evolutionary algorithms in intelligent diagnosis of diseases. *Computers in Biology and Medicine*, *124*, 103935. DOI: 10.1016/j.compbiomed.2020.103935

Khan, S., Yairi, T., & Torres, J. (2020). A review on machine learning algorithms for the health domain. *Health and Technology*, *10*(5), 1087–1109. DOI: 10.1007/s12553-019-00365

Kumar, A., & Sharma, R. (2023). Deep Q-networks in healthcare: A review of applications and challenges. *Journal of Healthcare Informatics Research, 7*(2), 123–138. DOI: 10.1007/s41666-023-001234

LeCun, Y., Bengio, Y., & Hinton, G. (2015). Deep learning. *Nature, 521*(7553), 436–444. DOI: 10.1038/nature14539 PMID: 26017442

Lee, H., Park, J., & Kim, S. (2024). Computational intelligence for smart healthcare decision-making: Integrating deep reinforcement learning and clinical data. *Healthcare Analytics, 5*, 100123. DOI: 10.1016/j.health.2024.100123

Li, C., Hu, Y., & Deng, Y. (2020). Deep reinforcement learning: Fundamentals, research and applications. *IEEE Access: Practical Innovations, Open Solutions, 8*, 135354–135381. DOI: 10.1109/ACCESS.2020.3011375

Manocha, A. K., Singh, M., Jain, S., & Jain, V. (Eds.). (2022). *Smart computational intelligence in biomedical and health informatics*. CRC Press., https://www.routledge.com/Smart-Computational-Intelligence-in-Biomedical-and-Health-Informatics/KumarManocha-Singh-Jain-Jain/p/book/9780367624149

Reuters. (2024, March 25). Can artificial intelligence extend healthcare to all? Reuters. https://www.reuters.com/sustainability/can-artificial-intelligence-extend-healthcare-all-2024-03-25/

Shen, R. (2024). The transformative impact of artificial intelligence in healthcare: Innovations, applications, and future prospects. SHS Web of Conferences, 207, 03018. https://doi.org/DOI: 10.1051/shsconf/202420703018

University of Pittsburgh & Leidos. (2025, April 18). Pitt, Leidos use AI to fight cancer and health disparities. Axios. https://www.axios.com/local/pittsburgh/2025/04/18/pitt-leidos-use-ai-to-fight-cancer-and-health-disparities

Chapter 3
# AI-Powered Healthcare Solutions:
## Bridging the Medical Gap in Underserved Communities Worldwide

**Leelawati Pokhrel**
https://orcid.org/0009-0005-2675-1720
*SAITM, India*

**Mohd Arsalan**
*SAITM, India*

**Priyanka Rani**
*GITAM University, India*

**Puneet Garg**
https://orcid.org/0000-0002-4635-546X
*KIET Group of Institutions, India*

**Placido Rogerio Pinheiro**
https://orcid.org/0000-0002-1718-1712
*University of Fortaleza, Brazil*

## ABSTRACT

*This chapter examines the transformative ability of artificial intelligence when it comes to dealing with global health challenges with a specific attention to developing countries. However, the implementation of AI in developing countries is facing unique challenges, including moral ideas around infrastructure limits, data short-*

DOI: 10.4018/979-8-3373-3311-3.ch003

*ages, regulatory structure and rights and inclusion. Through the extensive analysis of case studies, new technologies and political structure, this book examines both opportunities and obstacles that are effective in global health contexts. It provides a roadmap for researchers, decision makers, health professionals and technology developers to ensure that these innovations meet local needs, respect cultural references and promote the health care system. AI contributes to the on-going discourse on the role of technology in achieving sustainable development and universal health coverage by investigating the intersection of global health and development.*

## 1. INTRODUCTION

Artificial intelligence (AI) represents one of the most important technological innovations in modern times, with intensive implications to address global health inequalities. In the context of developing countries, where the health care system often struggles with basic infrastructure and resource challenges, AI not only provides step-by-step improvements, but potentially transformative solutions that can help reduce traditional development (WHO 2021).The use of AI in global health includes a wide range of techniques ranging from relatively simple rules - based systems to refined deep learning algorithms, which are able to process huge amounts of unnecessary data. These techniques are distributed in the continuity of the health care system from-from-from-from-by-from-the-time community services and community-based interventions to clinical diagnosis, treatment of treatment and health system management (Gill et al., 2024)

The speed of detecting AIS's ability in this domain comes from many convergence factors. First, frequent health inequalities between high-or-more and lower/ intermediate countries are ready despite decades of development efforts. While global health indicators have, overall, corrected, the progress varies dramatically in areas, many developing countries still have a high burden of preventive and healing conditions. According to the World Bank, maternal mortality in countries with low income is about 40 times higher than high -income countries, while child mortality shows similar inequalities (World Bank, 2023).Secondly, many developing countries have a significant reduction in health professionals which estimates the global lack of 18 million health workers by 2030, with the largest health requirements with the most serious deficit (WHO, 20223).

The AI system can offer mechanisms to increase and expand the possibilities of existing health professionals, so that work transfers and more efficient use of limited human resources (Saini et al., 2023.).Third, fast digitalisation creates in development areas in development areas in development areas for wide use of mobile technologies for AC capable health intervention. Even in remote areas with limited infrastructure, mobile penetration often exceeds 80%, forming a potential channel for AI-controlled delivery of health services (GSMA, 2022).However, the introduction of AI technologies in these contexts raises complex questions about fitness, stability and equity. Developed technologies can first and foremost fail in high resources when transplanted in the atmosphere with different obstacles, disease profiles and cultural references. In addition, there are legitimate concerns that can increase the existing inequalities implemented in a bad way, leading to "digital division" leading to further damage (Kumar et al., 2024).

This chapter examines these opportunities and challenges through an interdisciplinary objective, and draws on the approach to global health, computer science, morality and implementation science. It considers both technical aspects of AI applications in resource transactions and broad social, economic and political views that will determine their impact. Overall, analysis is based in the basic principle that technology should serve human needs and values, especially in contexts where basic health rights remain incomplete for many people. By seriously examining the new evidence and preliminary implementation, the purpose of this chapter is to provide a nice understanding of how AI can contribute more justified, accessible and impactin developing nations, while acknowledging the significant barriers that must be overcome to realize this potential.

*Figure 1. Global health scenario in developing countries*

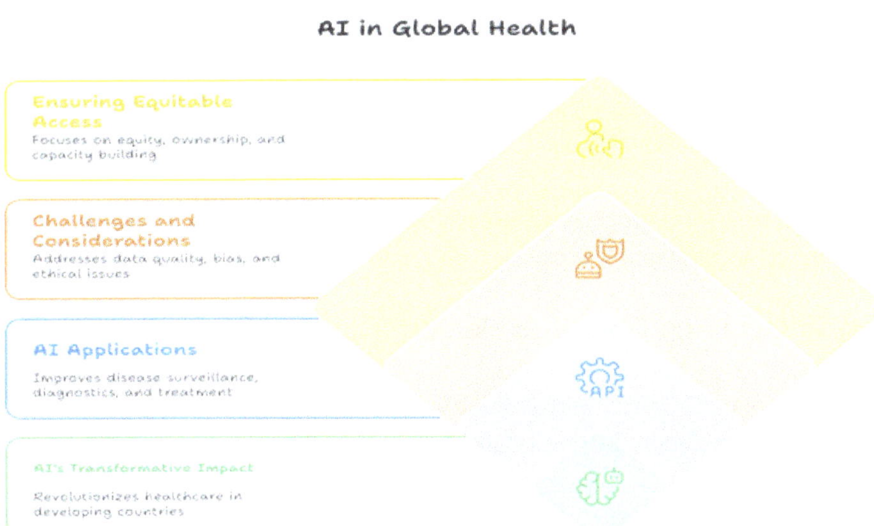

In many developing countries, the health care system faces sufficient challenges, including:

- Restricted workforce for health services (doctor, nurse, specialist)
- Inadequate infrastructure for health care, especially in rural areas
- Economic obstacles and resource restrictions
- High load of both infectious and non-infectious diseases
- Limited access to clinical technologies and treatments

## 1.1. Infectious Disease

### 1.1.1. HIV/AIDS, TB and Malaria

- Accounts for 67% of global HIV cases (UNAIDS 2023) in Africa Under by.
- India has 27% TB cases of the world (WHO 2024).
- Malaria deaths in Nigeria, DRC and Mozambique are high.

### 1.1.2. Emerging Epidemic (Zika, Ebola, Dengue, Cholera)

- Slight monitoring system delays outbreak reactions.
- Climate change expands mosquito -borne diseases (e.g. Dengue in Bangladesh, Brazil).

### 1.1.3. Non-Infected Disease (NCD)

- Heart disease, diabetes and cancer now cause 71% of deaths (WHOS) globally.
- Urbanization and processed diets operate overweight and high blood pressure in India, Mexico and Egypt.

### 1.1.4. Mothers And Children's Health

- Africa south of Sahara and South Asia has the highest maternal mortality.
- Malnutrition affects 149 million children under the age of 5 (UNICEF).

### 1.1.5. Health Access and Inequality

- Rural-Urban Division: 50% of Africans deficiency when basic health services.
- High expenses for package push families into poverty (eg India's Ayushman Bharat helps, but retains the holes).

### 1.1.6. Stories of Progress And Success

A. Vaccination and extinction of diseases
    - Polio near-action (Pakistan and Afghanistan remains spatial).
    - HPV vaccine rolls in Rwanda, Bangladesh reduce the risk of cervical cancer.

### 1.1.7. Mobile Health Innovation

- M-Pesa Fund Emergency Healthcare of Kenya.
- Essennivani telemedicine of India serves 100m+ patients.

### 1.1.8. Global Participation

- GAVI, the vaccine coalition immunized 500 meters+ children since 2000.
- Global Fund saved 50 meters+ lifetime from HIV, TB and Malaria

According to the World Health Organization, almost half of the world's population lacks access to essential health services, with a majority with low and medium -sized income countries (WHO, 2021). This Start reality creates an urgent need for innovative approaches that can maximize limited resources.

## 2. AI APPLICATIONS IN GLOBAL HEALTH

### 2.1. Disease Diagnosis And Screening

AI-powered diagnostic tools can significantly enhance the accuracy and speed of disease detection, particularly in areas with limited access to specialized health-care professionals. • Detection of tuberculosis (TB): AI algorithms, for example developed by cure. Analyse the chest radiographs to detect high accuracy TB, which enables initial diagnosis in remote areas.

For example:

AI-driven clinical equipment can significantly increase the accuracy and speed of the disease, especially in areas limited to special health professionals.

*Figure 2. Malaria diagnosis: AI-driven microscopy equipment, such as Zebra Medical View, detects malaria parasites in blood tests, can reduce the dependence on effective technicians*

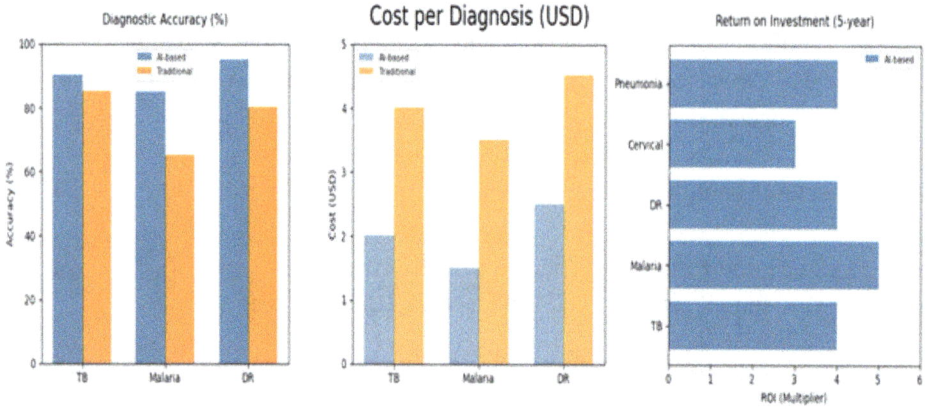


## 2.2. Future Analysis For Outbreak Of Diseases

AI models can analyse large amounts of data including climate patterns, population movements and health records to predict the outbreak of the disease. For example:

Pose-pandemic prognosis: Use platform AI as a blueot and track and predict the spread of infectious diseases, such as COVID-19, which enables time intervention (Garg, P. et al., 2023).

## 2.3. Personal Treatment and Drug Search

The AI -Eit patients can accelerate drug discovery and tailor -made treatment, which is particularly valuable in handling diseases such as HIV/AIDS and cancer. For example:

AI in HIV treatment: Tools that IBM Watson for Clinical Testing helps identify the optimal treatment regimens for HIV patients in low resource settings(Gill, A. et al., 2024).

Medication reporting: AI platforms, such as Benevolantai, identify existing medicines that can be presented for new treatment, which reduces the time and cost of drug development(Soni et al., 2022).

## 2.4. Telemedicine and Distance Monitoring

AI-operated telemedicine platforms enable consultation and continuous monitoring of patients, reduces the gap between health care and underlined population.

*Figure 3. Remote access of telemedicine*

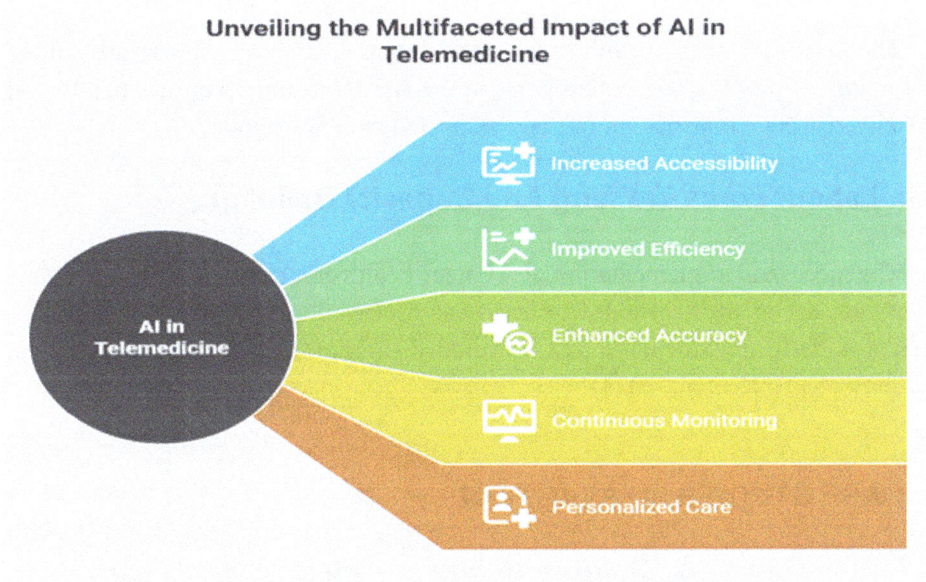


For example:

Babylon Health: This AI-driven platform provides virtual counselling and health evaluation, making the health care system available in rural and remote areas.

# 3. CHALLENGES TO IMPLEMENT AI IN DEVELOPING COUNTRIES

## 3.1. Infrastructure and Resource Barriers

Many developing countries require infrastructure to support AI technologies, such as reliable internet connection and power shortage. In addition, the high cost of the AI system may be a barrier to adoption.

## 3.2. Data Availability And Quality

The AI model requires high quality data sets for training and verification. In many developing countries, health data is often incomplete, fragmented or non-existent, which limits the effectiveness of AI solutions (Chauhan.S et al., 2021).

## 3.3. Ethical and Privacy Problem

The use of AI in the health care system improves moral issues related to the possibility of privacy, consent and bias in the AI algorithm. To ensure that the AI systems respect a transparent, fair and respected patient's rights.

## 3.4. Labour Force Training And Capacity Building

The successful implementation of AI in the health care system requires a trained workforce in both medical and technical domains. Developing countries often have a lack of skilled professionals who can develop, distribute and maintain the AI system (Ramasamy, L. K. et al., 2024)

# 4. CASE STUDIES: IN AI ACTION

## 4.1. AI for Morse & Children Health in Africa South Sahara

In countries such as Kenya and Nigeria, applications of AI-Mobile Mobile Health are used to improve health results and children. For example, the Mom connect initiative in South Africa uses AI to provide pregnant women for personal health information and birth care (Ansari, A., et al., 2022).

*Figure 4. The cycle of enabling the environment*

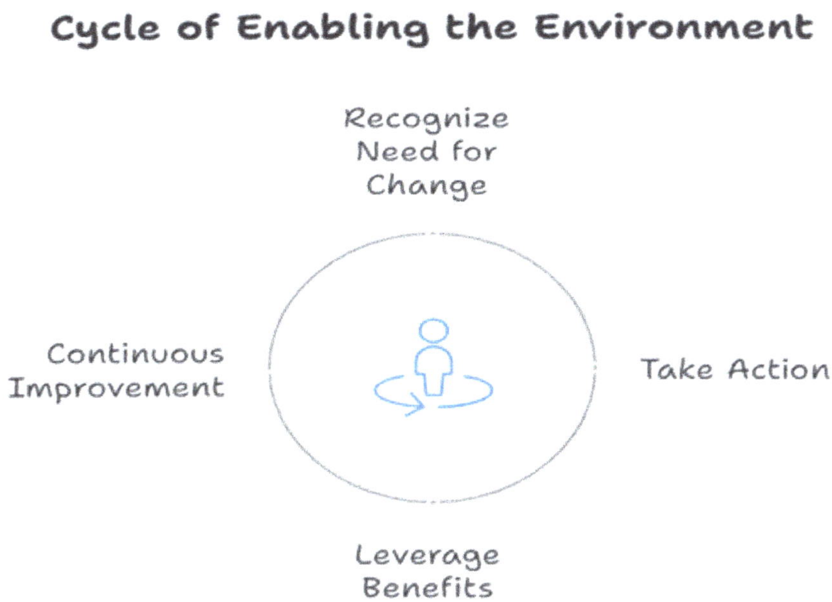


## 4.2. AI in Combating Neglected Tropical Diseases(NTDs)

AI gets the benefit of fighting NTDs such as leprosy and schistosomiasis. In Brazil, AI algorithm is used to analyse satellite images and predict the spread of shistosomiasis to enable targeted interventions.

## 4.3. AI for Mental Health In Countries With Low Incomes

AI-operated catboats, such as Wysa, are used to provide mental health care in low-income countries, where mental health is limited to professionals. These catboats provide cognitive behavioural therapy (CBT) and other interventions to help individuals deal with stress, anxiety and depression.According to the World Health Organization (WHO), mental health disorder is a growing global crisis, affecting 1 in 4 people at some point in their lives. In low -income countries (LIC), limited health care infrastructure, stigma and lack of mental health professionals are even more serious. For example, Africa south of Sahara has less than 2 psychiatrists per 100,000 people, compared to 60 per 100,000 per 100,000 people. Artificial Intelligence (AI) provides a transformative opportunity to bridge this difference by providing scalable, cheap and available mental health solutions. However, the process limitation settings bring to implement AI-controlled mental health protection with unique challenges, including digital divisions, moral concerns and obstacles to infrastructure. This analysis suggests how AI can revolutionize mental health care in LIC, and address these obstacles (Gill, A. et al., 2024).

### 4.3.1. High Circulation, Low Treatment Speed

- Depression and anxiety affects over 300 million people globally, untreated with 75% cases in low and moderate-or-II land (LMIC).
- Suicide rates in countries such as Lesotho, Guyana and India are dangerously high, where mental health services are rare.
- Post-match region (eg Syria, South Sudan) faces a high rate of PTSD, but trauma is a lack of doctor.

### 4.3.2. Hinder Mental Health Care

- Stigma and cultural beliefs: Many communities view mental illness as a spiritual or moral failure, and discourages people from seeking help.
- Lack of professionals: There are less than 10 psychiatrists in countries such as Zambia and Uganda.
- Cost and access: Therapy is often urban-centred, which reduces the countryside.

### 4.3.3 How AI LIC Can Change Mental Health Care

AI can democratization of mental health care through automatic diagnosis, chatbots, predictive analysis and telemedicine. Below are the most important applications:

#### *4.3.3.1. AI-Vagnet Screening Of Mental Health*

- Mobile application and SMS-based tools:
- WHO "Step-by-step" program uses AI-oriented CBT (cognitive behavioral therapy) through basic phones.
- Shim, an AI chatbot, Swahili-Language provides mental health care in Kenya.
- Voice and text analysis:
- AI can detect depression and anxiety through the speech pattern (eg vocal biomarks of Sonde Health).

#### *4.3.3.2. Chabot's and Virtual Therapist*

- Chabot (used in Rwanda and Nigeria): An AI chat boat that distributes CBT techniques through WhatsApp.
- Wysa (pilot in India): An emotionally intelligent fine that helps with stress and insomnia.

*Figure 5. Limited mental healthcare access in low-income countries*

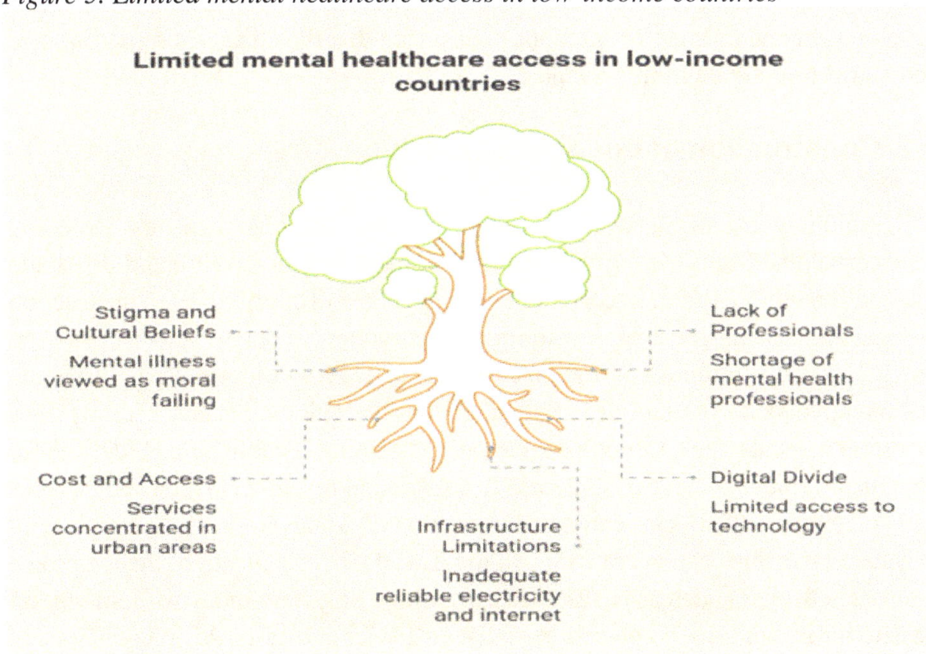


## 5. ETHICAL CONSIDERATIONS AND FUTURE DIRECTIONS

### 5.1. Secure Equity and Inclusive

The AI solutions should be designed for equity, and ensure that they benefit all areas of the population, including marginalized and weak groups. This requires addressing prejudice in the AI algorithms and ensuring that AI technologies are available to those who need them most(Gupta, M et al., 2024). Integration of artificial intelligence (AI) into the Global Health provides unique opportunities to improve the health care system, especially in low resource settings. However, it also increases important moral concerns that need to be addressed to ensure fair and inclusive implementation. One of the most important challenges is the risk of algorithm bias, where trained AI systems on datasets in high-or-in-the-high-country cannot represent the right population in countries with countries with low and medium-sized revenues (LMIC). This can lead to increasing existing health inequalities, recommendations on incorrect treatment or inadequate treatment recommendations. For example, a mental health chatbott developed using data mainly from the western population is unable to recognize the culturally specific expressions of the crisis in African or Asian contexts. To reduce this, it is necessary to involve local communities in the development and training of AI models, ensuring that the dataset is representative and algorithms are culturally adapted.

## 5.2. Construction of Local AI Capacity

Developing countries should invest in building local AI capacity including educational and training programs, to ensure that they can develop and distribute AI solutions that fit their specific health challenges (Topol, 2019). Construction of local AI capacity involves developing infrastructure, expertise and sketching to provide local communities or organizations to create AI solutions that fit, distribute and maintain local communities or organizations that suit their needs. This includes investing in local talents through education and training, establishing guidelines for data management and ensuring access to calculation resources. Open source tools and collaborative platforms can democratization of AI development, while public-private partnerships can operate innovation. Local AI capacity strengthens to solve unique challenges - such as health care, agriculture or governance - without relying on external institutions. By promoting self -confidence and moral AI practice, society can use AI's ability, and reduce risks such as prejudice and addiction.

## 5.3. Associated with Approach

Global cooperation is necessary to utilize AI's full capacity for global health. Partnerships between governments, international organizations, academics and the private sector can facilitate the sharing of knowledge, resources and best practicesN. (Puri et al., 2022)

## 5.4. Regulatory Structures

It is important to develop strong regulatory structures to ensure safe and moral use of AI in the health care system. These frameworks should address problems such as data privacy, algorithm transparency and responsibility.Rapid integration of artificial intelligence (AI) in the health care system provides transformation opportunities - from the detection of early illness to personal treatment schemes. However, without a strong regulatory structure, AI adoption also leads to significant risk, including data violations, algorithm bias, lack of transparency and responsibilities. In order to ensure that AI is used safely and morally, authorities, health institutions and international bodies must have legally implemented rules that deal with data hood, algorithm transparency, accountability and equity (Gill, A. et. al, 2024).. This report examines the most important components of the effective AI regime in the health care system and proposes action -rich strategies for decision makers.The effective regulatory structure should be done on five basic principles:

### 5.4.1. Data Privacy and Security

- Patient's consent: The AI system must obtain clearly, informed consent before collecting or processing health data (eg GDPR -SAMSE).
- Anishanization and encryption: Mandate-identity technique to prevent the transient of sensitive patient records.
- Violation of fracture: Strict punishment is necessary for unauthorized data leaks (e.g. HIPAA in the United States).

### 5.4.2 Algorithm Transparency And Clarity

- Right to clarification: Patients and doctors should understand how an A-rich diagnosis or treatment recommendations are made.
- Open Source Audit: Supervisory authorities must have access to AI source code for bias testing (e.g. the AI Act to the EU).
- Development of performance: Developers must publish the accuracy rate, error cases and demographic prejudice (similar to the FDA drug experiment).

### 5.4.3 Responsibility and Responsibility

- Clear chain of responsibility: Determine whether AI developers, hospitals or doctors are responsible for errors related to AI (Kumar, R. et al., 2024).
- Human overview Mandate: Doctor-in-loop system requires where AI supports-like replacement medicine decisions.
- Death insurance: Expand coverage to include an A-assisted caring accident.

### 5.4.4 Equity and Prejudice Relocities

- Various training data: AI models must be validated in race, gender, age and socio -economic groups.
- Prejudice audit: Independent third party (eg WHO, NIH) should consider AI units before distribution.
- Evaluation of equity assessment: Values on AI are expanded or reduce inequalities in the health care system.

### 5.4.5 Global Harmony

- Criminal standard: Adjust regulations with WHO guidelines, EU AI ACT and American FDA AI/ML Framework.
- Associated inspection: International bodies (e.g. WHO, OECD) should monitor the global health effects of AI.

## 6. THE EFFECT OF AI OPERATED CLINICAL EQUIPMENT IN RESOURCE LIMIT SETTINGS CAN BE DETERMINED THROUGH SEVERAL MAIN STUDIES AND IMPLEMENTATION

The effect of A-controlled clinical units in resource-limited settings is shown through several main studies and implementation of the real world, which highlights the opportunity to improve the health care distribution despite infrastructure and economic obstacles. In the low resource environment, where the lack of trained medical personnel and clinical equipment is widespread, AI-operated equipment has shown a promise to increase accuracy, efficiency and access. For example, a 2020 study evaluated in Nature Digital Medicine evaluated the AI-based ultrasound system in the rural Kenya, where the minimum-trained heroes used tools to detect high-risk pregnancies.The AI-assisted screening achieved 95% accuracy by identifying complications such as fatal errors compared to 78% with traditional methods, significantly reduced mother and newborn mortality. Similarly, Google's AI Diabetic Retinopathy Screening Tool Distributed in Thailand and India showed that AI could match the clinical accuracy of ophthalmologists, which can enable early intervention in areas with a serious lack of experts, and detect Blind-Tea-Tea-Tay conditions.Another important implementation is an AI-powered portable ex-ray system equipped with tuberculosis (TB) detection algorithms tested in South Africa and Peru. The 2021 WHO -Backed test found that these devices reduced the time for TB diagnosis from weeks to minutes, with 88%sensitivity, even when run by social health workers. This approach proved to be particularly valuable in remote areas with a lack of radiologists. In addition, those developed by AI-driven ECG equipment, such as Student, have been used to diagnose arrhythmia in Africa south of Sahara, with a study shown 30% improvement in prices compared to manual interpretation of general doctors.Despite these successes, challenges, including internet addiction, high starting costs and resistance to adoption. Innovations such as offline AI models (e.g. Swipe senses for Transition Control in Uganda) and public-private financing models address these obstacles. Overall, evidence indicates that A-in-controlled clinical equipment can bridge significant intervals in resource-limiting environments, but sustainable scaling requires local training, infrastructure support and only policy structure.

## 6.1. Tuberculosis Detection

AI revolutionizes tuberculosis (TB), especially in resource -limited environments where radiologists and laboratory functions are forced. Deep learning algorithms can analyze the x-rays with the breast with high accuracy, identify TB terms such as cavities, infiltration and pleural drivers that can be remembered by superior health professionals. The study suggests that the AI system receives a sensitivity rate of 85–95% in TB detection, similar to expert radiologist. Portable AI solutions such as QXR and CAD4TB enable rapid screening in social settings, and reduce diagnostic delays from weeks to minutes.These systems are particularly valuable for high-risk population, including HIV-positive patients and living conditions. AI also improves the sputum butter microscopian analysis, more frequently of acid-fasting base than manual methods of automated systems. WHO has supported several AI-based TB detection tools for use in primary care settings, and recognizes their ability to expand the screening coverage. However, challenges remain, including the requirement for different training data sets to ensure accuracy in ethnic groups and integration of AI into the existing workflow for the health care system. When combined with molecular clinical units such as Genexpert, AI-operated radiography creates a strong screening diagnostic cascade that can accelerate the global tuberculosis setting effort (Puri et al., 2022).

- A deep learning system developed by rimre.ai for tuberculosis screening achieved 95% sensitivity and 92% specificity when tested in more than 1.5 million coffins X -rays from 22 places (Raj Raman et al., 2020) in 14 countries(World Health Organization (WHO., 2021).
- In the implementation of a region in the Philippines, the AI-Huzmented screening increased by 32% in the detection of the TB case, while comparing to standard attitudes by reducing the cost of the TB case by \$ 312 to \$ 168 (Panicer et al., 2022).

- The placement of STOP TB partnership of AI-AI-driven mobile X-rays in Vietnam treated around 15,000 scans per month in 2023, and identified 1,870 TB cases, which will remain unintentional (STOP TB Partnership, 2023) (Gill et al., 2024)

These technologies demonstrate particular promise in high-burden countries like India, South Africa, and Indonesia, where they're helping to address critical gaps in TB detection capacity while maintaining affordability - some solutions cost less than $1 per screening. As AI systems continue to improve through federated learning approaches that incorporate data from multiple regions, their role in TB control programs is expected to expand significantly in coming years.

*Figure 6. AI-Driven Tuberculosis Detection*

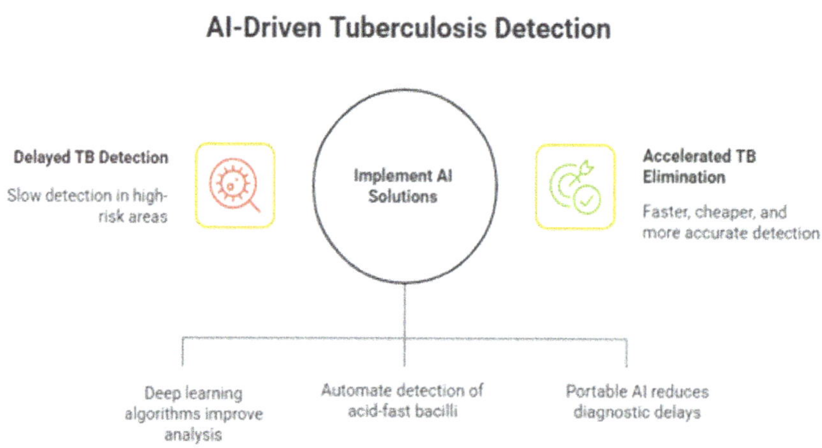


## 6.2. Malaria Diagnosis

AI also changes malaria diagnosis by enabling fast, accurate detection in low resources settings. Deep learning algorithm can analyze digital images of blood voting with 95–98% accuracy, which reduces the diagnosis time for rival specialist microscopists from 30 minutes to 60 seconds. Portable AI-operated devices such as “Autocopes” are integrated with standard microscope, identifying and counting plasmodium parasites in blood tests with minimal exercise. Field samples in Uganda and Kenya demonstrated these systems, which also maintain high sensitivity (97%) with humiliated samples, and address an important challenge in distance clinics.

- A smartphone -based deep learning system to detect malaria achieved 93.4% accuracy in 2,750 blood outbound tests in the rural Tanzania, compared to trained microscopists (97.1%), but available to a fraction of costs ($ 0.27 per test vs. $ 3.4) .
- Sector test in Uganda showed that health workers in society who use AI-assisted diagnostics properly identified malaria parasites in 88.6% of cases compared to 61.3% without AI help, probably 420 cases of inappropriate treatment of 1000 patients were prevented(Garg, P. et al., 2023)

Smartphone-based AI app allows health care workers to take blood-voting images and get immediate clinical results without internet connection, especially valuable in mobile health campaigns. These technologies also address human factors - the AI system does not experience fatigue or variability in interpretation, and produces frequent results in thousands of samples. WHO has recognized AI's ability to bridge the global lack of 3 million malaria clinics, which have discovered a 40% faster case in outbreak areas with pilot programs. While challenges remain in maintaining devices and ensuring quality control, AI-Mango diagnosis represents a scalable solution that can prevent 50,000 unnecessary deaths in advance, especially to detect more accurate detections, especially in children under five years of age for the mortality of malaria.

## 6.3. Diabetes Retinopathy

- Google-developed AI system for screening diabetic retinopathy performed 98.1% sensitivity and 92.3% specificity in 11,711 patients in Thailand, where the screening costs reduced the screening costs compared to expert reference (Raumvibunsuz et al., 2019) to 74%.
- In India, the implementation of the Medios AI system in 301 primary care centres examined more than 78,000 patients over a year, identifying 12,500 cases of synthinopathy, which required intervention, with an estimated cost of $ 4.2 million (Kumar, R. et al., 2024)

Diabetic retinopathy is a complexity of a diabetes that damages the retina and causes visual loss or blindness when not treated. High blood sugar levels weaken the blood vessels of the retina, causing leakage, swelling or abnormal growth. The initial phase (non-promoted) cannot show any symptoms, while the advanced phase (proliferative) includes bleeding and scar tissue. Risk factors include poor glycaemic control, hypertension and prolonged diabetes duration. Diagnosis includes retina examination, florescent angiography or optical Co-oresce Tomography (OCT). Severe cases in management include strict blood sugar control, laser treatment, anti-weighing injection or vitrectomy. Regular screening is important for early discovery and prevention of vision loss in diabetic patients.

## 6.4. Cervical Cancer

- An AI-based visual assessment algorithm for cervical cancer screening tested in 4,128 Women in Nigeria Achieved 91.7% Sensitivity and Specificity of 84.1%, Both Visual Inspections Were Screened With Acetic (Sensitivity: 75.4%) (Hu Aal, 2020) Did.
- Mobile-based cervical cancer screening system that was posted in rural South Africa, examined 11,452 women in 2022, and identified 1,873 high-risk cases for further evaluation, saving $ 121 compared to $ 295 for traditional screening programs.

*Figure 7. Advancements in Cervical Cancer Screening*

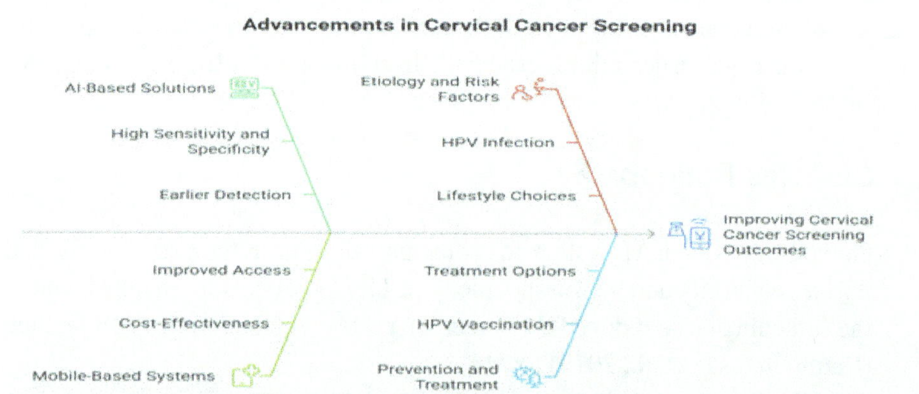


Cervical cancer is a viciousness of the cervix, mainly due to frequent infections with high -risk human papillomavirus (HPV) types, especially HPV -16 and HPV -18. It develops gradually, often develops from the previous wounds (CIN) over the years. Risk factors include early sexual activity, more partners, smoking and immune suppression. Early stages can be tangible, but advanced cases can cause abnormal bleeding, pelvic pain or discharge. The screening through PAP lubrication and HPV testing enables rapid detection, while vaccination (e.g. Gardassil, Cervarix)

HPV-Prevents related cervical cancer. The treatment depends on the phase and may include surgery, radiation, chemotherapy or targeted therapy. In low resources settings contribute limited access to screening to high mortality. The global initiative, such as WHO is 90-70–90 strategy, aims to vaccinate, screen and treat to eliminate cervical cancer by 2030. Consciousness, prevention and timely intervention are important to reduce the burden.

## 6.5. Pneumonia in Children

- An intensive teaching algorithm to detect children's parties from the chest X -rays achieved 96.2% accuracy when tested in 5 232 X -rays from five hospitals in Bangladesh and Pakistan, which reduced the wrong diagnosis of 38% compared to Junior Doctors (Rahman et al., 2020).
- In a possible study in 14 primary care functions in Tanzania, AI-assisted diagnosis improved proper antibiotics from 29.3% and reduced unnecessary references by 41.7%, with properly diagnosed with estimated savings of $ 4.32 per child .

Pneumonia is an important cause of disease and mortality in children under five, especially in low resources. It is an acute respiratory infection affecting the lungs, caused by bacteria (eg streptococcus pneumonia, homophiles flu), virus (e.g. RSV, flu) or fungi. Symptoms include fever, cough, fast or labour -intensive breathing, breast integration and in severe cases, cyanosis or lethargy. Risk factors include malnutrition, low birth weight, incomplete vaccination, indoor air pollution and overload. The diagnosis is primarily clinical, which is supported by fast tests in pulse asymmetry, chest x -rays or advanced settings. Handling depends on severity: Light cases are treated at home with oral antibiotics (e.g. amoxicillin), while severe pneumonia requires hospitalization, oxygen therapy and intravenous antibiotics. Prevention strategies include breastfeeding, vaccination (PCV, HIB, measles and whooping cough), reduce air pollution and promote hygiene.

WHO's guidelines for the treatment of child disease (IMCI) help the front health workers identify and treat pneumonia quickly. Although they are prevented and treated, pneumonia is still an important public health challenge, where timely intervention is important to reduce child mortality.

## 6.6. Cost-Effectiveness Analysis

- A systematic review of 18 AI diagnostic implementations in sub-Saharan Africa found an average cost-effectiveness ratio of $734 per disability-adjusted life year (DALY) averted, well below the WHO threshold for "highly cost-effective" interventions in most countries studied (Joshi et al., 2023).

- Economic modelling suggests that scaling AI diagnostic tools for the top five high-burden diseases across 47 low-income countries could prevent 3.4 million deaths annually by 2030 while generating net savings of $2.7 billion in healthcare costs, primarily through earlier intervention and reduced hospital admissions (McKinsey Global Institute, 2022).

## 6.7. Workforce Multiplication Effects

- In Rwanda, the distribution of AI diagnostic support tools at 41 rural health stations effectively multiply expert capacity by being able to make initial screening for seven common conditions with 87.3% accuracy compared to expert assessment, effectively available for expert level diagnostics for another 1.2 million people (Saini, P. et al.,, 2023).
- Analysis of 24 implementation sites in Ghana, Kenya and Uganda found that each AI system is distributed for diagnostic support, for effectively expanded expert coverage with a factor of 3.7, about 11% cost (World Economic Forum and Boston Counselling Group, 2022) are equal to 1,75(Wahl, B. et al., 2018). These numerical conclusions show both technical effect and practical effects of the AI-operated diagnostic tools, when resource-wide settings are implemented in the settings, then the ability to address their ability to address significant holes in health access, and generate sufficient cost savings(Rajput, R et al., 2024).

# 7. CASE STUDIES

## 7.1. Robot: AI-Powered Mental Health Chabot

### 7.1.1 Background

Developed by Psychologists at Stanford University, Robot is an AI-driven Chabot that distributes cognitive behavioural therapy (CBT) techniques through cognitive interaction. It helps users to handle anxiety, depression and stress by offering daily check -in, mood tracking and evidence -based copying strategies.

### 7.1.2 Success Story

A 2017 study published in JMIR Mental Health found that for two weeks, participants who use Robot experienced a significant reduction in signs of depression and anxiety compared to a control group. Immediate AI's ability to provide decision -free support made it especially effective for young adults in search of traditional medicine.

### 7.1.3 Impact

- **24/7 accessibility** for users in crisis.
- **Reduced stigma** by offering anonymous support.
- **Scalability**, reaching thousands of users globally.

## 8. KINTSUGI: AI FOR EARLY DEPRESSION DETECTION

Kintasugi is an AI voice analysis tool that analyses the speech pattern and detects signs of anxiety and anxiety - such as Tone, Roll and Word Choice –DuringRoutine Healthcare Calls (Singh et al., 2024).

### 8.1. Success Story

The pilot study in 2022 with an American health care provider found that Kintsugi identified cases of unmarried depression with 80% accuracy, leading to initial intervention. In one case, a patient who discussed chronic pain was flagged for symptoms of depression, causing timely referral to mental health.

### 8.2. Effect

- Inactive screening without the need for direct investigation.
- Integration into Telethon platforms for spontaneous identity.
- Reduction in health care costs by stopping growth.

## 9. MIND STRONG: AI FOR BEHAVIOURAL HEALTH MONITORING

### 9.1. Background

Mind strong uses smartphone interactions (writing speed, roller patterns and apps) to assess mental health in real time. AI discovers changes in mood and cognitive work displacements in AI depression, PTSD and schizophrenia (Mittal et al., 2024).

### 9.2. Success Story

A 2020 study involving Giants with PTSD has shown that Minestrones AI already predicted relay episode for 7-10 days so doctors could meet treatment plans. The worsening symptoms of a veteran were detected through slow writing, and motivated an intervention that prevents a crisis.

### 9.3. Effect

- Uses continuous monitoring without input.
- Early alert system for high risk patients.
- Adjustment of personal care based on real -time data.

## 10. TESS: AI FOR SCALABLE MENTAL HEALTH SUPPORT

### 10.1. Background

TESS is a psychologist AI assistant who provides personal mental health care through the text message. It uses Natural Language Processing (NLP) to provide copy strategies, psychoanalysis and crisis resources.

### 10.2. Success Story

In the distribution in 2018 in the university environment, it was found that students using TESS reported 30% lower stress levels after four weeks. A student who struggled with the concern for the exam received daily CBT-based messages, which significantly improved their copying ability.

### 10.3. Effect

- Low costs Mental health care for low population.
- Burnout low physician by handling routine check -in.
- Detected efficiency in the workplace and academic surroundings.

## 11. REPLIKA: AI FOR EMOTIONAL SUPPORT & COMPANIONSHIP

### 11.1. Background

The replica is an AI Companion app designed to provide emotional support through interaction, which imitates experienced dialogue to learn from user inputs.

### 11.2. Success Story

Users' admirers highlight cases where replication helped people with social anxiety or gave rest during the depressive episode. A 2021 survey found that 78% of users felt less lonely after regular use.

### 11.3. Effect

- Non-law emotional expiry.
- Support for crisis for isolated individuals.
- Medical practice for social skills.

### 11.4. Challenges and Moral Thoughts

While AI provides ground-breaking benefits, challenges remain:

- Data privacy anxiety (e.g. speech and behavioural tracking).
- More dependence on AI against human physician.
- Algorithms bias when diagnosed with different populations.

## 12. APPROPRIATE TECHNOLOGY DEVELOPMENT

Artificial intelligence (AI) has the ability to revolutionize global health, especially in developing countries where the health care system faces challenges such as limited infrastructure, labour shortages and economic obstacles (Holmes et al., 2004) However, in order for AI to be truly effective in these settings, it must be developed as an appropriate technique - which means that it must be cheap, accessible, culturally relevant and durable. Contrary to high resources, where AI focuses on advanced applications such as robotic surgery or advanced diagnosis, AI should prioritize practical, scalable solutions in low and between -oriented countries (LMICS), which address immediate health services while gaining control over obstacles such as poor internet connection, low digital control (Esteva et al., 2017).A large region where AI can have a significant impact is the clinical support. In areas with a lack of trained medical professionals, AI-controlled equipment can help health workers in society in the diagnosis of diseases such as tuberculosis, malaria and diabetes retinopathy using cheap depiction devices. For example, Google's AI has been distributed in India for screening diabetic retinopathy, analyzing Retina images to detect early signs of blindness in diabetic patients, which also enables timely intervention in rural clinics with limited experts (Garg et al., 2024). Similarly, people developed by AI-powered ultrasound tools such as butterfly networks are laptop, affordable imaging solutions, which can be used to monitor pregnancy and reduce maternal mortality of midwives in remote areas.Another important application is the prognosis analysis for the outbreak of the disease. AI models that analyze data from sources such as the use of mobile phones, satellite images and social media can predict the spread of infectious diseases such as cholera or dengue before growing (Garg, P. et al., 2022). For example, the promoted mail, an enhanced Global Outbreak monitoring system, helps identify the first warning signals of the epidemic so that governments and voluntary organizations can allocate resources more efficiently.

AI solutions for developing countries should be designed for the local obstacles, priority:

- Low power consumption
- Offline functionality
- Compatibility with existing systems
- Minimum maintenance requirements
- Local language support

In Africa, AI-controlled platforms such as MTRAC SMS-based reporting to track the trend of real-time disease from the health workers in society, improving the reaction time in areas with poor health information systems(Malik, A. et al., 2023). However, these techniques should be designed to function with offline or low bandwidth, as Internet use is inconsistent in many development areas. A hand-to-hand-hygiene monitoring system used in Uganda shows projects such as Swipe-sense, how AI can be reconciled with single, low-technical equipment (in this case

Bluetooth-Soap Dispenser) to reduce hospital-produced infections without continuous connection.Beyond the diagnosis and monitoring, AI can increase personal treatment and farming support (Puri, N. et al., 2022). Among countries with high HIV/AIDS -circulating, AI -Chatbots as Babil's virtual health assistant in Rwanda offers drug performers and answers the patient's questions in local languages, improving compliance with treatment. Mental health is another area where AI can bridge the interval, used in Mental Health Chatbott, Wisa, refugee camps, where trauma is consulted for psychologists (Yadav, P. S., et al., 2022).. However, in order for such units to be effective, they should be culturally adapted to the stigma around local faith, language and some diseases. A size-pass-up AI model trained on Western data cannot identify relevant symptoms or communication styles for other population, leading to incorrect diagnosis or resolution.A major challenge in distributing AI for global health is to ensure local capacity building instead of making dependence on foreign technical companies (Varshney et al., 2022). Permanent AI solutions require local developers, health professionals and decision makers to adapt and maintain these systems. Initiatives such as AI4D Africa promote Homerun AI talent by supporting African researchers in developing reference-specific health algorithms. Similarly, it enables the AI platforms such as Tensor flow and Fast Healthcare Interoperability Resources (FHIRS) local innovative on existing equipment without prohibition costs. Another obstacle is a lack of data - many AI models depend on large data sets, but LMIC often lacks digitized health records. Cooperative efforts such as Radiology AI model for Evevan (Raime), as anonymity imaging data from many low -income countries, help train more representative algorithms.Finally, moral ideas will guide the distribution of AI in global health. Problems such as data, algorithm bias and informed consent are particularly important in the weaker population(Garg, P.et al., 2025).. For example, AI, the identity of the face identity used in the patient's identity should avoid racial bias, and the future model should not strengthen the existing differences in the health care system. Organizations such as the World Health Organization (WHO) develop guidelines for moral AI in health, and emphasize openness, equity and responsibility. Public-Private Partnership can also play a role board, voluntary organizations and technology companies should work together to ensure that the AI solution is in accordance with national health preferences instead of just operating after profits.

## 13. CONCLUSION

AI has the ability to revolutionize global health, especially in developing countries where the challenges of health care are the most intense. By taking advantage of AI for disease diagnosis, future indication analysis, personal treatment and telemedicine, we can improve health results and reduce inequalities. However, there is a need to meet challenges related to infrastructure, data quality, morality and labour capacity to feel this ability. With the right investment, collaboration and regulatory structure, AI can become a powerful tool for obtaining equity and improving millions of people around the world.Finally, AI provides many promises to improve health services in developing countries, but the success depends on the right technology development solutions that are low costs, adaptable and designed to keep in mind the local needs. By focusing on clinical support, prediction of the disease, adherence to treatment and capacity building, AI can help to bridge health intervals and strengthen local communities to achieve better health results, and address moral and infrastructure challenges. The future of AI in global health is not in mimicking high -income models, but in the innovation of lean, flexible systems, which work within the obstacles to resource -limited environments, and ensures that technological development comes all, not just privileges.

This chapter provides a comprehensive overview of the role of AI in global health, with a focus on developing nations. It highlights the potential of AI to address critical health challenges while also acknowledging the barriers that must be overcome to ensure its effective and ethical implementation.

## 14. REFERENCES


Ansari, A., Kaur, B., Rakhra, M., Singh, A., & Singh, D. (2022, December). Handwritten text recognition using deep learning algorithms. In *2022 4th International Conference on Artificial Intelligence and Speech Technology (AIST)* (pp. 1-6). IEEE.

Chauhan, S., Singh, M., &Garg, P. (2021). Rapid forecasting of pandemic outbreak using machine learning. *Enabling Healthcare 4.0 for Pandemics: A Roadmap Using AI, Machine Learning, IoT and Cognitive Technologies*, 59-73.

Esteva, A., Kuprel, B., Novoa, R. A., Ko, J., Swetter, S. M., Blau, H. M., &Thrun, S. (2017). Dermatologist-level classification of skin cancer with deep neural networks. *nature, 542*(7639), 115-118.

Garg, P. (2024). Prediction of female pregnancy complication using artificial intelligence. In *Artificial Intelligence and Machine Learning for Women's Health Issues* (pp. 17–35). Academic Press.

Garg, P. (2025). Explainable AI & Model Interpretability in Healthcare: Challenges & Future Directions. *EKSPLORIUM-BULETIN PUSAT TEKNOLOGI BAHAN GALIAN NUKLIR, 46*(1), 104–133.

Garg, P., Dixit, A., & Sethi, P. (2022). (Forthcoming). Ml-fresh: Novel routing protocol in opportunistic networks using machine learning. *Computer Systems Science and Engineering*.

Garg, P., Srivastava, A. K., Anas, A., Gupta, B., & Mishra, C. (2023). Pneumonia Detection Through X-Ray Images Using Convolution Neural Network. In *Advancements in Bio-Medical Image Processing and Authentication in Telemedicine* (pp. 201–218). IGI Global.

Gautam, V. K., Gupta, S., & Garg, P. (2024, March). Automatic Irrigation System using IoT. In *2024 International Conference on Automation and Computation (AUTOCOM)* (pp. 100-103). IEEE.

Gill, A., Jain, D., Sharma, J., Kumar, A., & Garg, P. (2024, May). Deep learning approach for facial identification for online transactions. In *2024 International Conference on Emerging Innovations and Advanced Computing (INNOCOMP)* (pp. 715-722). IEEE.

Gupta, M., Garg, P., & Malik, C. (2024). Ensemble learning-based analysis of perinatal disorders in women. In *Artificial Intelligence and Machine Learning for Women's Health Issues* (pp. 91–105). Academic Press.

Holmes, J., Sacchi, L., & Bellazzi, R. (2004). Artificial intelligence in medicine. *Annals of the Royal College of Surgeons of England*, *86*, 334–338. PMID: 15333167

Kumar, R., Das, R., Garg, P., & Pandita, N. (2024, April). Duplicate Node Detection Method for Wireless Sensors. In *2024 Sixth International Conference on Computational Intelligence and Communication Technologies (CCICT)* (pp. 512-515). IEEE.

Malik, A., Nandal, D., Gupta, V., Garg, P., &Nandal, V. INTELLIGENT SYSTEMS AND APPLICATIONS IN ENGINEERING.

Malik, M., Garg, P., & Malik, C. (2024). Artificial intelligence-based prediction of health risks among women during menopause. *Artificial Intelligence and Machine Learning for Women's Health Issues*, 137-150.

Malik, T., Nandal, V., & Garg, P. (2024, May). Deep Learning-Based Classification of Diabetic Retinopathy: Leveraging the Power of VGG-19. In *2024 International Conference on Emerging Innovations and Advanced Computing (INNOCOMP)* (pp. 645-651). IEEE.

Mittal, H. K., Dalal, P., Garg, P., & Joon, R. (2024, May). Forecasting Pollution Trends: Comparing Linear, Logistic Regression, and Neural Networks. In *2024 International Conference on Emerging Innovations and Advanced Computing (INNOCOMP)* (pp. 411-419). IEEE.

Puri, N., Saggar, P., Kaur, A., & Garg, P. (2022, July). Application of ensemble Machine Learning models for phishing detection on web networks. In *2022 Fifth International Conference on Computational Intelligence and Communication Technologies (CCICT)* (pp. 296-303). IEEE.

Rajput, R., Sukumar, V., Patnaik, P., Garg, P., & Ranjan, M. (2024, March). The Cognitive Analysis for an Approach to Neuroscience. In *2024 International Conference on Automation and Computation (AUTOCOM)* (pp. 524-528). IEEE.

Ramasamy, L. K., Khan, F., Joghee, S., Dempere, J., & Garg, P. (2024, March). Forecast of Students' Mental Health Combining an Artificial Intelligence Technique and Fuzzy Inference System. In *2024 International Conference on Automation and Computation (AUTOCOM)* (pp. 85-90). IEEE.

Saini, P., Nagpal, B., Garg, P., & Kumar, S. (2023). CNN-BI-LSTM-CYP: A deep learning approach for sugarcane yield prediction. *Sustainable Energy Technologies and Assessments*, *57*, 103263.

Sharma, R., Gupta, S., & Garg, P. (2022, July). Model for predicting cardiac health using deep learning classifier. In *2022 Fifth International Conference on Computational Intelligence and Communication Technologies (CCICT)* (pp. 25-30). IEEE.

Singh, M., Garg, P., Srivastava, S., & Saggu, A. K. (2024, April). Revolutionizing Arrhythmia Classification: Unleashing the Power of Machine Learning and Data Amplification for Precision Healthcare. In *2024 Sixth International Conference on Computational Intelligence and Communication Technologies (CCICT)* (pp. 516-522). IEEE.

Soni, E., Nagpal, A., Garg, P., & Pinheiro, P. R. (2022). Assessment of compressed and decompressed ECG databases for telecardiology applying a convolution neural network. *Electronics (Basel)*, *11*(17), 2708.

Srivastava, A. K., Verma, I., & Garg, P. (2024, May). Improvements in Recommendation Systems Using Graph Neural Networks. In *2024 International Conference on Emerging Innovations and Advanced Computing (INNOCOMP)* (pp. 668-672). IEEE.

Topol, E. J. (2019). *Deep Medicine: How Artificial Intelligence Can Make Healthcare Human Again*. Basic Books.Topol, E. J. (2019). *Deep medicine: How artificial intelligence can make healthcare human again*. Basic Books.

Varshney, A., Lamba, S., & Garg, P. (2022, July). A Comprehensive Survey on Event Analysis Using Deep Learning. In *2022 Fifth International Conference on Computational Intelligence and Communication Technologies (CCICT)* (pp. 146-150). IEEE.

Wahl, B., Cossy-Gantner, A., Germann, S., & Schwalbe, N. R. (2018). Artificial intelligence (AI) and global health: How can AI contribute to health in resource-poor settings? *BMJ Global Health*, *3*(4), e000798. PMID: 30233828

World Health Organization. (2021). Ethics and governance of artificial intelligence for health: WHO guidance: executive summary. In *Ethics and governance of artificial intelligence for health: WHO guidance: executive summary.*

Yadav, P. S., Khan, S., Singh, Y. V., Garg, P., & Singh, R. S. (2022). A Lightweight Deep Learning-Based Approach for Jazz Music Generation in MIDI Format. *Computational Intelligence and Neuroscience*, *2022*(1), 2140895. PMID: 36035841

Chapter 4

# Machine Learning and Computational Intelligence for Smart Healthcare: Advancing Diagnosis and Treatment

**Siva Subramanian R.**
https://orcid.org/0000-0002-7509-9223
*SRM Institute of Science and Technology, India*

**R. Asha**
*Sathyabama Institute of Science and Technology, India*

**J. Sangeetha**
*S.A. Engineering College, India*

**A. Adaikkammai**
*RMD Engineering College, India*

**T. Thilagam**
https://orcid.org/0000-0002-7657-0726
*Vel Tech Rangarajan Dr. Sagunthala R&D Institute of Science and Technology, India*

**P. Aparna**
https://orcid.org/0009-0007-7510-2561
*RMK College of Engineering and Technology, India*

## ABSTRACT

*Machine Learning (ML) and Computational Intelligence (CI) are revolutionizing the healthcare sector by enhancing diagnostic accuracy, personalizing treatments, and optimizing healthcare delivery. This chapter explores the applications, challenges, and emerging trends of ML and CI in smart healthcare, focusing on areas such as medical imaging, disease prediction, personalized medicine, and treatment recommendations. Key challenges such as data quality, algorithmic bias, and mod-*

DOI: 10.4018/979-8-3373-3311-3.ch004

*el interpretability are discussed, alongside emerging technologies like federated learning, explainable AI, and digital twins. The integration of ML and CI with clinical workflows promises to improve patient outcomes, reduce costs, and foster a more personalized approach to healthcare. The future of smart healthcare lies in developing transparent, collaborative, and scalable AI systems that enhance human expertise while preserving patient privacy and safety.*

## 1. INTRODUCTION

### 1.1 Motivation: The Rise of Smart Healthcare Technologies

The healthcare system of the world has evolved significantly in the last decade due to the progression of the information technology, increased availability of information, and the focus on patient-centric treatment. While traditional healthcare care delivery models have been poorly endowed with resources, were largely paper-based, and had traditionally relied on a reactive approach in patient care, traditional care delivery systems are gradually transforming into smart connected system where data, devices and decision support tools interconnect in a system (Boopathi, S & Khang, A. 2023). This approach is also known as smart healthcare and seeks to bring about changes in the patient care delivery system in a bid to increase the quality of service delivery and efficiency in the delivery of medical services while at the same time lowering the costs. This change is due to several factors including; rise in incidences of chronic diseases, increase in population life expectancy, increased costs of healthcare and the recent global health crises including the current COVID-19. They have revealed the shortcomings of conventional approaches and made a case for intelligent solutions that will allow the execution of certain tasks, risk evaluation, and the prevention of undesirable occurrences. With this in mind, Machine Learning (ML) and Computational Intelligence (CI) have proved to be effective tools in enhancing clinical efficiency and effectiveness, as well as in optimizing the value of the health care data (Sikdar & Guha, 2020).

### 1.2 Role of Machine Learning and Computational Intelligence

Machine Learning and Computational Intelligence serve as the technological backbone of smart healthcare initiatives. Machine Learning, which is a branch of artificial intelligence, is the process by which a system takes data, finds out correlations and makes predictions based on data without having to being programmed(Kaur, J. 2024). In healthcare, there have been brilliant outcomes recorded on the usefulness of ML algorithms across various applications such as diagnostic images analysis, predictive modeling, treatment planning, and patient monitoring (Gopi et al., 2024). On the other hand, Computational Intelligence is a set of methodologies which are based on the principles of natural world for solving complex, non-linear and often, uncertain systems such as fuzzy logic, evolutionary algorithms and artificial neural networks. These approaches are particularly useful in health care where uncertainty, vagueness and heterogeneity are inherent in data as well as in decision making. For example, fuzzy logic systems are able to interpret rather imprecise medical terms, and on the other hand, evolutionary algorithms are able to find the best course of treatment from a large solution space. Thus, both ML and CI are synergistic as they supplement each other's strengths. Although, ML is good at handling large scale structured and unstructured data, CI techniques are more reliable in uncertain or low data condition. Their combination is making it possible to develop intelligent health care applications that are accurate, scalable and more importantly adaptive and robust (Khang 2023).

## 1.3 Scope and Objectives of the Chapter

The purpose of this chapter is to provide an insight on how Machine Learning and Computational Intelligence are being used to enhance smart healthcare, especially in diagnostic and therapeutic areas. It also captures the latest advancements, and defines the approaches that are behind the modern advancements. The subject of the survey is generic as well as innovative and covers both concepts that are fundamental to the field and those that are currently in development. It is applied in numerous healthcare areas, but not merely, such as diagnostic imaging, disease risk estimation, clinical decision-making, drug development, and individualized medicine. The chapter also discusses how both ML and CI are applied not only to support the clinicians but to improve the healthcare process through automation, optimization and real time analysis.

## 1.4 Contributions of the Chapter

The following are the major contributions of this chapter to the field of smart healthcare research:

1. Well-organized Classification: It provides a comprehensive classification of ML and CI techniques against the applications in the healthcare domain like diagnostic, planning, and decision-making.
2. Multidisciplinary Approach: The chapter has a multidisciplinary approach to the problem, which is important for creating comprehensive solutions to the challenges in the field of medicine, data analysis, and artificial intelligence.

3. In addition to the methods and applications, it also assesses their performance, interpretability, scalability, and ethics in a critical manner hence offering the users, both researchers and practitioners with a better understanding.
4. Thus, while there are numerous surveys that discuss AI in healthcare in general, this chapter aims at examining the two most effective areas of AI application: diagnosis and treatment.
5. Future Trends: This chapter presents trends like explainable AI, federated learning, and digital twins while providing a reference for future development that combines technology and clinical practice as well as patients' safety.

In conclusion, the introduction provides a background to the detailed analysis of the topic that is ML, CI, and healthcare and their interactions in the current world. In this context, it can be stated that identifying the potential of intelligent algorithms and their integration into healthcare systems and processes is not only relevant but also highly important for the future development of medicine.

## 2. BACKGROUND AND FOUNDATIONS

### 2.1 Overview of Smart Healthcare Systems

Smart health can be described as the integration of latest information technology and medical services to create patient-oriented, informed and preventive type of medical care. Smart healthcare is also proactive, as opposed to the conventional systems that only respond to health issues and are usually uncoordinated. This is achieved through the use of technology like Electronic Health Record (EHR), Mobile Health (mHealth), Wearable technology, Telemedicine, etc(Vigneswari & Yamini, 2024). These components help to form an integrated healthcare system with the flow of large amounts of data from various sources and its processing and analysis in real time. The rise of IoT contributes to this change because it is through heart monitors, blood glucose monitors, smartwatches, and other devices it is possible to track people's physiology and behavior outside of clinical settings(Ponnuviji, N. P et al., 2023). The use of such technologies, coupled with cloud computing in addition to real time analytics enables the clinicians to remotely supervise the patients, diagnose early signs of the diseases and make informed decisions(Dhinakaran et al., 2025; Ponnuviji et al., 2025)). This is a clear shift from episodic care models which are quite traditional and categorizes smart healthcare as a fluid, adaptable and sustainable model of the future of medicine (Keerthika et al., 2023).

*Figure 1. Overview of Smart Healthcare Systems*

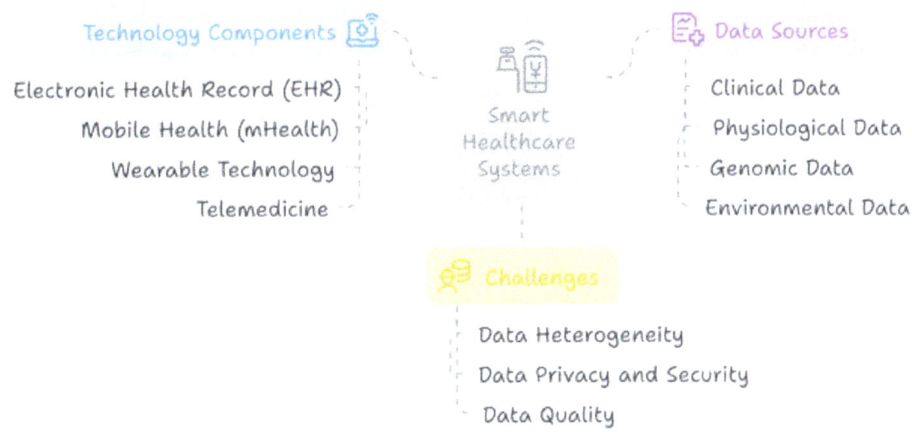


## 2.2 Basics of Machine Learning and Computational Intelligence

Thus, the essence of smart healthcare is in intelligent computing models capable of analyzing vast and intricate data to provide valuable information. The following capabilities are endowed through two fundamental fields namely machine learning (ML) and computational intelligence (CI). Artificial intelligence is the use of algorithms that constantly learn from experience of historical data to make decisions and make observations(Lakumarapu, S et al., 2024). It is generally divided into three categories namely supervised learning, unsupervised learning and reinforcement learning. Supervised learning techniques which uses labeled data are common in health care, where they are used in disease diagnosis, patient prognosis, or for image analysis. For instance, X-ray images tagged with annotations of some shapes can successfully identify diseases such as tumors or even fractures. Unsupervised learning, in contrast, involves the identification of structures in data that have not been labeled, for example, grouping of patients according to the risk level or distinguishing new diseases based on the genetic characteristics of patients. Reinforcement learning is quite suitable for decision making that occurs in a step by step manner and an agent learns to make the best choices through trial and error. In the field of health care, it has been used in cases like the choice of treatment for a particular patient or planning for robotic surgery. Computational intelligence is an enhancement of ML that integrates concepts that mimic the features of biological and nature systems, which can deal with ambiguity, vagueness, and problem-solving. Neural networks, especially deep neural networks are adopted in this field and have been proven efficient for data that are in the nature of images and sounds. Fuzzy logic systems which mimic human decision making are useful in clinical problems areas where vagueness is often observed for example in the assessment of symptoms or the patient's complaints. Genetic algorithms and particle swarm optimization are two of the evolutionary algorithms which are based on the natural selection process. They are especially beneficial in medical cases where other optimization techniques do not work, for instance, determining the right drug regimen or the right dosage of radiotherapy. The combination of both, ML and CI, makes it possible for healthcare systems not only to predict outcomes but also to learn from new, changing data in a clinical setting (Yamini et al., 2023).

## 2.3 Data in Smart Healthcare

The basis of intelligent healthcare is the data that it utilizes and analyzes. Smart healthcare data is big, complex and in constant production from various sources. Electronic health records are the primary source of records that hold complete information on the patient's health history and records, lab results, prescriptions, and clinical notes. X-ray, MRI, CT scan images and ultrasounds offer visual information that is important for diagnosis(Maithili, K et al.,2024). Simultaneously, smart wearables and smartphone applications log data obtained from physiological signals like heart rate, blood pressure, glucose level, and sleeping or physical activity. Genomic and proteomic data, due to development in bioinformatics, provide molecular aspects of precision medicine which is the crucial step in the development of precision medicine. Also, environmental and behavioral data gathered through the application, GPS or social media gives patient information on his/her lifestyle and the social factors affecting health. Nonetheless, the healthcare data or any data as a source of knowledge has its own drawbacks and challenges that make a direct approach to learning and applying it difficult in machine learning and computational intelligence systems. The first of them is data heterogeneity. The clinical data is available in different forms such as numerics, text, images, and time series sensor data. Combining and coordinating these modalities is a challenging task which usually involves non-trivial preprocessing pipeline. The last key issue would be of data privacy and security. Any data related to medical field is highly sensitive and there are many strict rules that should be followed. It is thus challenging to ensure that the model training is compliant and at the same time accessible. There is still the problem of data quality, where many datasets contain missing values, data that are entered incorrectly due to errors, malfunctioning equipment or where data was collected at different times with different methods. Additionally, supervised learning methods rely on having large amounts of clean labeled data which are often difficult to obtain in healthcare due to the time and costs associated with obtaining expert labels. To overcome these issues, there are methods such as data imputation, augmentation, and transformation that are being adopted by researchers. Federated learning is slowly becoming popular as an option that promises to train the model across a number of systems without necessarily consolidating the data (Antunes et al., 2022 ; Nguyen et al., 2022). There are also other techniques that are being used to address the issue of limited labeled data including transfer learning and semi-supervised learning. All these developments in data management and computation provide the foundation for the smart healthcare systems on which diagnostic tools, therapeutic planning and practical and real-time clinical decision support systems are being developed.

## 3. ML AND CI TECHNIQUES IN DIAGNOSIS

### 3.1 Medical Imaging Analysis

Medical imaging is one of the most promising fields in the healthcare domain where machine learning and computational intelligence have been making a great contribution to increasing diagnostic accuracy and rate. Deep learning, especially CNNs have greatly impacted the analysis of radiological, pathological, and dermatological images. CNNs are good at learning the hierarchy in the image data and can be used to identify the subtle patterns or abnormalities in the X-ray, MRI, CT scan, and histopathological images. In radiology, deep learning models can be trained to diagnose, for example, fractures, lung nodules or signs of pneumonia at the level of accuracy that is comparable to that of radiologists. In a similar way, in dermatology, CNNs have been applied in the diagnosis of skin lesions and distinguishing between benign and malignant tumors using dermoscopic images, and sometimes even outcompeting general practitioners. Apart from CNNs, GANs have proved to be useful in medical imaging applications. GANs can be used to synthesize new medical images that can be used for data augmentation due to the shortage of labelled training data. They are applied also in applications like image filtering, deblurring, or in translating scans from one modality to another, such as MRI to CT scan. Most recently, the transformer based models which were earlier designed for natural language processing tasks have been used in vision tasks in healthcare. ViTs can be beneficial in medical image analysis as they capture global information about the image and are useful in analyzing image features of certain complexity or high resolution. These advances assist in automated image-based diagnosis and help the clinicians in early diagnosis of the diseases as well as minimizes diagnostic errors and delays.

## 3.2 Disease Prediction and Risk Assessment

Disease diagnosis and risk assessment of the patients are the major determinants of the preventative and precision medicine, and the roles of the ML and CI techniques in these procedures are being expanded continually. Based on factors like demographics data, lifestyle data and clinical history, there can be developed an accurate prognosis of such diseases as diabetes, cardiovascular diseases, and various kinds of cancer. For example, it can use blood pressure and cholesterol records of a patient from the past years to predict the likelihood of heart disease and act accordingly. There are several types of machine learning algorithm that can be applied in this process. SVMs are useful for two-class discrimination and have been used in the diagnosis of diseases, including breast cancer, using records and images. Random forests are an efficient machine learning technique derived from the so-called bagging and boosting methods and have a high accuracy and noise immunity, which makes them quite suitable for risk assessment and determine the importance of features in clinical data sets. DNNs are especially useful when working with a large and complex dataset as they are comprised of multiple layers. These models can learn feature representations at a high level, which do not need to be designed by hand, which enhances the accuracy of the prediction in various diagnosis. Moreover, the disease progression models are now including temporal and longitudinal data which look at the patient's disease progression over time. Recurrent neural networks (RNN) and Long Short Term Memory (LSTM) networks are being employed in sequential data analysis for instance the progression of the kidney function or the risks of hospitalization based on previous admissions and therapies. These models make it possible for the clinician to have a prediction of the individual patient needs, and this makes it easier to avoid complications and readmissions.

*Figure 2. ML and CI Techniques in Diagnosis*

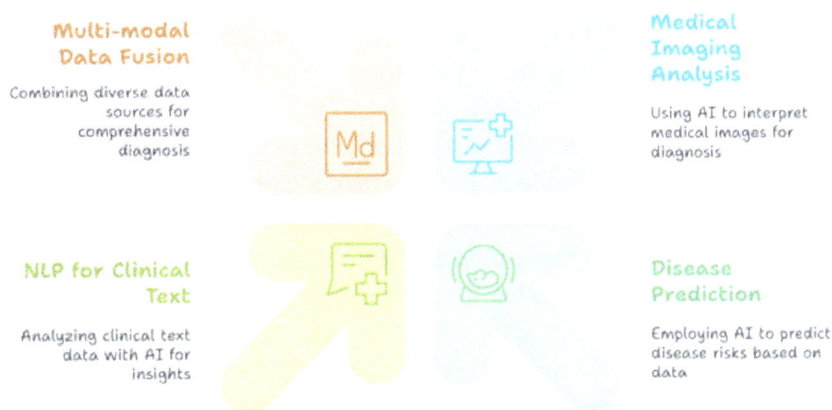


## 3.3 Natural Language Processing for Clinical Text

Most of the healthcare knowledge is contained in unstructured text documents, for instance, electronic medical records, discharge summaries, pathology reports, and clinical notes. NLP tools are required for the analysis of these documents as they contain lot of information that can be useful. Previous methods of clinical NLP included rule-based and keyword extraction, while the latest trends in deep learning and transformers have improved the results. Information extraction is one of the important NLP tasks in the healthcare field, which aims at extracting structured data including symptoms, diagnoses, medications, laboratory values, etc from the unstructured text. NER models identify these concepts, whereas relation extraction models reveal their relationship, for instance, a certain symptom with a diagnosis or a treatment. They also help in identifying the cohort, coding for billing and real time clinical decision support where important patient details are highlighted during consultations. Likewise, with the help of SA and TM, one can analyze patient feedback and physician's notes to check the overall healthcare quality and first signs of either patients' dissatisfaction or physicians' burnout. NLP can be said to greatly enhance the role of machine learning in diagnostics because it can turn unstructured data into usable and analysable data.

## 3.4 Multi-modal Data Fusion for Diagnosis

In real world scenario, there is no single type of data that can provide a complete picture of patient's health status. For an accurate diagnosis, information may be gathered from imaging, genomics, lab, and clinical notes among others. These are the different data sources that are used in the diagnosis of a patient's condition; and the process of combining them is known as multi-modal data fusion. This is a field where the use of the advanced ML and CI techniques has the possibility of showing a lot of promise. This chapter presents some of the approaches to the fusion of multi-modal data. Early fusion is the process of fusing the raw data from various sources before the feature extraction process while late fusion is the fusion of the results from different individually trained models from each modality. Intermediate or hybrid fusion takes place during the model training where learned features are combined. For instance, integrating radiological images with genes, clinical data, and others has enhanced the diagnosis of tumors and recommendation of the right treatment. Likewise, in neurology, integration of patient's brain scan with clinical and neuropsychological tests and genetic data aids in early diagnosis of Alzheimer's disease. However, there are some difficulties in multi-modal fusion. Often the data are collected at different formats, resolution, and sampling frequency in different modalities, thus alignment of data can be challenging. Also, it is not always possible to get all types of data for a particular patient due to certain reasons. To deal with these issues, data preprocessing, data imputation, and the model design that can work with incomplete or temporally inconsistent data are needed. However, with the recent developments in the federated learning, attention mechanisms and cross-modal transformers, the multi-modal fusion is becoming more realistic, which will further enhance the development of more accurate and contextual diagnostic systems.

# 4. ML AND CI IN TREATMENT AND PERSONALIZED MEDICINE

## 4.1 Treatment Recommendation Systems

*Figure 3. ML and CI in Treatment and Personalized Medicine*

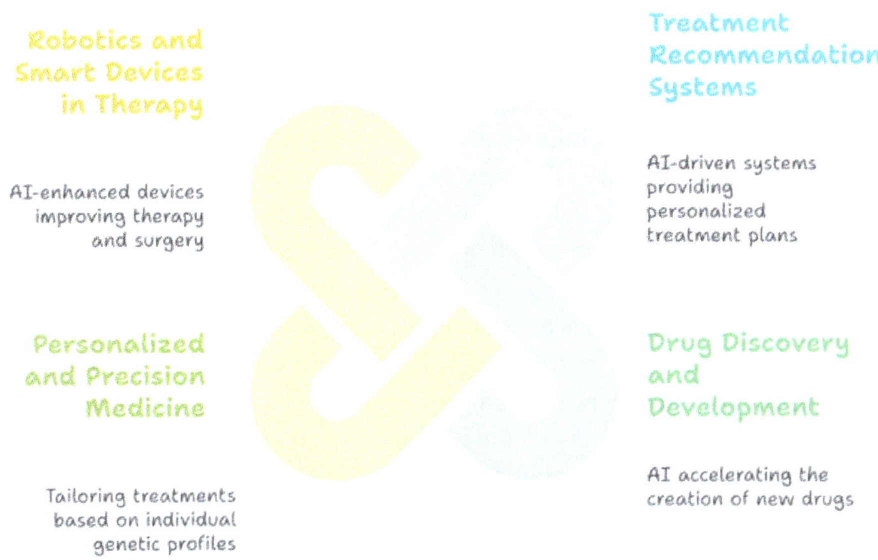


The most significant change that has been brought about by Machine learning (ML) and computational intelligence (CI) is the formation of treatment recommendation systems. These systems help clinicians by providing recommendations of the probable therapeutic treatment plans that are most likely to yield good results in light of the patient's characteristics. At its core of this effort is the Clinical Decision Support Systems (CDSS) that use the ML algorithms and also suggest the moderated treatment plans that are evidence based, inform the drug interactions, and signal out possible adverse results. CDSSs are being integrated into electronic health record systems in which the systems provide treatment regimens based on a patient's medical history, presenting signs and symptoms and diagnostic data. This not only relieves the physician burden but also guarantees greater standardization and safety of the patient care process. Specifically, RL, a branch of ML that finds applications in sequential decision making, is being increasingly used in modeling adaptive therapy. Unlike most of the other models that utilize some pre-defined inputs and outputs, the RL agents learn their actions by experiencing the environment and then learning from the results either in terms of rewards or penalties. In the treatment planning it creates the possibility of changes in the approach depending on the changes of a patient's condition. For instance, RL has been applied in dosing the chemotherapy cycles, in diabetes to individualise insulin therapy and in rehabilitation exercises based on patients' improvement. Such applications show how, through time, it is possible to create models that would adapt the treatments to the patients' needs and, thus, have better results with less side effects.

## 4.2 Drug Discovery and Development

Drug discovery is one of the most lengthy and costly processes, which can take over ten years and several billions of dollars to develop a new drug. ML and CI are transforming this field in that they are being applied to different phases of the drug development process, starting from molecular design to preclinical evaluation. Another promising approach is generative models including VAEs and GANs that can be used for creation of new drug-like molecules. These models can obtain the distribution of known chemical compounds and generate new ones that possess preferable characteristics, such as high binding velocity or low toxicity. GNNs have been of great importance in cheminformatics due to the fact that molecules can be represented naturally as graphs of atoms bonded together by chemical bonds. GNNs can learn more accurate and detailed representations of the molecules, thus making them capable of predicting the drug's efficacy, bioavailability, and possible side effects. When these models are used in combination with high-throughput screening data as well as the data on protein-ligand interaction, they will help in identifying better drug candidates faster than the conventional approaches. In addition, there is the application of ML in drug repositioning, which involves using already existing drugs to treat new diseases. Therefore, using antiviral activity as one of the search criteria, during the COVID-19 situation, for instance, available ML models were used to screen known compounds, thus, showcasing flexibility that AI provides when there is an urgent need for approaches to drug discovery. Moreover, computational intelligence is also applied to virtual screening and pharmacokinetics which in turn cuts the need for expensive and time-consuming laboratory experiments.

## 4.3 Personalized and Precision Medicine

This relatively new medical model of care aims at abandoning the strategy of treating patients all the same way and instead focusing on meaningful variations between patients in terms of their genotypes and phenotypes and environmental-genetic ones. ML is instrumental in this process, particularly in the high-dimensional data such as the genomics data. Said models can find biomarkers to categorize patients into subgroups displaying similar risk of a disease or similarity of treatment outcomes from analysis of whole-genome sequencing, transcriptomics, proteomics, and other -omics techniques. This stratification is important in cancers for instance, different patients present the similar symptoms and so may react differently to the general treatment. It is possible to use ML models to determine which genetic mutations are related to drug resistance or drug sensitivity and use this information for the development of individual treatment plans. It is also applied in the prediction of side effects of drugs so that the clinician can either avoid the use of such drugs or prescribe them at a certain dosage level. In addition, it is used in the development of polygenic risk scores that is a score derived from multiple genetic markers to predict the risk of certain diseases in an individual. These scores are increasingly being employed in primary prevention, counselling or screening prior to the development of disease. Since the multi-omics datasets are increasingly integrated, there are meaningful expectations and opportunities for the increased effectiveness of individualized medicine for increasing the efficiency of treatments and decreasing the costs of the healthcare sector.

## 4.4 Robotics and Smart Devices in Therapy

Apart from decision making and drug making, the combination of both ML and CI is revolutionizing physical therapy and surgeries using robotic and intelligent devices. Self-learning prosthetic legs enable a user's real time interaction with the environment and lifestyle routines of the amputee by providing better, flexible and comfortable movement. These systems adapt themselves from the feedback received from the user as well as the environment and thus are less cumbersome and the rehabilitation time is considerably less in these systems. The second is the surgical systems like the da Vinci systems which are a complex area that relies on computational intelligence in making them functional. These robots help surgeons in performing precise movements that are stable and less invasive to the human body and thus fastens the recovery period. These systems are improved through ML by analyzing intraoperative data and making decision support for real-time decision making such as pointing out anatomic features or possible risks. Another area that has value in the application of adaptive intelligent systems is rehabilitation. They utilize sensors and ML in order to track the progress of the patient and to adapt the corresponding exercises. It not only makes the therapy more individualized but also encourages the patients with interactive and gaming feedback systems. Moreover, portable rehabilitation instruments that are fitted with feedback systems allow for constant observation beyond the clinic, which is a link between inpatient and outpatient rehabilitation. In conclusion, merging of ML and CI in treatment and personalized medicine can greatly enhance the health care by anticipating, diagnosing and treating diseases and illnesses in a more efficient and personalized manner. The indicated technologies, continuing to develop, will surely transform many aspects of health treatment and care across specialties, including chronic illness management, pharmacotherapy, surgeries and rehabilitation.

# 5. COMPUTATIONAL INTELLIGENCE FOR HEALTHCARE OPTIMIZATION

## 5.1 Evolutionary Algorithms in Treatment Planning

The focus of this chapter is on the application of a type of optimization algorithms called evolutionary algorithms (EAs) in dynamic environment of healthcare, and more specifically, in treatment planning. These algorithms work through generation of a population of solutions through generation and applying operations such as mutation, crossover and selection to arrive at a near optimal solution. In the case of smart healthcare, EAs are often used in radiotherapy planning where the goal is to maximize the dose to tumors while minimizing the dose to the healthy tissues. This entails operating in a constrained and a multi-objective domain – something that is well within the realm of evolutionary approaches. For instance, GAs have been applied to optimize beam angles, intensity and dose distributions in IMRT. Such optimizations help in controlling the tumor and reducing the side effects that are detrimental to the body. In a similar manner in surgical planning, evolutionary algorithms help in decision making on the best path to take or orientation to adopt in the surgical procedure taking into consideration the degree of invasiveness and protection of essential structures in the anatomy. This is very applicable for conditions that require surgery in the cranium or for those less invasive procedures such as the laparoscopic surgeries that call for perfection. It also means that EAs can also be used to develop patient-specific treatment plans due to its flexibility. Such algorithms can adapt the treatment procedures within a few seconds thanks to the introduction of patient data like anatomical imaging and physiological parameters. They are also used in determining the optimal design of wearable health care devices or implantable sensors regarding comfortability and accuracy of data acquisition. These applications clearly show how evolutionary computing is useful not only to increase the effectiveness of the treatment but also to minimize the risks of the procedure and the costs of the healthcare.

## 5.2 Fuzzy Logic Systems in Diagnosis

Healthcare decision-making is always associated with risks due to uncertainty, vagueness, incompleteness, or ambiguity of data, symptoms, or interpretations.

Fuzzy logic systems, which are one of the computational intelligence techniques, are most useful in handling such uncertainty. Fuzzy logic is different from binary logic as it allows for the use of degrees of truth while binary logic requires precise input data with precise results. This makes it ideal for diagnosis in cases where patients' signs and symptoms and test results do not fit any textbook descriptions. In fuzzy logic systems, knowledge is incorporated into rule base that reflects human way of reasoning as clinicians. For example, a rule might say "If the blood pressure is high and cholesterol is very high, then the likelihood of getting a heart disease is high." These rules are then tested with membership functions that assign the input variables to fuzzy sets such as low, moderate, and high according to certain values. The above rules are accumulated and then de-fuzzed in the system to generate the risk score or the diagnosis recommendation. Fuzzy diagnostic systems have been used in various fields, for instance, cardiovascular risk assessment, diabetes, liver disease, and neurological disorders. Their advantage is that they can deal with vagueness of physiological data and natural language that is typical for clinical practice. Also, it is applied in wearable devices and mobile health since physiological data is often continuous and noisy, and soft decision-making models are needed. The openness of the fuzzy logic, which gives the clinicians the ability to see what the system is doing and how it arrived at a given decision, also increases the level of trust in the AI applications for healthcare. This interpretability is particularly important in medical decisions where one needs to justify the decision and ensure the decision made is clinically accurate. Therefore, fuzzy logic remains the most effective way of integrating medical expertise and translating humanlike behavior into an algorithmic form.

## 5.3 Hybrid Systems

Although, each of the computational intelligence techniques have been found to be very effective when applied in the health care system, integrated system which include more than one computational intelligence technique have been found to be more effective. These systems make use of features of different paradigms; the neural network to recognize patterns, the fuzzy logic to make easy interpretation and the evolutionary algorithms to optimize the models. One of such hybrids is the neuro-fuzzy system that combines the learning ability of the artificial neural networks (ANNs) with the fuzzy logic that mimics the human reasoning. However, in a neuro-fuzzy system, the neural network extracts fuzzy rules and membership functions from data and does not need to be programmed. This makes the system to be dynamic and learn from new evidence in clinical practice in order to enhance the diagnostic or predictive capacities. Such models have been used in cancer identification, prognosis of the patient, and chronic diseases like asthma and hypertension.

They are more useful when the input data is of mixed type whereby some of the inputs could be numerical while others could be categorical or textual in nature. Another rather promising subclass of algorithms is a subclass which blends the concepts of evolutionary algorithms with deep learning. In such blended scenarios, EAs are employed to fine tune the hyperparameters, features or architectures of deep learning models, in a way that automates the model development process. For instance, when using personalized medicine, hybrid evolutionary-deep learning systems may accurately choose suitable characteristics such as genetic profiles or imaging characteristics among many for personalization of the predictive models to the subgroups of customers. These systems are especially helpful when one is working with high-dimensional data and the noise in the data set is very high since it would take a lot of time to do it manually. Multi-modal data integration is also supported by hybrid models through the integration of the neural network ability to represent the data and the fuzzy system or EA's rule-based or optimization ability. In clinical decision making, these systems have the advantage of high accuracy and at the same time are easy to interpret and meet technical and legal requirements. Also, their ability to operate in noisy, incomplete or conflicting data environment makes them ideal for real life health care environment where perfect data input environment is the exception rather than the norm. In sum, computational intelligence can be considered as a multipurpose tool for managing the healthcare processes starting from the diagnosis and up to the individualized treatment. Evolutionary algorithms work great at solving optimization problems, fuzzy logic tries to emulate human's decision-making process and merge it into system, and hybrid systems combine two or more methods providing both strength and versatility. These techniques are still developing and are becoming closely associated with advanced technologies and are likely to revolutionize health care systems, making them more intelligent, self-organizing, and patient-centered.

## 6. CHALLENGES AND OPEN ISSUES

Although a lot of advancements have been made in the integration of ML and CI in the smart healthcare system, several challenges and issues remain to be solved that prevent widespread implementation and integration. These issues lie in the technical, ethical, operational, and regulatory levels and in each, there are potential challenges to patient safety, data management, and clinical outcomes. Overcoming these challenges is critical for creating the intelligent healthcare systems full potential.

## 6.1 Data Availability and Quality

In the context of using ML and CI in healthcare, one of the main obstacles that can be identified is the data issue. Healthcare information is scattered across various facilities and systems, and may be in different structures, completeness, and accuracy. Some of the data may be missing, a particular field may contain different values and entries made manually may also be wrong. However, information that comes from wearable devices and mobile health applications can be unreliable or non-standardized in most cases. Primary annotated datasets, and in particular, datasets suitable for training a supervised learning model are scarce in many medical domains. Data labelling is a tedious process that involves human input and is time-consuming and expensive as it requires professionals in the clinical field. Moreover, owing to regulations like HIPAA and GDPR, data cannot move freely between institutions and jurisdictions; it leads to data provinces. Despite that, federated learning and privacy-preserving methods present themselves as viable solutions, their application creates more difficulties in model training and distributive implementation (Banabilah et al., 2022). In conclusion, making clean, diverse, and representatively labelled data available can be viewed as one of the main challenges potentially blocking the way to creating high-quality healthcare AI systems.

## 6.2 Model Interpretability and Explainability

Another drawback often associated with ML & CI is rather the lack of interpretability of the models, especially those created using deep learning. Although these models are usually more accurate than traditional models, they are often described as the 'black box' because of their internal structure. In clinical environments, where decisions are required to be traceable and explainable, lack of understanding of how a given decision was made can lead to a lack of trust and therefore, the model will not be used. Clinicians require explanations that are in the format of medical reasoning especially when the decisions made by the AI are counterintuitive to clinical or logical reasoning or when they are against the recommended standard procedures. It should be noted that Explanatory AI (XAI) tries to address this issue by proposing ways of producing feature visualizations, decision paths or counterfactuals. However, many of these techniques are still emerging and may not be very useful to the healthcare practitioners. Moreover, the complexity of the model is another issue that may come with the interpretability problem where models with low complexity are easier to interpret but have less accuracy compared to deep neural networks. The problem of how to achieve good interpretability while maintaining high performance is still an active topic of research, which must be addressed before models can be used in clinical settings.

## 6.3 Ethical Concerns and Bias in Algorithms

Ethical concerns are always relevant in the health care practice, and there is no exemption of ML/CI systems from bias, fairness, and discrimination. These systems are trained to learn from data, and therefore, might be continually trained on data that contains structural bias inherited in our systems or society, where there are differences in health care provision and treatment. Consequently, the developed AI models can perpetuate or facilitative discrimination. For instance, models trained from the data obtained from urban areas may not work well in the rural areas or areas with low representation of patients. Likewise, the models that do not consider the demographic differences may provide the wrong or even detrimental advice for minorities. Another form of bias can be related to the samples used in the study whereby some conditions, treatments, or populations are not well represented. This is especially the case in rare diseases or pediatric care, where data are scarce to begin with. To achieve ethical AI, it is necessary to said efforts like bias checking, fairness preserving learning algorithms, and proper dataset selection in this regard. Furthermore, there is a need to address the issues related to the informed consent, patient privacy, and data ownership as the key ethical principles that have to be considered throughout the AI life cycle. The management of such issues can be done through the formation of ethical standards and multi-disciplinary committees.

## 6.4 Integration with Clinical Workflows

If the ML and CI tools are to be useful, they need to be incorporated into the current clinical processes. But, the problem is that most of these AI systems are designed and developed away from the clinical practice settings, and as a result, they often have poor usability, interfere with the workflow, and are not embraced by the clinicians. The clinicians are busy people with little time to spare, who are exposed to a lot of information and high stakes, which makes any adjunct have to demonstrate straightforward, accurate, and time-saving advantages. For effective implementation, there must be easily accessible interfaces, compatibility with other HISs, and real-time functionality that can be used at the patient's bedside. In addition, there should be ways by which clinicians can contribute their opinion and make changes to the AI recommendation if needed. In addition, it is also important to educate and train the medical personnel on the effectiveness of using the AI tools in their practice. There is a need to involve the users in the design process of AI through human-centered design and participatory design methods to ensure that AI supports the delivery of clinical care.

Regulatory and Standardization Issues: Last but not least, the areas of regulation and standardization seem to present the key impediments, with regard to scale and scope, to the adoption of both ML and CI in the field of healthcare. As compared to conventional medical devices or drugs, the AI-based systems are adaptive, data-driven and stochastic in nature and hence non-deterministic in many cases, thus posing challenges to assess and qualify them according to the existing regulatory frameworks. Currently, no specific guidelines have been developed by agencies like the FDA and EMA regarding the approval process, post-market regulation, and update procedures of AI tools in the healthcare sector. It is also the case with data formats, assessment criteria, and reporting. This has a disadvantage of reducing the possibility of interoperability, reproducibility, and collaboration across different institutions. It is crucial to have standardization in annotating data, validating models and benchmarking the performances to build trust and to meet the regulatory requirements. In addition, legal norms should answer the following questions: Who is responsible for the consequences arising from the use of AI? Who owns the rights to the models developed by an AI? What rights do patients have in relation to an AI system making decisions about them? In conclusion, it is possible to state that both ML and CI have the potential to revolutionize smart healthcare, but their application is accompanied by numerous difficulties. The problems of data quality, model interpretability, ethical concerns, clinical practicality, and regulatory compliance should be solved to develop beneficial, fair, and effective AI systems in the healthcare domain. The future development would depend on a convergence of technologists, clinicians, ethicists and policymakers that will employ the values of the practice of medicine - safety, humanity and putting patients first.

## 7. EMERGING TRENDS AND FUTURE DIRECTIONS

The healthcare delivery system awaits even more revolution with the advancing of technologies such as, Machine Learning (ML) and Computational Intelligence (CI). A new wave of innovations is emerging and is already changing the ways in which intelligent systems are created, deployed and implemented in the clinical setting. These emerging trends do not only help to overcome some of the current issues but also create the new opportunities for the development of the personalized, more transparent, and integrated healthcare model. In this part, we overview several trends affecting the development of the smart healthcare systems that ranges from secure data protection to patient's digital avatars.

Federated Learning and Privacy-Preserving AI

The first one is the federated learning, a paradigm that is expected to solve the problem of data privacy and the presence of institutional silos. Centralized machine learning techniques involve data centralization and mostly leads to several challenges such as data breach and regulation problems. On the other hand, federated learning allows various healthcare centers to train the AI models without data sharing (Bashir et al., 2023). However, the model is trained at each site in parallel, and the parameters or gradients obtained from the training are exchanged and combined at the center. It greatly improves data privacy, which is crucial when it comes to abiding by the HIPAA and GDPR, and encourages cooperation between hospitals, labs, and countries. From a more operational perspective, federated learning makes it possible to train models on various data while preserving the patient's anonymity. It is especially useful in the case of rare diseases, where there is limited information and the data are located in various institutions. It is anticipated that as the technology advances, it will be a key component in building big-scale PHE systems in healthcare. There are also other methods that are getting a rise in the interest they receive are: Differential Privacy, Homomorphic Encryption, and Secure Multi-Party Computation. These techniques prevent data leakage but allow AI model training and provide mathematical guarantee of the same. Incorporation of these methods in clinical models of artificial intelligence can be seen as the first steps toward creating reliable and safe smart health.

Explainable AI (XAI) in Clinical Settings

Another important direction is the introduction and use of the methods of explainable artificial intelligence (XAI) designed for the clinical environment. Although the focus was on the model performance, the importance of interpretability in the decision-making process in the medical field has also been realized. The future actions of clinicians or regulators and the patients must be acquainted with the reason behind the AI models making some of the predictions especially when the predictions made are about their future diagnoses, treatment or any other life-changing plans. XAI methods try to explain what led to a particular decision by pointing to the features that contributed, presenting decision rules, or using diagrams that mimic human thought. For example, heatmaps derived from gradient-based approaches in clinical imaging can identify which particular areas of an MRI or X-ray were used to make a diagnosis by the model. In textual analysis, care can be taken to draw attention to segments of the patient history in the decision-making process. Aside from these tools, designing ways of presenting these in a metaphoric and clinically informative manner for the end-users remains an area of improvement. It is not only important to meet the requirements of the regulation and ethics but also to provide useful information to health care professionals. Subsequent systems will probably be designed to include real-time explainability, which means that the clinicians will be able to engage with the AI system and question its recommendations, which will help to build the trust and the accountability. Human-in-the-Loop Systems and Collaborative Intelligence. So, full automation of medicine is not a feasible and ethically acceptable goal today, but the human-in-the-loop systems are more realistic and effective. These systems are cooperative systems that involve integration of the AI systems with the human experts, where the two work hand in hand. While AI is capable of handling great volumes of data and fine analyzes of such data within a short span of time, humans are endowed with contextual information, moral compass, and emotions. In diagnosis, there is the integration of human intelligence where the clinicians can confirm, modify or reject the outputs of the AI models (Saraswat et al., 2022).

In treatment planning, they endorse the concept of the decision support where the AI provides the patient with viable treatment plans, and the physician incorporates patient preferences and clinical factors. Such frameworks are especially useful in the conditions where the decision-making process has to occur in the conditions of uncertainty and time pressure, as it is the case in emergency medicine or critical care. The term 'collaborative intelligence' means that the role of AI is not to replace clinicians, but rather enhance it. It is believed that the next steps in the development of such systems will include their ability to learn from the users' feedback, modify themselves based on the users' behavior, and provide highly individualized help to the practitioners. This paradigm ensures safety, usability, and ethical aspects in the implementation of artificial intelligence in health care.

Digital Twins and Virtual Patients

Digital Twins – another innovation of the IT sector and medical industry, virtual representations of objects, processes and phenomena in the outside world – are becoming quite promising in the context of the sphere of personalized medicine. In healthcare, digital twins are being created to mirror patient information from electronic health records, genome, wearable devices, and images, etc. Such models can represent diseases development, forecast treatment outcomes and even conduct trials and evaluations virtually before taking them to reality. For instance, in the field of cardiology, there are digital heart models that can show the impact of a particular drug or surgical procedure before the actual application of such treatment plan. In oncology, virtual tumors can be applied to evaluate the effectiveness of chemotherapy regimens depending on a patient's molecular characteristics. With the enhancement of computing power and data integration, the concept of digital twins is going to transform not only the individual patient care but also the medical research, drug trials, and simulations of public health. Thus, there are several challenges that need to be addressed when creating clinically validated digital twins, such as high fidelity modeling, real-time data synchronization, and validation. However, they are an exciting and innovative concept for the development of smart healthcare in the future (Lavanya et al., 2025).

## 8. CONCLUSION

This chapter has aimed to find out how Machine Learning (ML) and Computational Intelligence (CI) can help in improving smart healthcare in terms of diagnosis, treatment, and individualized care. The conclusions made in this review reveal some of the benefits of adopting these technologies to enhance the delivery of health care services, but they also point to the current limitations. It has been established that both ML and CI have shown their efficiency in handling huge amounts of data from various sources, diagnosis, treatment, and patient care. For example, deep learning for diagnosis of illness through imaging analysis, chronic diseases progression prognosis, and reinforcement learning of treatment are already beneficial in practice today. Nevertheless, there are some challenges that remain the following: data quality and availability, the issue of interpretability of the given models and, finally, integrating technologies into clinical practice. Ethical problems such as data protection, bias in the algorithms, and other ethical issues do not disappear as AI is being integrated in actual healthcare settings. It is therefore important to ensure that these systems are transparent and fair and conform to clinical decision-making processes to gain the confidence of the healthcare professionals and patients. The increasing popularity of HITL models and XAI shows that AI should enhance rather than replace the decisions made by the healthcare workers. The significance of introducing ML and CI in the healthcare sector is immense. They are contributing towards the development of personalized healthcare in which treatment and diagnosis are made based on the patient's characteristics. This is a shift that is making health care more personal, productive and productive especially in chronic diseases, cancer and complicated diseases. Also, Federal learning, Digital twin, along with real-world evidence will bring additional improvements in cultivating the smart healthcare systems' scalability, privacy, and flexibility. The future of smart healthcare in the next generation is to advance AI and CI as the symbiosis with human resources. The future healthcare systems will be more complex, open and adaptive, which will be learning from the actual implementation. Due to technological improvements in privacy preservation, combined intelligence, and post-implementation surveillance, AI will help in delivering timely, personalized, safer, and efficient treatment. The integration of these technologies has the future of transforming healthcare into more fair, effective, and patient-oriented system.

## REFERENCES


Antunes, R. S., André da Costa, C., Küderle, A., Yari, I. A., & Eskofier, B. (2022). Federated learning for healthcare: Systematic review and architecture proposal. [TIST]. *ACM Transactions on Intelligent Systems and Technology*, *13*(4), 1–23.

Banabilah, S., Aloqaily, M., Alsayed, E., Malik, N., & Jararweh, Y. (2022). Federated learning review: Fundamentals, enabling technologies, and future applications. *Information Processing & Management*, *59*(6), 103061.

Bashir, A. K., Victor, N., Bhattacharya, S., Huynh-The, T., Chengoden, R., Yenduri, G., & Liyanage, M. (2023). Federated learning for the healthcare metaverse: Concepts, applications, challenges, and future directions. *IEEE Internet of Things Journal*, *10*(24), 21873–21891.

Boopathi, S., & Khang, A. (2023). AI-integrated technology for a secure and ethical healthcare ecosystem. In *AI and IoT-Based Technologies for Precision Medicine* (pp. 36–59). IGI Global.

Dhinakaran, D., Kumar, N. J., & Ponnuviji, N. P. (2025). Safeguarding confidentiality and privacy in cloud-enabled healthcare systems with spectrasafe encryption and dynamic k-anonymity algorithm. *Expert Systems with Applications*, *279*, 127584.

Gopi, B., Kokila, M. S., Bibin, C. V., Sasikala, D., Howard, E., & Boopathi, S. (2024). Distributed Technologies Using AI/ML Techniques for Healthcare Applications. In Social Innovations in Education, Environment, and Healthcare (pp. 375-396). IGI Global.

Kaur, J. (2024). Smart Solutions for Health: Computational Intelligence Reshaping the Industry 4.0 Healthcare Paradigm. In Advances in Computational Intelligence for the Healthcare Industry 4.0 (pp. 194-211). IGI Global Scientific Publishing.

Keerthika, K., Kannan, M., & Khang, A. (2023). Medical data analytics: Roles, challenges, and analytical tools. In *AI and IoT-Based Technologies for Precision Medicine* (pp. 1–15). IGI Global.

Khang, A. (Ed.). (2023). *AI and IoT-based technologies for precision medicine*. IGI Global.

Lakumarapu, S., Nithyanandhan, R., Bhargavi, V. S., & TP, A. (2024, August). Machine Learning Approaches for Liver Disease Prediction: A Comparative Analysis. In 2024 5th International Conference on Electronics and Sustainable Communication Systems (ICESC) (pp. 159-164). IEEE.

Lavanya, M., Ashwini, A., & Balasubramaniam, S. (2025). The Virtual Revolution of Digital Twins in Chronic Healthcare Management. In AI-Powered Digital Twins for Predictive Healthcare: Creating Virtual Replicas of Humans (pp. 169-200). IGI Global Scientific Publishing.

Maithili, K., Ponmalar, A., Yamini, B., Karthikeyan, M., Anish, T. P., Maheswari, B., & Subramanian, R. S. (2024). Advances in AI and Machine Learning for Healthcare Informatics. In Machine Learning and Generative AI in Smart Healthcare (pp. 1-22). IGI Global.

Nguyen, D. C., Pham, Q. V., Pathirana, P. N., Ding, M., Seneviratne, A., Lin, Z., & Hwang, W. J. (2022). Federated learning for smart healthcare: A survey. *ACM Computing Surveys*, *55*(3), 1–37.

Ponnuviji, N. P., Nirmala, G., Kokila, M. S., & Priyadharshini, S. I. (2025). Optimizing Image Retrieval in Cloud Servers with TN-AGW: A Secure and Efficient Approach. Journal of The Institution of Engineers (India): Series B, 106(2), 459-473.

Ponnuviji, N. P., Sumaiya Begum, A., Gnanasekaran, T., Rajendiran, M., & Shenbaga Ezhil, S. (2023, April). Leveraging Random Forest for Intelligent IoT Systems in Industrial Environments. In International Conference on Internet of Things (pp. 46-57). Cham: Springer Nature Switzerland.

Saraswat, D., Bhattacharya, P., Verma, A., Prasad, V. K., Tanwar, S., Sharma, G., & Sharma, R. (2022). Explainable AI for healthcare 5.0: Opportunities and challenges. *IEEE Access : Practical Innovations, Open Solutions*, *10*, 84486–84517.

Sikdar, S., & Guha, S. (2020). Advancements of healthcare technologies: Paradigm towards smart healthcare systems. In *Recent trends in image and signal processing in computer vision* (pp. 113–132). Springer Singapore.

Vigneswari, J., & Yamini, B. (2024, November). Smart Health Monitoring System Using IoT Sensors in Cloud Environment. In *2024 International Conference on Smart Technologies for Sustainable Development Goals (ICSTSDG)* (pp. 1-5). IEEE.

Yamini, B., Sudha, K., Nalini, M., Kavitha, G., Subramanian, R. S., & Sugumar, R. (2023, June). Predictive modelling for lung cancer detection using machine learning techniques. In 2023 8th International Conference on Communication and Electronics Systems (ICCES) (pp. 1220-1226). IEEE.

Chapter 5

# Advancing Healthcare With Predictive Analytics for Disease Diagnosis and Risk Assessment


**Siva Subramanian R.**
*SRM Institute of Science and Technology, India*

**Subhash Chandra N.**
*CVR College of Engineering, India*

**S. Vijayaselvarani**
*Veltech Tech Multi Tech Dr. Rangarajan Dr. Sakunthala Engineering College, India*

**Anand Babu R.**
*Panimalar Engineering College, India*

**Anto Gracious L. A.**
https://orcid.org/0000-0003-2386-9182
*R.M.K. College of Engineering and Technology, India*

**K. Jeyakarthika**
*Ramco Institute of Technology, India*

**D. Raja**
*Thiagarajar College of Engineering, India*



## ABSTRACT

*Predictive analytics has emerged as a transformative tool in healthcare, enabling early disease diagnosis, risk assessment, and personalized treatment. This chapter examines the application of machine learning and statistical models in clinical settings, highlighting their impact on disease prediction and prevention. Key data sources such as electronic health records (EHRs), medical imaging, genomics, and wearable devices are explored, alongside methods including deep learning,*



DOI: 10.4018/979-8-3373-3311-3.ch005

*ensemble techniques, and statistical models. The chapter also addresses challenges such as data quality, bias, and privacy concerns, while discussing emerging trends like federated learning, real-time analytics, and integration with wearable devices.*

# 1. INTRODUCTION

## 1.1 Background and Motivation

In the past few years, the healthcare sector has seen a need for new approaches to deal with rising costs, more elderly people, and more cases of chronic diseases (Ali et al., 2023). The increased number of diabetes, cardiovascular disease, cancer, and neurodegenerative disorders around the world is putting a lot of stress on healthcare systems. As a result of these issues, researchers and clinicians are looking for tools that make it easier to diagnose diseases early and to decide which treatment plan works best for each patient. If at-risk groups are identified early and diseases are spotted before any symptoms, the number of sick, deaths, and costs can all be reduced. The use of digital health technologies has led to a major change in how healthcare data is now created, gathered, and studied. Due to EHRs, wearable devices, medical imaging, genomic sequencing, and real-time monitoring, there is now an incredible amount of health data, often known as big data. As a result of this surge, AI and ML techniques are being used more in healthcare analytics. Doctors are increasingly using predictive analytics in AI to help guide their choices and decisions in patient care. It makes it possible for healthcare professionals to identify potential diseases, assess the risk for each patient, use resources in the most efficient way, and design affordable and patient-friendly preventive plans. The combination of up-to-date computer methods with a wide range of healthcare data is changing the way diseases are diagnosed and treated. Still, while there has been a lot of advancement, issues like data quality, making sense of AI models, ethical aspects, and proving their use in the real world prevent AI from being used everywhere (Ambhika, C et al., 2024). To solve these problems, you need to know about modern predictive analytics, how they are used in medical practice, and what obstacles stand in the way of their effective use.

## 1.2 Scope and Objectives of the Survey

The goal of this survey is to outline the state of predictive analytics as it relates to diagnosing diseases and assessing risks. The chapter brings out the various uses of data in healthcare to derive useful information, especially on how diseases can be diagnosed better, and the most at-risk individuals to a given condition. The aim is to relate the concepts of predictive models to their practical application of the models in hospitals and health care facilities. The area of interest includes an in-depth examination of the various forms of data that are utilized in predictive healthcare analytics, such as EHRs, imaging records, lab results, genomic findings, and data captured by wearable devices. It investigates how such datasets can be used to construct machine learning and deep learning models (Sreelakshmi, S et al., 2024). Moreover, it examines different kinds of algorithms, including outdated statistical solutions and newer forms of AI and examines their effectiveness in different health environments. Besides explaining the use of predictive analytics, the survey examines the field in which it has been of great use, which include cardiovascular risks prediction, cancer detection, diagnosis of neurological disorders, and prediction of the emergence of infectious diseases.

### 1.3 Structure of the Chapter

The chapter is organized from this point on as explained below: Section 2 deals with the fundamentals of predictive analytics and healthcare data including their definitions, types, and the issues that are generally associated with them. The section 3 is concerned with machine learning and statistics applied to predictive modeling, sorted by their usage and purpose. In section 4, several case studies and examples of the use of predictive analytics in the diagnosis of diseases are mentioned. Section 5 explains how models are being used to assess and sort risks, demonstrating how this can be done at the population and individual level. Section 6 covers using the right evaluation measures, understanding how the systems work, and achieving clinical validation, all of which are vital for deploying predictive systems effectively. It lists some of the continuous problems, such as the quality of data, ethical dilemmas, and rules that may limit progress. This section highlights a number of new trends and future pathways, including the rise of federated learning, multimodal analytics, and privacy-preserving technologies. Section 9 brings the chapter to a close with a recap of the most important points and a request for further teamwork to improve using predictive analytics in healthcare.

## 2. BASICS OF PREDICTIVE ANALYTICS IN THE HEALTHCARE FIELD

### 2.1 Definitions and Key Concepts

Predictive analytics is part of data science that looks at past data, uses statistics, and machine learning to make predictions about what will happen in the future (Kumar, V., & Garg, M. L. 2018). When it comes to healthcare, predictive analytics tries to forecast conditions such as diseases starting, their development, and the patient's response to treatment by studying patient data. It is not the same as descriptive analytics, which looks at old data to spot trends, and prescriptive analytics, which offers useful tips based on what the data predicts. It helps link what happened in the past with the decisions to be made in the future. The main ideas in healthcare predictive analytics are diagnosis of illnesses and evaluation of risks. To diagnose a disease or condition, doctors look at symptoms, test results, and other data from patient examinations. This includes spotting illnesses that have not yet been diagnosed or predicting an upcoming illness by looking at early symptoms. In the other way, risk assessment aims to estimate what the chances are for a person to develop a certain health condition within a certain time span. Often, demographics, their lifestyle, family history, and other conditions are used to determine which patients are at high risk of the disease. Taking care of patients, planning resources, and choosing the best interventions all require accurate assessments of risk (Mishra, N., & Silakari, S. 2012).

## 2.2 Types of Healthcare Data

How well predictive models work in healthcare is mostly influenced by the quality and range of information they receive. There are many types of healthcare data, each one giving us different information about patient health. Doctors rely heavily on the Electronic Health Record (EHR) as a data source. Information stored in EHRs includes patient demographics, their diagnoses, what medications they are on, lab test results, notes made by doctors, and their medical history(Dhinakaran, D et al., 2025). The reason EHR data is used for predictive analytics in many cases is because it covers the full course of a patient's medical information. Medical imaging is an important type of data that includes X-rays, MRI, CT scans, and ultrasound among other modalities. They help us see what is happening inside the body and, due to computer vision, deep learning models can now detect signs of illnesses like cancer, stroke, and pneumonia. Genomic data lets us see the health of a patient at the molecular level. Because genome sequencing is becoming more affordable, genetic information can now be included in models to determine a person's risk of disease, find mutations, and shape personal treatments. Genomic data is particularly effective at helping predict chronic diseases, for example diabetes and cardiovascular issues. Wearable and sensor data gathered from things like smartwatches, fitness trackers, and continuous glucose monitors help to continually monitor heart rate, activity levels, sleep, and blood glucose. It helps identify unusual changes in health, which allows for earlier and more active care for those with chronic illnesses. In addition, looking at social and behavioral factors such as socioeconomic status, mental health, nutrition, how active a person is, and the environment plays an important role in assessing a patient's risks. While these factors are not always considered in clinical care, they are now being acknowledged for greatly affecting health results.

### 2.3 Challenges in Healthcare Data

Even though there is a lot of healthcare data, many issues make it difficult to use that data for predictive analytics. Missing data is a big problem that occurs in clinical data sets all the time. It is possible to have missing values because of inconsistent notes, incomplete medical records, or if patients decide not to continue with the study. Missing data should be dealt with using strong imputation methods, as it can greatly change how accurately the model works. Data heterogeneity poses another challenge. The data in healthcare comes in a range of different forms, from different sources, and is coded with various standards and terminologies. When using different types of data together, it is important to preprocess, standardize, and harmonize the information before building a predictive model. With patient information being sensitive, privacy and security become very important in healthcare. Laws now dictate strict rules for how data can be used, who it can be shared with, and how it is stored. In order to maintain the privacy of data and still build a model, innovative methods such as de-identification, federated learning, and differential privacy are needed. Interpretability of the models is also a major issue to consider. If a model makes a prediction, clinicians should know the reasons behind it to rely on its results. While logistic regression allows us to understand how it works, most deep learning algorithms are not transparent and work in a hidden way. It is important to design explainable AI approaches to ensure AI can be used in clinical settings and ethically (Kashyap, R., & Piersson, A. D., 2018).

## 3. MACHINE LEARNING AND STATISTICAL METHODS

### 3.1 Classical Machine Learning Models

Predictive analytics in healthcare relies heavily on the base provided by classical machine learning (ML) models (Subha, S et al., 2025). Because of their simplicity and low computational needs, these models are often used on structured data like lab results, demographic information, and codes used for diagnoses (Nanehkaran et al., 2023). Many medical predictions rely on logistic regression, due to its simple and clear working process. It determines the odds of the outcome happening or not by adding and combining the values of the input features. While it cannot deal well with non-linear situations, the model is still widely used in clinical research (Kocher,

G., & Kumar, G., 2021). Decision trees divide the data step by step, using different thresholds along the way, and end up with a tree-like structure. They are simple to understand and use, but they can easily overfit the data. Support Vector Machines (SVMs) are useful for working with large amounts of data and perform best when the task is to sort items into two categories (Bansal, M et al., 2022). They try to find the best line that can separate the classes with the biggest distance between them. K-nearest neighbors (k-NN) is a method that classifies a new instance by looking at the most common class among its 'k' closest neighbors. Although easy to use, k-NN can take a lot of computing power and be easily affected by noise. When many decision trees are combined into a random forest, their collective results help to avoid overfitting and reduce the amount of variance in the model. Their robustness and ease of use keep these classical models a key part of clinical risk prediction tools.

*Figure 1.* **Machine Learning and Statistical Methods**

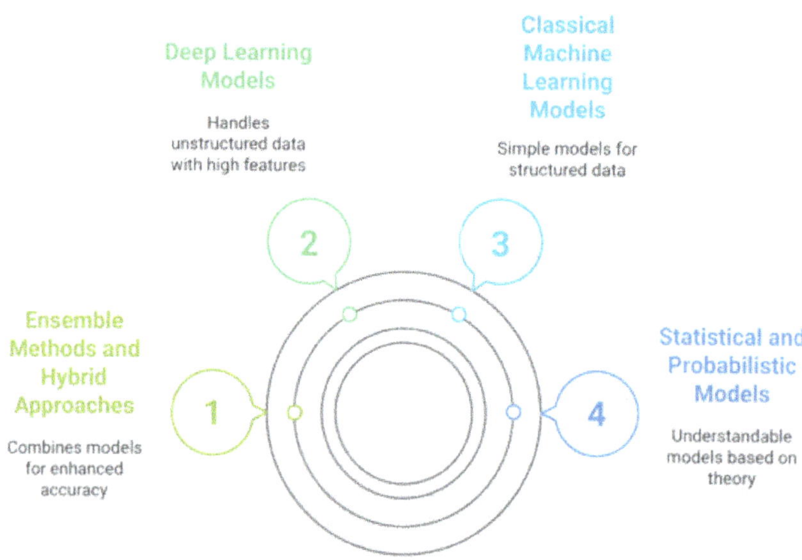


## 3.2 Deep Learning Models

With deep learning, healthcare analytics is now able to handle data that is unstructured and has a high number of features such as medical images, text, and signals over time. CNNs are designed to work effectively on visual information (Bhatt et al., 2021). They have been extensively applied in radiology and pathology in the identification of patterns in X-ray films, MRIs and tissue samples. CNNs are able to detect correlations between image components and thus are excellent in tasks such as cancer detection and detecting diabetic retinopathy. When it comes to time-series data in healthcare, the most popular models to work with are Recurrent Neural Networks (RNNs) and Long Short-Term Memory (LSTM) networks, (Babu Vimala, B et al., 2023; Priyadharshini, S et al., 2025). They are good at observing the changes in patient vitals, medicines, and EHR logs over a time period. They are used to project hospital readmissions, changes in a patient's disease, and the results of various treatments. In recent years, models based on Transformers, which were first built for natural language processing, have found use in healthcare. By using self-attention, Transformers are able to study entire sequences all at once and learn context more efficiently than RNNs. They allow for better accuracy and flexibility, but they also need vast sets of data and are sometimes criticized for being hard to understand[Boopathi, S. 2023].

### 3.3 Ensemble Methods and Hybrid Approaches

Using different models together in an ensemble helps the prediction become more accurate and reliable. Bagging involves forming a number of models from different bootstrap versions of the training set and then averaging their predictions. Random forests are an excellent case of bagging used on decision trees. Unlike training, boosting builds models step by step, trying to correct the mistakes made by the previous models. Algorithms such as AdaBoost, GBM, and XGBoost have been used in healthcare for things like predicting mortality and identifying different diseases.

By stacking generalization, ensemble learning adds further value by combining many different models to produce a better outcome. Combining classical ML with deep learning is a new trend in the field. CNNs can be used to extract features, while the last step is to classify the data using gradient boosting. They help in making predictions and can adjust to work with different types of data.

### 3.4 Statistical and Probabilistic Models

In many situations, where it is important for models to be simple to understand, accurate, and solidly based on theory, traditional statistical models are still used. Bayesian networks show how variables may be related to each other using a directed acyclic graph. They help explain how different factors cause a disease and deal with uncertainties in diagnosing a patient. It is especially useful in medicine that Bayesian inference takes into account knowledge that is already available.

Survival analysis is a method that helps model the time it takes for an event to occur, for example, the time until disease appears or a person dies. The Cox proportional hazards model is a common technique for both risk estimation and comparing different treatments in clinical research. Markov models are also used, mainly to describe the development of diseases and the shifts in a patient's health state over a period of time. They are often used in health economics and decision analysis to analyze future effects and the value for money.

## 4. APPLICATIONS IN DISEASE DIAGNOSIS

### 4.1 Cardiovascular Diseases

Since cardiovascular diseases (CVDs) are the number one cause of death around the world, it is very important to spot and assess the risks early in predictive healthcare. Through the use of large patient data, including different measurements, predictive analytics has helped improve the diagnosis of CVD. These types of models use logistic regression or ensemble methods to look at blood pressure, cholesterol, smoking, and family history to predict the chance of upcoming heart problems. Additionally, using echocardiograms, CT angiography, and MRI with CNNs has allowed for the automatic recognition of heart problems that might be caused by diseases of the heart and arteries. Additionally, with deep learning, especially RNNs and 1D CNNs, ECG analysis can automatically discover arrhythmias, myocardial infarctions, and similar electrical issues, helping to speed up and improve the accuracy of medical care in emergencies and remote locations.

### 4.2 Cancer Detection and Diagnosis

By using predictive analytics, it is now possible to catch cancer early, predict the outcome, and design the best treatment strategy. Machine learning and deep learning are widely applied to look at medical images, biopsy reports, and genomic data. CNNs have demonstrated excellent performance at early detection by looking at mammograms for breast cancer, CT scans for lung cancer, and MRIs for prostate cancer. They have the ability to detect small patterns that might escape the eye of a human radiologist. In addition, genomic information is being used to make predictions, especially in targeted cancer care. Studying gene expression and the mutations in a person's DNA allows the models to predict their likelihood of getting certain cancers, the behavior of the tumors, and the best therapies for them (Mangairkarasi, S et al., 2025). For example, combining genomic information with clinical records has made it possible to group tumors and predict their response to therapy, helping to guide more personalized ways of caring for patients.

*Figure 2.* **Applications in Disease Diagnosis**

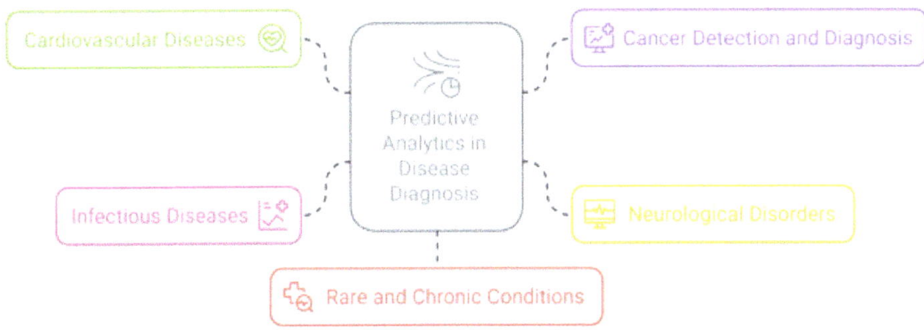


## 4.3 Neurological Disorders

The use of predictive analytics has made it much easier to diagnose diseases such as Alzheimer's disease, Parkinson's disease, and epilepsy. Most of these conditions need to be monitored over a long period, and this is best achieved using time-series or sequential data analysis. For example, the identification of Alzheimer's has improved through models that use results from brain scans, tests of cognitive ability, and electronic health records. It is possible to identify early signs of brain shrinkage using CNNs or 3D deep learning, which often come before any clinical symptoms. Wearable sensors have been used to monitor movement in people with Parkinson's, and machine learning has helped identify patterns linked to how severe and fast the disease is progressing. By using EEG signals, trained models can spot and even anticipate seizures in epilepsy, helping improve both safety and wellbeing of patients. They prove that using imaging, physiological data, and a patient's story together supports better diagnosis of neurological diseases.

## 4.4 Infectious Diseases

It was during the COVID-19 pandemic that predictive analytics really came to the fore, as models were used to help diagnose, predict outcomes, and track the spread of the virus. To help with the diagnosis of COVID-19, deep learning was used to analyze chest X-rays and CT scans, making it possible to detect the disease quickly even where resources are limited. They also helped hospitals make better use of their resources by using demographic and medical data to predict the risk of severe outcomes for patients. Besides helping individuals, predictive models made it possible to quickly model the risk of an outbreak by using information on the virus's spread and people's movement. Much like with COVID-19, similar methods have been used for influenza, dengue, and other infectious diseases, helping public health respond more actively.

### 4.5 Rare and Chronic Conditions

It has been found that predictive analytics is highly effective at detecting both rare and chronic diseases, as they are often missed due to their hardly noticeable symptoms. As a result, it is now much easier and more accurate to diagnose diabetic retinopathy in non-specialist settings due to deep learning models on retinal images. In CKD, doctors use lab readings on glomerular filtration rate, serum creatinine, and urine protein to look for early kidney problems and determine if the disease will advance to end-stage renal disease. Just like for heart issues, asthma diagnosis and management use inputs from wearables and environmental sensors to help predict risks of an asthma attack for each patient. With the help of continuous and multiple types of data, predictive analytics allows for earlier support and better control of diseases for patients with ongoing health problems.

## 5. RISK ASSESSMENT AND STRATIFICATION MODELS

### 5.1 Population Risk Prediction

These models are significant in public health and preventive medicine as they aid in identifying individuals within a community who are at the highest risk of contracting some diseases. The models are likely to utilize demographic, clinical, as well as behavioral information in estimating the probability of the occurrence. The Framingham Risk Score is a common instrument which is a product of the Framingham Heart Study and is used to forecast the risk of a heart issue of an individual in the subsequent 10 years. Polygenic Risk Scores (PRS) have been identified as a novel method of measuring population risk based on genomic information in the last couple of years. PRS are a combination of influences of several genes distributed across the genome, each of which has a low effect on the risk of disease. It allows determining the opportunity to better comprehend the risks of an individual to develop heart disease, diabetes type 2, or various types of cancer. The scores can be used to enhance screening regulations and guide interventions to the individuals who are at risk of contracting the disease because of their genes when they are incorporated in population health tools.

## 5.2 Personalized Risk Assessment

In addition to group analysis, personalized risk analysis compares forecasts with personal characteristics, and this increases the precision of medical care. It bases the evaluation on the genomic data, occupation, family history, and the surrounding environment. The inclusion of data on wearable sensors such as physical activity, heart rate, and sleep can provide a more informed picture of the health of an individual. With these two data sources, risk profiling may be dynamic and continuous, rather than a one-time practice. Blood sugar monitoring, coupled with data on what people with diabetes eat and how they exercise, can help people with diabetes predict and prevent high and low blood sugar problems. AI models can also be trained to adjust risk ratings when new information is available and thus they become more accurate with time. They enable clinicians and the patients to make decisions together and therefore people are more empowered to act in order to avert health issues that are brought about by their personal risk factors.

## 5.3 Predictive Models in Preventive Care

With the help of predictive analytics, health professionals will be able to identify individuals, who are likely to develop certain health issues and intervene in the process earlier than ever before. Based on the risk of someone, predictive models are applied to recommend when and how frequently various kinds of screening ought to be conducted. In this manner of working, the preventive services are effective and fewer unnecessary treatments are made.

Also, the predictive tools may motivate individuals to make the necessary changes in their lifestyle. Therefore, in case the model indicates that a person is more likely to develop hypertension or type 2 diabetes, physicians can discuss diet, physical activity, and smoking cessation earlier. Due to this fact, nowadays models are available in online health systems and wellness applications that help the users to remain on course with their behaviors. In some cases, such solutions include gamification or reminders to encourage users to adopt preventive measures.

In medical care, predictive models are applied to make decisions regarding vaccinations, e.g. selecting those patients who are most likely to experience complications of influenza or COVID-19. These models will make people take care of their health in advance and relieve the burden on the healthcare system due to their predictions.

## 5.5 The Use of Tools and Dashboards in Clinical Environments

The success of using risk assessment in the clinic is mainly influenced by the ease of use and design of the tools and dashboards. Risk calculators, for example, the

ASCVD risk estimator and the Gail model, are often used by doctors to help discuss patients' health and plan treatments. To use these tools, doctors put in information about the patient, and the system provides a risk estimate, often showing the result with graphs or percentile charts.

The latest Clinical Decision Support Systems (CDSS) are built right into EHR platforms, which provides immediate risk alerts and tips to healthcare providers. They can mark patients at risk, propose tests for diagnosis, and advise on evidence-based treatments. For example, CDSSs use vital signs and laboratory values to spot patients who might have sepsis and recommend early action that could help save their lives.

True AI-powered tools are designed to be easy to understand and use, so healthcare professionals can rely on the findings. Healthcare organizations can also use visual dashboards to monitor population-level risks and decide on the most effective ways to manage and use resources(Shiny Irene et al., 2025).

## 6. MODEL EVALUATION AND CLINICAL VALIDATION

### 6.1 Performance Metrics

In healthcare, it is important to look past accuracy when evaluating predictive models, since doctors may need to understand how the model works in detail. Evidently, accuracy can be misinterpreted when dealing with datasets where some classes are much rarer than others, which is often the case in medicine. As a result, Area Under the Receiver Operating Characteristic Curve (AUC-ROC) is often chosen as a better metric. AUC measures how well a model is able to tell classes apart with different cutoff values, so it is a common measure for binary prediction systems in healthcare.

Another important group of metrics is made up of precision and recall. Precision measures how well a test predicts positive results, especially so that we do not give a false positive, and recall (or sensitivity) measures how well it recognizes true positives, critical when it is risky to miss a positive diagnosis. The F1-score is calculated by averaging precision and recall, allowing for a balanced measurement. If the dataset is unbalanced, using AUC-PR can provide more useful information than using AUC-ROC.

In addition to grouping, calibration checks how close the predicted probabilities are to the outcomes. It is important for a model to produce risk scores that match real-world chances, as this helps healthcare workers decide on the best treatment. It is common to use Brier scores and calibration plots to measure this. It is also important to note that reclassification indices such as NRI measure how a new model does a better job at sorting patients into risk categories compared to an existing standard.

All of these metrics work together to assess how well the model distinguishes between groups, fits the data, and is useful for medical care.

## 6.2 Explainability and Interpretability

While performance measures the success of a model, interpretability helps us understand its reasoning, which is becoming increasingly significant in medical AI. It is important for clinicians to rely on and trust the predictions made by AI when making vital choices. Since neural networks are often seen as "black boxes," there has been a push to develop explainable AI methods.

SHAP is a framework that uses cooperative game theory to assign numbers to each feature showing its role in a prediction. SHAP values make it easier for clinicians to see which clinical factors had an impact on the predicted risk and by how much. In much the same way, LIME uses easy-to-understand models to help understand the predictions made by complex algorithms. They help to make the reasoning behind the model's assessment of a patient clear.

In image-based diagnostics, saliency maps and Grad-CAM point out parts of the medical image that played a key role in the model's results, making it easier for radiologists to confirm the model's decisions. A new way of looking at this is through counterfactual explanations, which point out how different input data could lead to new predictions. They help make the process clearer and ensure that predictions are in line with how doctors think.

Explainability should be considered as both a technical and an ethical issue. It ensures fairness, responsibility, and proper use of AI in healthcare services for people. It is possible that models that are not understood by clinicians may not win their approval or be accepted by regulators.

## 6.3 Clinical Trials and Real-World Validation

Creating a successful model in a computer is just the beginning of the process for using it in medicine. The model should be tested and proven through studies carried out both before and after its development. By testing it on historical data, retrospective validation helps to see if the model works, but can be affected by biases present in the set. Meanwhile, prospective validation puts the model to the test in real hospitals to make sure it functions properly in real life. As part of validation, the model is often put into use in clinical settings, and the results on patient care are measured. They evaluate how easy it is to use the technology, if clinicians like it, if there is too much alerting, and what impact it really has on diagnosis, treatment, or patient outcomes. In the case of sepsis, the model needs to flag patients who are at risk and also prompt actions that can prevent death. Nowadays, clinical trials often check the accuracy of predictive models, particularly when such models impact the decisions made about patients' treatment. These trials are carried out like drug trials, with randomization and control groups, so that we can see if the AI tool benefits patients. As a result, clinical validation makes certain that predictive models are effective and make a true difference in healthcare.

## 7. CHALLENGES AND LIMITATIONS

### 7.1 Data Quality and Standardization

The quality and standardization of data are among the biggest problems in predictive analytics for healthcare. Most of the time, healthcare data come from electronic health records, imaging systems, laboratory instruments, and wearable sensors and are saved in many different formats. Since there are so many different types of data, it is hard to bring them together and study them. In addition, EHRs may have incorrect, inconsistent, or missing data, which can lead to a poor performance of the model (Kokila et al., 2024). For example, if there are missing details about the patient's medications or the codes are not correct, the risk predictions may be incorrect. Even though standardizing data using HL7 FHIR (Fast Healthcare Interoperability Resources) is still in progress, its adoption varies from one healthcare system to another. You need to start with reliable and clean data for your models to work and scale.

### 7.2 Bias and Fairness in Predictive Models

Predictive models may unintentionally keep or increase the unfairness seen in the data used to train them for some populations. Bias in models is often caused by datasets in which certain age groups, genders, or ethnicities are present in very high numbers. As an illustration, if a cardiovascular risk model is mostly based on men's data, it might not work well for women and could result in the wrong diagnosis or less treatment. Also, income, education, and the location where people live may not be included properly or at all, which affects the fairness and equity of the model. To address these problems, we should use methods such as bias auditing, fairness-aware modeling, and use equal opportunity or demographic parity metrics when testing models. The need to share the sources of the data, the assumptions made in the model, and how each subgroup performs is vital to prevent harm and avoid making models that worsen health disparities.

## 7.3 Generalizability and Transferability

Many predictive models have a hard time being used in different clinical scenarios or for various patients. A model that was trained in a large medical center could not work well in a small community hospital or overseas, as there are differences in how medicine is practiced, who the patients are, or in the structure of their data. Because of this issue, predictive analytics cannot be widely applied and does not have a big impact in real life. Models ought to be tested using a range of datasets and should be updated frequently to keep up with new medical guidelines and trends in health. Using federated learning and domain adaptation, it is now possible to learn from different data sources while maintaining the privacy of patients. Nevertheless, it is still very difficult to make mobile phones truly portable.

*Figure 3.* **Challenges and Limitations**

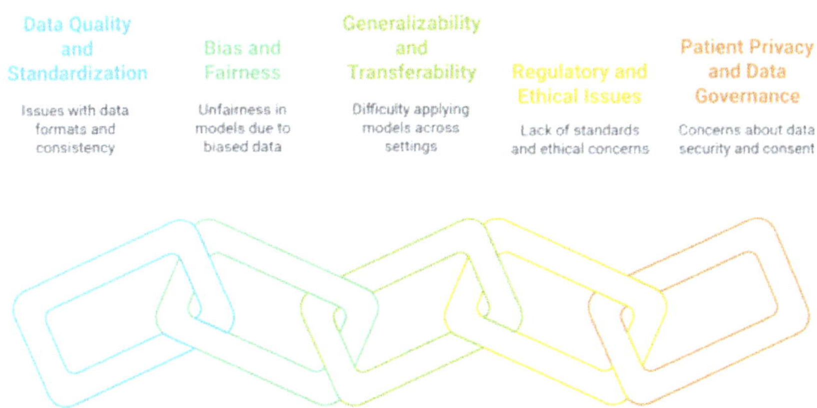


## 7.4 Regulatory and Ethical Issues

Regulatory rules for AI and predictive analytics in healthcare are still forming, and a lot of tools have not received approval from the FDA. There are no standard methods for validating, checking, and watching medical software after it is deployed. In addition, there are many ethical issues related to algorithms deciding important matters such as starting treatment or admitting a patient to the ICU. Some professionals are concerned that black-box models are difficult to understand, so they cannot explain to clinicians why a certain decision was made. Accountability, transparency, and the right to explanation from AI should be built into how predictive tools are created and put into practice. It is important for data scientists, clinicians, ethicists, and policymakers to work closely to address these issues and gain people's trust in AI-based healthcare systems.

### 7.5 Patient Privacy and Data Governance

Patient privacy, consent, and good data governance are all important issues because healthcare data are sensitive. It is important that predictive models have access to a lot of health information, and this information must be handled according to laws like HIPAA in the U.S. and GDPR in the EU. Still, when different types of information are combined, it can sometimes become possible to reverse the anonymization and de-identification methods and identify the data. More and more, questions are being raised about who owns the data, how it is shared, and if people have given their consent, as AI models make use of data collected from various devices. Making sure that data governance policies highlight patient autonomy, safe sharing of information, and clear use of data is essential. Differential privacy and homomorphic encryption are some of the promising ways to protect data in machine learning.

## 8. EMERGING TRENDS AND FUTURE DIRECTIONS

### 8.1 Federated Learning and Privacy-Preserving Analytics

As healthcare moves towards using data more, the issues of privacy, who can share data, and data being stored in isolated systems are still major obstacles. This new approach allows machine learning models to be developed in several institutions without sharing the original patient records. Algorithms are sent to various data sources in the community, trained on their own, and joined together at a central location. It ensures that patient data is hidden, and still, a larger and more diverse collection of data is used, which improves the model's ability to be used in different situations. International hospitals, which have to follow different regulations, can greatly benefit from federated learning. Meanwhile, differential privacy, secure multiparty computation, and homomorphic encryption are being investigated to ensure privacy as individuals and organizations get insights. These approaches will probably be key elements in the future of predictive healthcare.

## 8.2 Multimodal Learning

It is now common for doctors to look at a person's health as a whole when trying to diagnose diseases and foresee risks. Multimodal learning uses many forms of data, such as EHR records, images, DNA sequences, and medical notes, to make better and more accurate predictions. When the data sources are combined, models are able to detect patterns that are not clear from looking at them separately. As an example, bringing together histopathology images, genetic information, and a patient's clinical history can help doctors with both diagnosis and choosing the best treatment. Those deep learning architectures that rely on transformers and attention mechanisms have demonstrated good results in working with various types of data. It is also important for this method to help individualize medicine and explore disease pathways at a larger scale.

## 8.3 Real-Time Analytics with Edge Computing and IoT

Because of the spread of IoT, wearable health trackers, home monitoring systems, and smart implants, it is now much simpler to collect health data in real time. Nevertheless, sending the data to central servers all the time causes issues with bandwidth, latency, and privacy. Doing the data processing on the device or nearby means real-time analysis and decision-making becomes possible. In emergency and critical care, edge-enabled models can sense risk quickly, as they can identify a cardiac event from a wearable ECG monitor. These skills are especially helpful in regions that do not have much access to the cloud. The combination of edge computing and predictive analytics increases the system's speed and encourages equal and decentralized health services(Ponnuviji, N. P et al., 2024).

## 8.4 Integration with Wearable Devices and Mobile Apps

Because of consumer-grade wearable devices and health-related mobile apps, individuals now play a bigger role in their own health care. They are always collecting information about physical activity, heart rate, sleep, oxygen levels, glucose, and many other things. When used with predictive models, this kind of data can support early identification of health risks, constant tracking of chronic health problems, and flexible ways to manage them.

AI in mobile apps can give users personal recommendations for health, warnings, and reminders to change their behaviors. In this way, a person with diabetes could be given diet advice in real time when their glucose levels are shown by the monitor. Besides, these platforms make it easier for patients to be monitored remotely, relieving the pressure on healthcare facilities and increasing patient involvement.

With better sensor technology, wearables are likely to play an even bigger role in preventive and precision medicine.

## 8.5 Regulatory Frameworks and Responsible AI

Since predictive analytics play a role in healthcare, it is necessary to have strict regulations to make sure everything is safe, effective, and ethical. This means that it is necessary to ensure transparency, explainable models, ongoing monitoring after deployment, and continuous check of performance. At the same time, those working in healthcare are recommending the creation of responsible AI guidelines that put a strong focus on fairness, responsibility, and human control. Topics that are most discussed in policies today include algorithmic bias, model governance, and informed consent. It is important for clinicians, data scientists, ethicists, and regulators to team up and develop guidelines that promote new ideas and protect the public. In the future, the mixing of advanced analytics, real data, and clear regulations will lead to predictive models being part of clinical decision-making. When technologies improve and standards are set, we can expect healthcare to move in the direction of being customized, proactive, and fair for all.

# 9. CONCLUSION

Predictive analytics is quickly revolutionizing healthcare today by making it easier to diagnose diseases, measure risks, and provide customized treatment. We have looked at the main ideas, data types, machine learning and statistics, medical applications, and evaluation systems that characterize this area of study. From the traditional logistic regression to the latest deep learning and federated learning, many approaches are being used to enhance diagnosis, group patients by risk, and decide on early interventions. Predictive models are shown to help in cardiovascular diseases, cancer, neurological problems, infectious diseases, and chronic conditions when adopted in the clinic. The greatest benefit of predictive analytics comes from its ability to make sense of huge, complicated sets of data and reveal insights that was not possible before. They are expected to make it possible for detection and treatment to happen sooner, and also for resources to be used more effectively and patients to benefit more. Even so, to achieve this potential, it is important to deal with key challenges such as quality of data, biased models, privacy concerns, the ability to be used in many situations, and making sure AI is ethical. As predictive analytics progresses, it will be important to put in place strong rules and governance systems that care for patients. Going ahead, predictive analytics in healthcare will rely a lot on people from different fields working together. Clinicians, data scientists, engineers, ethicists, and policymakers need to team up to build and test models that are accurate and at the same time fair, interpretable, and suitable for healthcare. Besides, people must ensure that new inventions are guided by ethics and fairness. Through teamwork and use of technology, predictive analytics can bring about a new era of healthcare that serves people well and precisely around the world.

## REFERENCES


Ali, O., Abdelbaki, W., Shrestha, A., Elbasi, E., Alryalat, M. A. A., & Dwivedi, Y. K. (2023). A systematic literature review of artificial intelligence in the healthcare sector: Benefits, challenges, methodologies, and functionalities. *Journal of Innovation & Knowledge*, *8*(1), 100333.

Ambhika, C., Gayathri, S., & Sheena, B. G. (2024, August). Enhancing predictive modeling in high dimensional data using hybrid feature selection. In 2024 5th International Conference on Electronics and Sustainable Communication Systems (ICESC) (pp. 873-879). IEEE.

Babu Vimala, B., Srinivasan, S., & Mathivanan, S. K., Mahalakshmi, Jayagopal, P., & Dalu, G. T. (2023). Detection and classification of brain tumor using hybrid deep learning models. *Scientific Reports*, *13*(1), 23029. PMID: 38155247

Bansal, M., Goyal, A., & Choudhary, A. (2022). A comparative analysis of K-nearest neighbor, genetic, support vector machine, decision tree, and long short term memory algorithms in machine learning. *Decision Analytics Journal*, *3*, 100071.

Bhatt, C., Kumar, I., Vijayakumar, V., Singh, K. U., & Kumar, A. (2021). The state of the art of deep learning models in medical science and their challenges. *Multimedia Systems*, *27*(4), 599–613.

Boopathi, S. (2023). Deep learning techniques applied for automatic sentence generation. In Promoting Diversity, Equity, and Inclusion in Language Learning Environments (pp. 255-273). IGI Global.

Dhinakaran, D., Kumar, N. J., & Ponnuviji, N. P. (2025). Safeguarding confidentiality and privacy in cloud-enabled healthcare systems with spectrasafe encryption and dynamic k-anonymity algorithm. *Expert Systems with Applications*, *279*, 127584.

Kashyap, R., & Piersson, A. D. (2018). Big data challenges and solutions in the medical industries. In *Handbook of Research on Pattern Engineering System Development for Big Data Analytics* (pp. 1–24). IGI Global.

Kocher, G., & Kumar, G. (2021). Machine learning and deep learning methods for intrusion detection systems: Recent developments and challenges. *Soft Computing*, *25*(15), 9731–9763.

Kokila, M. S., Fenil, E., Ponnuviji, N. P., & Nirmala, G. (2024). Securing cloud-based medical data: An optimal dual kernal support vector approach for enhanced EHR management. *International Journal of System Assurance Engineering and Management*, *15*(7), 3495–3507.

Kumar, V., & Garg, M. L. (2018). Predictive analytics: A review of trends and techniques. *International Journal of Computer Applications*, *182*(1), 31–37.

Mangairkarasi, S., Ramana, T. V., Vaishnavi, R., Agalya, S., Sathya, V., & Subramanian, R. S. (2025). Advancing Healthcare Through Artificial Intelligence: Applications, Challenges, and Future Directions. In Responsible AI for Digital Health and Medical Analytics (pp. 113-134). IGI Global Scientific Publishing.

Mishra, N., & Silakari, S. (2012). Predictive analytics: A survey, trends, applications, oppurtunities & challenges. *International Journal of Computer Science and Information Technologies*, *3*(3), 4434–4438.

Nanehkaran, Y. A., Licai, Z., Chengyong, J., Chen, J., Anwar, S., Azarafza, M., & Derakhshani, R. (2023). Comparative analysis for slope stability by using machine learning methods. *Applied Sciences (Basel, Switzerland)*, *13*(3), 1555.

Ponnuviji, N. P., Elangovan, G., Sujatha, K., Jambulingam, U., Ganesan, I., & Lalitha, S. D. (2024). IoT-Enabled Assistive Technologies Approach for Personalized Geriatric Health Monitoring and Safety. In Future of AI in Biomedicine and Biotechnology (pp. 125-146). IGI Global.

Priyadharshini, S. I., Irene, D. S., Beulah, J. R., & Ponnuviji, N. P. (2025). Enhancing real-time health monitoring with hybrid recurrent long short-term tyrannosaurus search for menstrual cups. *Biomedical Signal Processing and Control*, *100*, 107065.

Shiny Irene, D., Ponnuviji, N. P., & Kalaivani, A. (2025). EHECA-HSWS: A Holistic Method for Improving Menstrual Health App User Experience. *Journal of the Institution of Electronics and Telecommunication Engineers*, •••, 1–12.

Sreelakshmi, S., Babu, A. A., Lakshmipriya, C., Gracious, L. A., Nalini, M., & Subramanian, R. S. (2024, October). Enhancing Intrusion Detection Systems with Machine Learning. In 2024 2nd International Conference on Self Sustainable Artificial Intelligence Systems (ICSSAS) (pp. 557-564). IEEE.

Subha, S., Balakrishnan, C., & Anish, T. P. (2024, August). Optimizing Machine Learning Algorithms for Heart Disease Prediction in Healthcare: A Comparative Study. In 2024 5th International Conference on Electronics and Sustainable Communication Systems (ICESC) (pp. 866-872). IEEE.

Chapter 6

# Harnessing Predictive Analytics for Disease Diagnosis and Risk Assessment:

## Transforming Preventive Healthcare With AI


**Mukul Sharma**
https://orcid.org/0009-0009-5560-6257
*Swami Vivekanand Subharti University, Meerut, India*

**Vikas Sharma**
https://orcid.org/0000-0001-8173-4548
*SRM Institute of Science and Technology, Delhi, India*

**Shashiraj Teotia**
https://orcid.org/0000-0002-0849-3642
*Swami Vivekanand Subharti University, Meerut, India*

**Tarun Kumar Vashishth**
https://orcid.org/0000-0001-9916-9575
*IIMT University, Meerut, India*

**Vivek Aggarwal**
*Ajay Kumar Garg Engineering College, Ghaziabad, India*

**Barkha Samania**
https://orcid.org/0009-0006-7824-1658
*SRM Institute of Science and Technology, Delhi, India*


## ABSTRACT


*In healthcare, applying AI alongside predictive analytics is transforming disease diagnosis, risk assessment, and treatment management. This chapter addresses the multidisciplinary impact of algorithm and data model sophistication on early detection, outcome forecasting, and patient identification stratified by risk. Health predictive analytics offers numerous possibilities by deconstructing vast and intricate datasets like electronic health records, genomic information, and data from*



DOI: 10.4018/979-8-3373-3311-3.ch006

*wearables into actionable, anticipatory, tailored Healthcare-focused on proactive personal preventive intervention. Predictive models like logistic regression, decision trees, and ensemble and deep learning are covered, along with their use in chronic disease management, cancer risk forecasting, and cardiovascular risk assessment. The chapter also analyses critical data concerns such as accuracy, explainability, bias and fairness, usability, and integration into clinical workflows.*

## 1. INTRODUCTION

The increase in the prevalence of chronic and acute illnesses, in addition to soaring health expenditures, has highlighted the need for more forward-thinking and preventive medical care practices. Conventional methodologies of diagnosis and treatment often wait for symptomatic burning issues to become apparent and happen to employ only retrospective evaluations, which often results in poor health being provided at interventional-late stages. In contrast, new technologies like Artificial Intelligence (AI) and data science are making it possible to enable a shift from responsive rather reactive healthcare systems to prophylactic ones. The change is primarily spearheaded by predictive analytics, which utilizes both historical and real-time data to anticipate health-related events and risks prior to their occurrence (Khinvasara et al., 2024).

### 1.1 Overview of AI and Predictive Analytics In Healthcare

Predictive analytics is an important predictive approach that enables the transformation of healthcare from reactive to proactive, focusing on prevention and early intervention, which AI – Artificial Intelligence, is making possible by allowing machines to mimic human thinking (Vashishth et al., 2024). Predictive Analytics works by applying statistical modeling, machine learning algorithms, and advanced data analytics to estimate the future health outcomes using historical and current data. In relation to healthcare, the importance of predictive analytics lies in the ability to predict the possible onset, progression, or recurrence of a disease prior to clinical manifestations. In contrast to the common approach methods that treatment is only initiated post disease manifestation, with predictive analytics the clinician is able to make worthwhile decisions in advance, and is therefore far more likely to be successful. Such a change is particularly useful in the case of chronic diseases and other complex health conditions which, when detected early, have the capacity to dramatically change the patient's health. The healthcare industry creates vast amounts of data from electronic health records, medical imaging, genomic sequencing, and wearable devices that constantly track bodily changes (Govindaraj et al., 2024).

AI technology in predictive analytics can identify patterns in large and complex datasets, processes, and analyses data that is multilayered and complicated, finding meaningful relationships within the information. For instance, AI algorithms can utilize a combination of real-time monitoring data, genetic markers, medical histories, and lifestyle habits to assess an individual's risk for developing cardiovascular illnesses, diabetes, or cancer. Through these predictive capabilities, patients can be categorized based on their individual profiles, enabling healthcare providers to customize strategies tailored to each individual patient's needs. This stratification of risk allows proactive and anticipatory, personalized care to be optimized, meaning close attention and timely action can be dedicated to high-risk individuals while others may just receive helpful advice on lifestyle changes and prevention education. Additionally, the integration of AI insights into the workflow of clinical practice aids in making more accurate, faster diagnoses without excessive tests, maximized use of healthcare resources, and improved efficiency of practices that help eliminate redundant diagnostic sessions (Adeoye and Adams, 2024).

The blending of healthcare with AI powered prediction marks the birth of a more sophisticated, effective, and preventive modern healthcare system rooted on predictive analysis. This allows care givers predispose from standard and outdate methodologies and embrace a more intelligent structure inclined to early spotting, correct appraisal, and strategic therapy formulation tailored for specified patients. There stands no doubt that healthcare services and health results in the near future are bound to change though-in increasing number and diversely throughout the population as development of the aforementioned technology.

## 1.2 Significance of Early Detection And Preventive Care

The modern clinical healthcare's core may rely on early detection and preventive care services especially considering the ever-growing burden of chronic and life-threatening diseases. For years, healthcare systems have taken a reactive approach—waiting to provide care until an illness is present, leading to late detection, high intensity treatment, and increased costs. Identifying definable health risks has started to shift towards a more proactive approach of attempting to identify possible ailments before the physical symptoms become glaringly obvious. The potential to identify early-stage illnesses, especially during the most treatable phase, can drastically improve outcomes and decrease long-term healthcare costs. Early detection provides intervention opportunities during the critical time when diseases are considered full preventable, or easier to manage. Hypertension, diabetes, and some cancerous conditions often portray biological or behavioural signs sufficient to warrant intervention way prior to any noticeable symptoms. Modern healthcare seeks to harness these subtle indicators through advanced diagnostic tools, enabling providers and patients to take proactive measures that do not just confine to the pausing or curing of diseases, but rather reversal of the condition altogether. For the case of cancer, the chronic condition is most often curable and treatable when detected at the initial stages as it is associated with a less severe treatment, improved Quality of Life (QoL), and greater likelihood of survival (Kuppuswamy et al., 2024).

Along with early detection, capturing preventive care enhances health by stopping disease before it starts. There is a problem when people don't have access to these services, whether it is routine screenings, guidance on lifestyle choices, vaccinations, or teaching people about health. Preventive care, when properly guided supported by advanced technology such predictive analytics and AI, becomes highly specific and meticulous, enhancing his/her efficiency. It is feasible to outline easily a patient's personalized preventive strategy tailored for these unique risks built using combinations of genetic information, environmental components, behavioural information, and medical history. Relieving the burden so many healthcare suffers raise the importance of integrating detection and preventive care into more clinical routine practice, which helps foster systemic efficiency. As stated in (Vashishth et al., 2023), hospitals and clinics can proactively manage potential health issues, which reduces the frequency of emergency room visits, intensive care unit admissions, and long-term treatments. This not only maximizes the efficient use of available resources, but also increases sustainability within the particular healthcare system. Developments in data analysis and wearable health technologies, as well as smartphone health applications, empower the shift towards proactive disease identification and prevention. Such applications provide real-time monitoring of a person's health, which allows for easy detection of deviations from the set norm and prompt action. In healthcare, the work of artificial intelligence makes the process easier because it merges information and presents them as actionable recommendations, which provides a more dynamic approach to care services delivery (Alam et al., 2024).

## 2. FOUNDATIONS OF PREDICTIVE ANALYTICS IN HEALTHCARE

The confluence of healthcare domain knowledge along with statistical science, data mining, and machine learning serves as the backbone for predictive analytics in healthcare. The main objective is to translate the data generated from various health records into actionable insights capable of estimating future medical occurrences, refining clinical judgments, and enabling early intervention in patient management. The power of predictive analytics is most felt when there is adequate, precise, and diverse data coupled with advanced computational models built to recognize patterns and make educated predictions about prospective outcomes. A world brimming with algorithms tailored for real-time data interpretation – wearables and mobile health apps – alongside genomic sequencing, diagnostic tests, electronic health records, and even medical imaging systems gives us an inexhaustible supply of data to tap into. The data sets are enormous and all-encompassing, stretching beyond clinical indicators such as lab values or blood pressure to include behavioural, social, and even environmental factors impacting health. The first step towards predictive analytics is invariably the data itself, which exists in heterogeneous forms, both structured and unstructured. Regardless of the source, it has one overriding characteristic – diversity. However, before any predictive modeling can take place, rigorous data preprocessing is a necessity, along with cleaning, normalization, missing value imputation, and system integration. After curating and cleaning the data, it's ready for exploration, as statistical models and machine learning algorithms are applied. Models are trained to understand intricate relationships between various components with the help of logistic regression, decision trees, support vector machines, ensemble methods like random forests and gradient boosting, and even deep learning neural networks. These models are then capable of predicting possible diagnoses, complications, or risks of readmission based on the learned historical data (Fatima, 2024).

*Figure 1. Predictive Analytics in Healthcare*

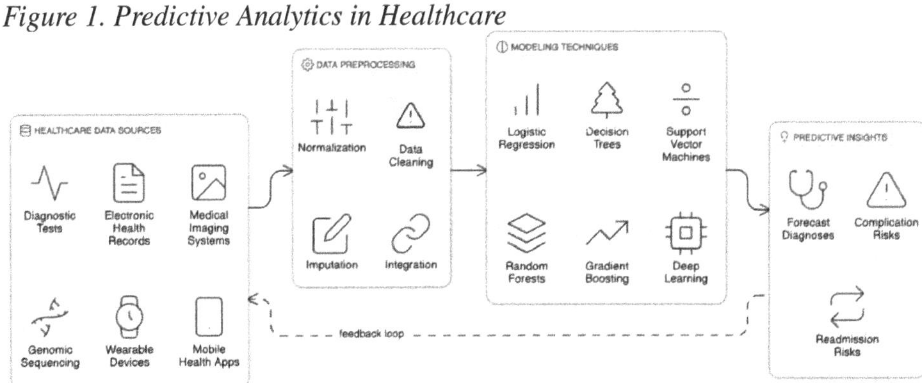


Take, for example, a model that is taught on thousands of patients with heart problems. It may be able to predict which of the new patients is most likely to suffer a heart attack within the year.

## 2.1 Definition and Key Principles Of Predictive Analytics

Forecasting future events or trends through the use of historical data, statistical algorithms, and machine learning techniques are called as predictive analytics. In healthcare, it is used to predict medical outcomes, perform risk assessments for diseases, optimize treatments, and facilitate clinical decision-making. It provides actionable insights from data which is unprocessed, disorganized, and intricately structured while enabling healthcare professionals to manage patient health proactively. Predictive analytics are conducted on the basis that the patterns and relationships in data from the past can accurate predictions about the future. Unlike descriptive and diagnostic analytics, this approach does not assess why events occurred in the past. Instead, it analyses future possibilities and possible interventions to influence desired outcomes (Yingngam et al., 2024).

There are a number of underlying principles when applying predictive analytics in healthcare:

1. **Data Driven Decision Making:** The analytics employed here rely entirely on data to make clinical decisions as opposed to instincts or singular pieces of clinical evidence. In healthcare, this translates to having access to data from different sources—electronic health records (EHRs), diagnostic imaging, as well as patient-reported data from mobile devices—to form a sound-based clinical decision. This principle of predictive analytics, provides assurance that healthcare trends and patterns are actionable and grounded to the reality, increasing the chances of receiving proper healthcare interventions (Tsai et al., 2025).
2. **Pattern Recognition:** Identifying useful patterns within collection of data is critical in appealing measures. A predictive approach depends on recognizing meaningful encounters in great datasets. Recognized patterns intersecting with certain diseases or eventualities can include symptoms, lab markers, genetic markers, lifestyle behaviours etc. For example, sustained increase of glucose levels in a patient alongside a sedentary lifestyle and high body mass index could indicate the presence of a muscle in diabetes. Timely recognition allows health care professionals to take appropriate action before the disease advance position greatly (Olalekan Kehinde, 2025).
3. **Risk Stratification:** Predictive techniques assign patients to different categories depending on the possibility of occurrence of specific medical events during a given period of time. Such measures make it possible to direct patient care phenomena for specific actions. In other terms, allocative efficiency is induced towards people considered high risk. These are people for whom immediate action, closer supervision for enhanced outcomes is feasible. For instance, in the setting of a hospital, predictive models can identify patients with a sufficiently high risk of readmission, prompting the care team to create tailored review processes or follow up recommendations to mitigate that risk (Ahmadi, 2024).
4. **Model Interpretability and Transparency:** Predictive models in clinical settings cannot be "black boxes." Providers need to grasp the reasoning behind a certain decision or prediction to act on it. Models interpret data in distinct

ways, which corresponds to the ability to outline the different aspects which influenced the patient's risk score · indeed, every model has its logic and can tell about it. Transparency allows for validation which is crucial for fostering clinical adoption alongside model troubleshooting and compliance with regulations (Gandhi and Prathyusha, 2025).

5. **Continuous Learning and Adaptation:** With the ever-changing new treatments, diseases, and patient populations, the healthcare ecosystem continuously evolves. Their predictive models should receive and act upon new data learning enabling those predictive models to adapt. This builds relevance for the models as standards, evidence, or patient characteristics change without losing reliability or accuracy.
6. **Privacy and Data Governance:** Sensitive data regarding healthcare should be treated with high care. Predictive analytics should function within frameworks that guarantee the upholding of data security, consent from the patient, and compliance with HIPAA or GDPR. Moreover, considerations of ethical nature arise, models should not strengthen pre-existing biases or act which infringes on the autonomy of patients.

## 2.2 Types of Healthcare Data: EHRs, Genomics, Wearable Sensors, etc.

Within predictive analytics, the accuracy and efficiency of models strongly depend on the quality and heterogeneity of available healthcare data. Data in healthcare is produced and recorded from different vantage points each day which and offers unique facets of a patient's health profile. The structured and unstructured types of data available form the backbone for accurate and proactive care methods. The following is data pertaining to healthcare:

1. **Electronic Health Records (EHRs):** One of the most comprehensive sources of healthcare data is the digital version of a patient's paper chart which is known as an EHR. EHR's contain patient demographics, medical history, medications, allergies, lab test results, imaging, treatment plans, and clinical notes. EHRs are captured at different times which allows for a longitudinal view of patient care. This longitudinal approach is useful for predicting the progression of diseases, evaluating treatment results, and identifying patients at risk. Incorporating EHRs into predictive models allows providers to make informed, data-backed decisions (Jayachandran et al., 2025).
2. **Genomic Data:** Information on an individual's genetic composition, including his or her DNA sequences, gene expression, and even genetic mutations, constitutes genomic data. This class of data assists in understanding familial

risks, certain predispositions, and even the possible reaction to selected drugs (pharmacogenomics). Utilized in predictive analytics, genomic data allows for more accurate and personalized health forecasts, especially concerning cancer, rare diseases, and some metabolic disorders (Recharla et al., 2025).

3. **Data from Wearable Sensors and Mobile Health Devices:** Technologies like smartwatches and fitness trackers actively monitor various physiological indicators, such as heart rate, sleep, physical activity, oxygen saturation, and glucose levels in real time. Along with biosensors, these devices enable remote patient monitoring and capture constant patient health data. Predictive models can process the vast streams of data to monitor performance metrics for anomaly detection, health event prognosis, and even provide timely intervention—particularly for chronic illness management and elderly patient care (Goyal et al., 2025).
4. **Medical Imaging Data:** Medical imaging refers to the X-ray, MRI, CT-scan, Ultrasound, and other form of imaging diagnostics that provide a non-invasive view into the human body. Image data, when analysed with AI algorithms, has the potential to expose patterns, sequences, and outlines that may be complicated to perceive with the naked eye. Applying analytics on images has the potential to aid in the early detection of diseases, classification of tumours, and even in foreseeing the advancement of diseases by evaluating visual changes over periods of time (Maha et al., 2024).
5. **Laboratory and Diagnostic Test Results:** Laboratory test data like blood work, urine tests, and pathology results provide important biochemical and cellular insights into the body's system. More often than not, these results are the first abnormal flag indicators that something in the body is or could potentially go wrong. Over time, the collection and analysis of lab data allows for the prediction of disease onset, monitoring of treatment efficiency, and detection of abnormal trends pre-clinically or before symptoms show up in a practical setting.
6. **Socioeconomic and Behavioural Data:** Health outcomes are substantially impacted by social determinants of health such as income, education, employment, housing arrangements, and lifestyle choices, which include smoking, alcohol consumption, and diet. Incorporating such data into predictive analytics improves understanding of the patient's health to make predictions that are not only more accurate, but also equitable by considering social, in addition to biological, risk factors.

## 2.3 Techniques of Data Preprocessing and Integration

Healthcare predictive analytics rarely starts with clean datasets. Raw data is seldom in a ideal format for direct application to analytical models. It comes from heterogeneous sources like EHRs, genomics, medical imaging, wearables, and is captured in different formats and with varying levels of quality. Therefore, ensuring accuracy, consistency, and usability for machine learning algorithms through data cleansing and integration are fundamental. These processes augment model performance, make results more interpretable, and mitigate risk for biased or erroneous predictions.

1. **Data Cleaning:** As discussed previously, the focus of this technique is filling missing or incomplete data, eliminating inconsistencies, mistakes, and duplicates whatsoever, hence why cleaning is the first step. In the domain of healthcare, the gap in value can be observed in patient records, lab results, or even in sensor data. In the case of data cleaning, these gaps can be filled by allotting certain values through statistical means. For example, in relation to data cleaning, averages (mean or median) can be calculated for continuous variables, while the most frequent value can be used for categorical ones. This process of data cleaning or filling gaps allows for more accurate predictions to be made, which strengthens the models put in place.
2. **Data Normalization/Standardization:** Standardization is recalibrating a set of values so that they lie between a specific minimum and maximum. In the case of healthcare, features such as reasoning, glucose levels, and even age can be observed through varying scales and units. If not well adjusted, larger numerical ranges might have a greater outcome than the predictive models, which without reason, would render them pointless. Standardization and normalization provide a common ground to balance out the features. In normalization, the goal is to make the values fall between the range of zero to one. In standardization instead of aiming for a specific range, aspiration would be for the mean to be zero while goal for the standard deviation would be one. Both actions serve the same purpose of ensuring the levels of all parts or variables to enhance model reliability and predictive accuracy.
3. **Data Transformation:** Unstructured healthcare data sources like clinical notes, medical imaging reports, or genetic sequencing contain raw data that require transformation and structure before being analysed. Techniques such as Natural Language Processing (NLP) can be utilized on clinical texts (doctor's notes, for example) to pull out structured data like symptoms, diagnoses, and treatment histories. Moreover, feature engineering methods such as creating a "comorbidity index" through a patient's medical history or converting drug dosage amounts into adherence scoring represent new variables derived from existing data. Transformative processes enable predictive models to analyze raw unstructured data through defined insights (Vashishth et al., 2024).
4. **Data Integration:** Integration involves combining datasets from different sources like EHRs, wearable sensors, genomic databases, and laboratory results into a

single cohesive view for advanced analysis and exploration. The various sources of healthcare data present differing formats, terminologies, and structures around them which pose a challenge to be integrated and analysed. Techniques like schema matching (aligning different data formats) and standardization with common coding systems like ICD (International Classification of Diseases) or SNOMED CT become imperative.

5. **Dimensionality Reduction:** It often happens in the case of genomic sequences as well as multi-feature EHRs that they contain a number of variables (features) which are not always required to be used for making predictions, and these is classified as high dimensional data. Reduction in dimensions with techniques like Principal Component Analysis (PCA) or t-distributed Stochastic Neighbour Embedding (t-SNE) can be performed to eliminate inconsequential information from the most critical. These methods assist in decluttering intricate datasets using sophisticated data techniques. Not only does the reduction of dimensions help to expedite the training process, but it also enhances the performance of the model by boosting accuracy through elimination of noise and inconsequential features.
6. **Data Validation:** Validation ensures that the pre-processed data is accurate and reliable, and ready for predictive modeling after the data has been altered, integrated, cleaned and transformed. Validation constitutes the final phase in the process of confirming reliability. Validation techniques usually involve analyzing integrated data against known benchmarks to compare the provided datasets, after asserting that all transformations have been executed, and conducting accuracy tests on value assumptions made. Data is examined to ascertain that there are no conflicts, inconsistencies and errors that may have been generated during preprocessing.

## 3. CORE PREDICTIVE MODELS IN DISEASE DIAGNOSIS

Through the use of predictive modeling, a proactive approach can now be taken in disease diagnosis, bringing a paradigm shift to the system. It utilizes patient data like history, symptoms, genetics, imaging studies, and EHRs to anticipate the likelihood of a disease, its progression, and other results. Predictive models will only work if sufficiently complex biomedical data is available for analysis because one of the most critical requirements is to recognize and discern patterns that indicate a healthy state or a diseased state (Vashishth et al., 2024).

## 3.1 Logistic Regression

Logistic Regression is a statistical method that is taught in the beginning stages of training. It has many applications, especially in binary classification such as in the identification of diseases. Unlike linear regression which deals with predicting the outcome of a continuous variable, logistic regression estimates the probability of occurrence of a condition like the presence or absence of a disease by fitting a logistic curve to the data. In other words, it predicts whether a set of independent factors (age, BMI, cholesterol, blood pressure) will result to a binary dependent variable—either diseased or healthy. By employing a logarithmic sigmoidal function on a linear model, a value from 0 to 1 can be assigned and thus, interpreted as probability (Singh et al., 2024).

*Figure 2. Logistic Regression Architectural Model*

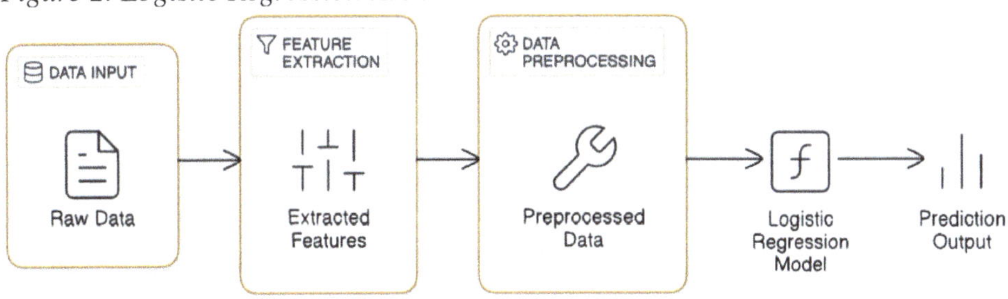


Because logistic regression is straightforward and interpretable, it is prevalent in the early detection of diabetes, heart conditions, and cancer in the medical field. Its advantages include the fact that the model coefficients are meaningful in determining the value of each predictor, hence useful for estimating the risk of the outcome, which is favourable for the clinicians. However, logistic regression has been known to have a major shortcoming – it assumes that there is a linear relationship between the independent variables and the log-odds of the dependent variable, which is often not the case in intricate medical data. Moreover, it has an inherent limitation when dealing with data that has non-linear relationships or interaction among the variables requiring higher order sophisticated models.

## 3.2 Decision Trees

Modeling the decisions related to conditions and diseases is one the most done works using trees. Unlike other classification works, disease or condition trees require understanding human decision making to effectively aid in mimicking it. A decision tree recursively partitions the data space based on feature values to create a tree structure of decisions culminating into one final prediction. Each feature under which a decision can be made in a tree is represented as a node while the outcomes that arise from the feature in question are branches, with final prediction being the leaf node. In our example of heart disease diagnosis, the decision tree is first told to look for a set cholesterol level where it will in turn check if the patient has high blood pressure, and if the patient meets the criteria will then look into age as well as lifestyle. The easiest example of model interpretable decision trees is found in the clinical algorithms used by doctors. Despite being simple models, decision trees possess the unique ability of handling both categorical and numerical inputs, making them pliable to complex healthcare datasets. Like all good things, these models come with a price as they struggle with over-fitting to a given dataset. This might result in poor generalization concerning unseen data. Accuracy and robustness can be enhanced using ensemble techniques like pruning, Random Forests, or Gradient Boosting.

## 4. APPLICATIONS ACROSS MEDICAL SPECIALTIES

The use of predictive analytics and AI across different verticals in healthcare is transforming how different specialties manage patient care. By utilizing the wealth of data available alongside powerful machine learning algorithms, healthcare systems can provide prior condition management, early diagnosis, and proper resource allocation. Each specialty has a unique experience with these technologies which improves the strategies aimed at managing the health of the populations as well as the health outcomes of individual patients.

### 4.1 Chronic Disease Management

Some chronic ailments that are quite common today are diabetes, and hypertension, along with chronic obstructive pulmonary disease (COPD) and chronic kidney disease (CKD). All of these are extremely impactful to the global health systems. For managing these conditions, there is predictive analytics which helps foresee which individual is most likely to be stricken with which disease, how will it advance, and what measures can be taken as a form of intervention. Through predictive analytics, models can be created using length-wise longitudinal health records, lifestyle patterns, biometric data from wearable sensors, as well as laboratory test results, enabling deviations from healthy baselines to be identified. For example, in diabetes management, algorithms are able to identify patterns in blood glucose levels and determine if the patient is at risk of hypoglycaemic episodes. Similarly, some hypertensive patients undergo blood pressure monitoring using machine learning which helps in programming recommendation structures, lifestyle change suggesters, and even dosage adjustments of medication. All of this aids in shifting the healthcare approach towards prevention instead of reactionary measures which drastically enhances the quality of life for patients while also minimizing hospital visits (Islam et al., 2025).

## 4.2 Cancer Detection and Prognosis

The predictive analysis of data impacts early detection, diagnosis, and prognosis of some common cancers such as breast, prostate, lung and colorectal cancer. AI models, powered by artificial intelligence, are capable of integrating imaging data, genomic data, and patient history in order to reveal hidden patterns, thus, broadening the scope of what is observable by human eyes. For example, mammograms can be analysed through deep learning algorithms which enables physicians to determine the existence of potential breast cancers at an earlier stage of detection. Furthermore, personalized treatment and screening methods are made possible through the incorporation of genomic data which identifies possible effacing mutation risks to an individual's own cancer. Additionally, predictive models that proportion survival estimates along with probability of recurrence and rate dependent on the patient's feedback and the tumour's traits are also made possible. All these factors increase the conviction of diagnosis and hence enable the oncologists to exercise better clinical choices substantiated with data clinched with sensible research (Patil and Shankar, 2023).

## 4.3 Cardiovascular Risk Prediction

Cardiovascular diseases (CVDs) are still the most significant cause of death all around the world. The application of predictive analytics gives a precise measure in evaluating the risk for heart attacks, strokes, and heart failures. Unlike traditional calculators that depend on age, cholesterol metrics, and blood pressure, AI models use more extensive and sophisticated data sets such as ECGs, echocardiograms, genetic data, and even data from lifestyle wearables. For instance, machine learning aids in early predictions of atrial fibrillation and heart failures which allows for proactive measures to be put in place. Those affected, as well as medical personnel, can receive alerts for anomalies thereby minimizing unwanted cardiac episodes. These approaches aid in the adoption of more focused proactive measures and improve efficiency in resource allocation within the health sector (Wable et al., 2024).

### 4.4 Infectious Disease Surveillance

The COVID-19 pandemic showcased magnificent increase in the need for timely and accurate surveillance systems for monitoring infectious diseases. As for today, predictive analytics plays an integral role in tracking and attempting to control the spread of diseases like influenza, tuberculosis, and other emerging viruses. Not only do electronic health records, public health databases, and mobile health apps provide a wealth of data to analyze, but additionally, public transport patterns and social media can be analysed to detect outbreak hotspots and estimate transmission rates. For instance, NLP can analyze clinical reports, news articles and other social media to pinpoint any developing disease clusters. With this information, numerous machine learning models can evaluate the feasible likelihood of an outbreak occurring and how impactful it could be. With this evaluation public health officials are able to make better and informed decisions on containment strategies. These functions help not only prepare for a potential medical crisis, but also allow efficient use of resources and precise action planning to target and combat the allocated diseases.

## 5. INTEGRATION WITH HEALTHCARE SYSTEMS

The successful implementation of healthcare analytics for prediction within the health care sector disproves the notion that algorithms are the primary consideration, and proves that system integration is a major key within predictive analytics. Even though fundamental concepts are given careful consideration, integrating predictive analytics with concrete systems provides tangible estimation that uplift decision-making possibilities and productivity.

### 5.1 Embedding Predictive Analytics Into Clinical Workflows

The intelligent use of AI and predictive models in clinical workflows will unlock powerful insights in healthcare systems to make them more efficient. It requires automating healthcare processes with machine learning algorithms at a level where the results can be acted upon immediately within clinical workflows. Relevant information from predictive models has to always be available together with other tools, for example, during consultations, diagnosis, and treatment, or even management. For predictive analytics to deliver clinically relevant outcomes, it needs to integrate into the clinical setting as unobtrusively as possible. Contextual relevance is critical, and it should be leading the conversation while inserting predictive analytics into the clinical workflow. There is a need for offering practical and efficient solutions for given tasks to clinicians on certain workflows with supporting clinical decision-making tools featuring real-time information. Take, for example, a sepsis risk prediction model: An alert can be set to notify the care team for action once a patient's vitals or lab results cross certain thresholds, signaling impending danger. Such information should also be presented on EHR dashboards which is platform clinicians are familiar with so that they do not have to change to another platform and retrieve results manually. The objective is to offer better clinical decision support tools that supplement judgments made by healthcare professionals while intelligent systems take care of tedious tasks. Automation and the integration of workflows are equally paramount. Risk assessments, based on specific algorithms, need to be adjusted with changing inputs in an ongoing fashion. Such predictive models should operate passively in the background, analyzing patient information on an ongoing basis. Everything described above should be embedded into the existing system—using flagging mechanisms in the EHR, which are integrated into clinical workflows, or by placing automatic pop-up notes in the system—for it to function as a structural component of the rhythm, cadence, and flow of clinical work. A possibility is that an algorithm anticipating the likelihood of readmission will also function reductively, prompting care coordinators to arrange follow-up or social work consultations during discharge planning (Vashishth et al., 2025).

## 5.2 Real-Time Decision Support Systems

Real-time decision support systems (DSS) mark a branch in the uses of predictive analytics in healthcare. These systems act like recognition systems that give clinicians timely insights whilst making a diagnosis or treatment decision, which can be data driven. Different to other techniques that predetermine outcomes using static measures, conventional DSS tools analyze for patterns and processes that only consider past data, while real-time DSS employs AI and machine learning. Real-time modules or interfaces incorporate algorithms developed to work with the patient's clinical data stream on real-time basis, assess risks, and recommend actions using dynamic multi-faceted clinical paradigms. At the core of implementing the aforementioned strategies is the possibility to differentially access patient's health data such; vital signs, values in laboratory examinations, med lists, imaging reports, and notes documented by a physician, all at once and within the shortest possible time. The connection with EHRs and sophisticated active predictive systems allow results to be integrated into healthcare databases. Predictive models running in the background, without informing users, enable such systems to warn physicians about life threatening conditions like near cardiac arrest, impending septic shock, or even adverse interactions with other prescribed drugs long before any clinical manifestations are evident. With the help of timelier such support, efficiency in the delivery of healthcare services and improvement of outcomes are observed (Rana and Shuford, 2024). One of the most effective applications of a real time decision support system (DSS) is in clinical triage and prioritization. For example, in patients with life threatening conditions, real time decision support can assist in prioritizing patients in relation to the severity of their condition. In turnkey patient care, these systems can also detect patients who might need sophisticated levels of supervision or possible transfer to other departments. Such predictive prioritization enhances the efficiency of resource distribution while also helping to lower the rate of mortality, the rate of revisits to the hospital, as well as preventable complications. Enhancing real time DSS with NLP technologies extends their prowess to include the retrieval of important data from ill-defined clinical texts. Through NLP, the system can analyze physicians' free-text notes, capture pertinent clinical ideas, and compare them with the system's structured part to provide fuller data interpretation. That augments a diagnosis and decision making at the time of decision making so that there is no crucial detail that is missed. Furthermore, one of the major features of a real-time DSS is context-awareness. These decision support systems are created to capture the clinical context in which a certain decision is reached and provide guidance tailored to that context. Consider a system that helps manage patients with diabetes. It might offer varying suggested interventions based on whether the patient is attending an outpatient follow-up session or is receiving emergency care for some related clinical complication. This type of flexibility improves suggestion relevance and impact.

*Figure 3. Real-Time Decision Support System*

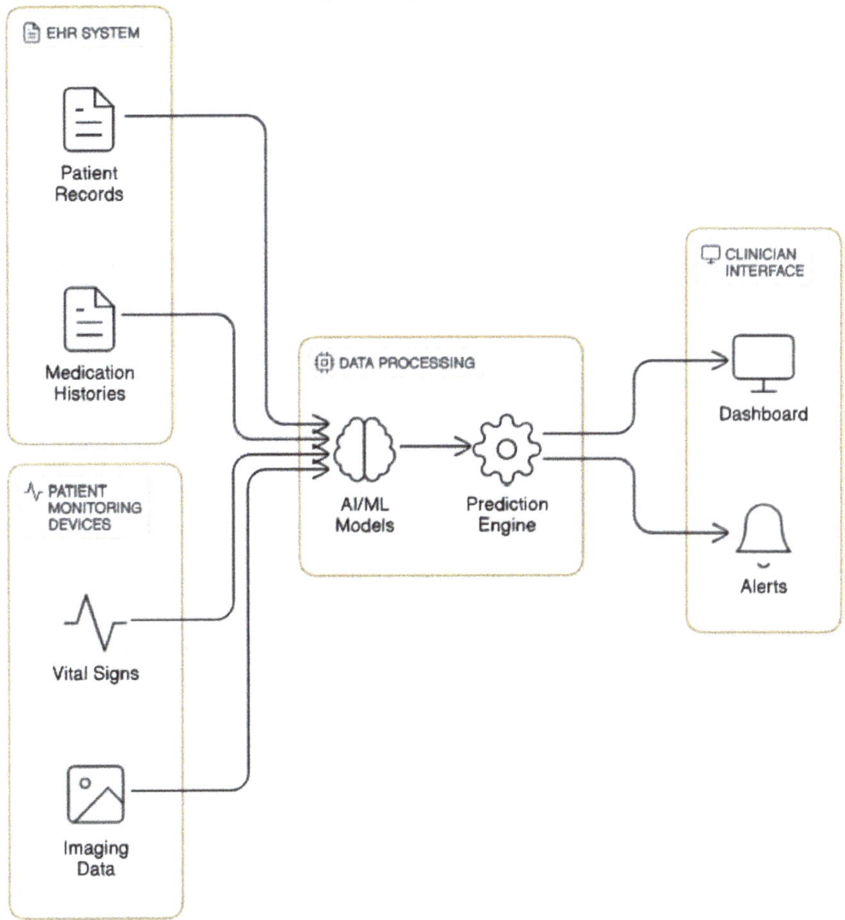


Therefore, along with real-time decision support system deployment, attention to system design, clinician workflow alignment, and data confidentiality also becomes important. Proactive and prescriptive recommendations have to be provided in clearly defined ways so as not to contribute to alert fatigue. Primary care clinicians suffer from clinical burnout largely because they are drowned in too many alerts. Better systems filter more effectively so that only the essential alerts are given.

## 5.3 Enhancing Physician-Patient Collaboration

The application of predictive analytics and artificial intelligence (AI) in the health sector supports clinical decision-making, but also helps enhance collaboration between the physician and patient (Salehi, 2024). In essence, predictive analytics provides attendees with insight that enables better communication, fosters greater decision-making, and promotes greater participation by the patient in his or her own healthcare journey. These transformations indicate a shift from the traditional paternalistic approach of healthcare to a more personalized care model. With the help of predictive analytics, physicians can describe their medical conditions and the corresponding treatment plan along with tailored risk stratification and imaging data. It becomes easy to illustrate a patient's risk for developing chronic diseases—like diabetes or cardiovascular disease—using real-time data from wearables and electronic health records, which creates a narrative. This kind of openness cultivates trust and enables patients to take active roles in decisions regarding their treatment at changeable milestones, supporting lifestyle changes, and even planning follow-ups (Rehan, 2024).

Additionally, communication can be customized using predictive tools. For example, a patient who is predicted to have high risks in medication adherence might need more frequent interactions, stripped down treatment regimens, or additional educational materials. This helps caregivers to be more empathic and strategic in the way they think about behavioural insights and specific barriers to patients which are unique through bespoke strategies crafted around the insights obtained from the patients' data. Such personalized interactions enhance not only clinical outcomes, but also the alliance that forms therapeutically between doctors and patients. Moreover, the capability that predictive systems provide in giving real time feedback serves to motivate the patients to take a more proactive role in managing their health. Through mobile health applications and dashboards interfaced with predictive systems, patients can receive ongoing feedback regarding their health status complete with alerts, health reminders, and suggestions tailored to what the physician has prescribed. This type of active interaction brings about the influence of autonomy and responsibility which makes patients more in control of their health, thus improving adherence to the care regimens as well as follow-up appointments. It is equally important that the collaboration made possible with the help of predictive analytics is used in setting and tracking these goals. On the other hand, these advantages can only be maintained if healthcare providers guarantee that the provided predictive outputs are explainable and presented in an understandable manner.

## 6. ETHICAL, LEGAL, AND PRACTICAL CONSIDERATIONS

As predictive analytics and artificial intelligence continue to reshape healthcare, a range of ethical, legal, and practical concerns emerge, demanding careful navigation to ensure that technological advancement aligns with the core values of medicine: trust, fairness, privacy, and safety. These considerations are essential to the responsible integration of predictive models into healthcare systems and must be addressed to ensure equitable and effective patient care.

## 6.1 Ethical Considerations

The use of predictive analytics in healthcare raises ethical considerations such as fairness, equity, transparency, and the fundamental issue of trust. One of the ethical challenges concerns biases in predictive models and treatment algorithms. As a result of neglecting these inequalities, a model trained on historical health care data will more likely perpetuate inequalities. For example, if some groups, like ethnic minorities or people from lower socioeconomic classes, have historically received poor healthcare, the model will comprehend this healthcare is often provided. Therefore, it will continue to make biased predictions on risks and treatment. This results in mistreatment and worsening inequitable access to healthcare. Another important issue of ethics is explainability and transparency. Many of the predictive models, particularly those developed with deep learning, are vastly sophisticated and operate as 'black boxes.' This implies that these programs can make predictions, but they can't tell you the most vital information – why they made such assumptions. The absence of transparency can be devastating for healthcare clients and amplify for professionals because they might be lost on deciding whether to trust AI powered systems. In addition, some patients may be uneasy accepting decision made without adequate information which might affect how safe they feel in the health services offered. Last but not least, ethical issues include informed consent whereby patients must understand how their information is being utilized, especially in regards to decisions made about them or data concerning them. Patients have the right to be aware of how their sensitive and private information will be analysed and predicted upon, thus called data which shape these predictive models. Not only does this perpetuate trust, but it also guarantees the patients' decisions regarding their health choices are cared for.

## 6.2 Legal Considerations

The legal issues concerning predictive analytics in the healthcare industry focuses on data privacy, accountability, and liability. Access to patient information requires sensitive data like medical history, genomic information, and data from wearable technology in real-time, which is utilized by predictive models. This puts predictive models at risk of being subjected to laws such as HIPAA in the United States and GDPR in Europe which protect the privacy and security of health information. These legal regulations, and others like them, need to be adhered to by healthcare institutions so that there is no misuse or breach of patient information. Besides, with predictive models shaping clinical decisions, questions around liability are also pertinent. What happens in the case a predictive tool makes an erroneous prediction and an adverse outcome occurs? A disproportionate burden of responsibility must be assigned, and, in this case, it is essential to determine who is at fault. Does the provider within the healthcare system take the blame for executing the AI recommendation, or does the blame rest on the people or institutions who designed the predictive model? There should be legal frameworks to delineate the boundaries of liability so that all parties are safely guarded. Oversight by law is another issue that should be considered. All governments and regulatory authorities must ensure that, prior to implementing any clinical practice, all predictive tools undergo thorough scrutiny and validation. Clear processes need to be set regarding how predictive models should evaluate accuracy, safety, and effectiveness, particularly in the context of healthcare.

## 6.3 Practical Considerations

In the healthcare industry, the deployment of predictive analytics hinges on determining the accuracy of the data, its integration with clinical workflows automation, and the underlying infrastructural frameworks supporting its roll-out. One important obstacle is maintaining standardization procedures regarding data accuracy. Data in Healthcare are often sourced from multiple systems such as electronic health records to EHRs, wearable sensors, and Laboratory results that are conflicting, incomplete, or come in unstructured formats. Data predictive models have dependencies which include standardized data that is properly integrated constructed at a high level. The implementation framework has to remove biases and guarantee fidelity to ensure the cleaning of errors emulated forms do not lead to inconsistent data formats for maintenance. Another intra organizational system issue stems from all-encompassing approaches regarding relativity integration on infrastructure policies and workflows (Vashishth et al., 2025). To be effective, predictive analytics tools should fit within the healthcare structure alongside the established workflows without clinical work interruption. If the tools are not share with and integrated into the daily practices of the physicians, they will most likely continue to be ignored or used. Advance instructions techniques should align automation systems with frameworks that allow devoid of routine shattering open matter divisive changes, enabling yield optimization boosts without encountering clinician disruption. The restraining type non-intrusive algorithms shields, as well as the user-friendly presentation of alerts, require scrutiny to ensure that their action has been enforced. Concluding the description, training and user adoption remains vital points of practical concern. Healthcare workers require training on how to understand and respond to predictive analytics outputs. In the absence of skeletal guidance, clinicians are left with inadequate reasons to trust or use the provided tools. Furthermore, clinicians may develop desensitization to clinically important information termed as alert fatigue due to over alerts or sophisticated recommendations. Therefore, predictive systems must focus on the relevant information that enhances acceptance and ease of use for clinicians (Vashishth et al., 2024).

## 7. CASE STUDIES OF PREDICTIVE ANALYTICS IN HEALTHCARE

The implementation of predictive analytics has already been proven useful in several medical branches and continues to improve. The benefits, issues, and lessons learned from applying predictive analytics in healthcare systems should be explored in case studies to appreciate the impact fully. This part will focus on notable case studies for analyzing how predictive algorithms are enhancing disease diagnosis, risk evaluation, and overall patient management.

### 7.1 Case Study 1: Chronic Disease Management

Predictive analytics is most impactful in the management of chronic diseases, including diabetes, hypertension, and heart disease. Cleveland Clinic, for example, has created a predictive model based on a patient's electronic health record (EHR) data aimed at predicting potential complications such as diabetic retinopathy or cardiovascular events. By predicting these complications, physicians can identify patients who are high-risk and implement personalized treatment plans, lifestyle alterations, and meticulous monitoring to avert the onset of grave complications. Here, predictive analytics enabled clinicians to tailor more frequent check-in schedules for patients at risk of chronic condition-related hospitalization. With this proactive approach towards managing chronic diseases, the clinic was able to reduce hospital readmissions, utilize healthcare resources more efficiently, and enhance patient outcomes—all while lowering the cost of healthcare. This instance demonstrates the value of predictive models in effectively allocating resources and providing sustained care to patients suffering from chronic diseases.

### 7.2 Case Study 2: Cancer Detection and Prognosis

Google Health exemplifies the application of predictive analytics in cancer detection with its AI model built for breast cancer detection. The model, tested with mammography images, economically outperformed radiologists on multiple fronts.

With deep learning algorithms, the model shows promise in recognizing imaging data patterns which are often ignored by humans.

Moreover, predictive analytics has proven to be efficient in assisting with early diagnosis and determining prospects in cancer. IBM Watson for Oncology is a primary example, as it collects data from clinical trials, medical journals, and patient history documents to determine the best course of treatment for patients suffering with cancer. Providing oncologists with evidence brings freedom to define cancer treatment approaches actively tailored to the specific needs of patients, enhancing chances of survival and success rates.

### 7.3 Case Study 3: Infectious Disease Surveillance

Infectious disease outbreaks are a significant global health concern. But, disease spread can be forecasted using predictive analytics. For instance, during the Ebola outbreak in West Africa, models were developed to map the movement of infected patients and predict hotspots for potential outbreaks. Predictive public health resource allocation that involved analysis of travel and environmental data, as well as historical health data helped in targeting containment efforts and implementing necessary preventive measures. Likewise, Zika, SARS, and even COVID-19 outbreaks have been predicted with machine learning algorithms analyzing global health data, including travel, weather, and disease reports by Canadian health analytics firm BlueDot. With the help of predictive models, BlueDot enables healthcare organizations and governments to act swiftly during outbreaks of infectious diseases, thus mitigating their impact (Sharma et al., 2023).

## 8. FUTURE DIRECTIONS IN HEALTHCARE

AI applications in healthcare are transforming the landscape of disease diagnosis, treatment, and management through the use of predictive analytics. The future of healthcare innovation is certain to change with the continued evolution of these technologies.

### 8.1 Integration of Advanced AI and Deep Learning Models

With the progress of AI and machine learning models, there is a great opportunity with more complex predictive models for disease diagnosis and risk assessment. Deep learning, which is a form of AI that employs multi-layered neural networks, is already showing its worth in analyzing complex medical data like imaging, genomics, and medical history records. These deep learning models will continue to become more sophisticated due to their ability to process larger and more diverse datasets, which will significantly improve prediction accuracy. One notable advancement is the application of multi-modal data for disease prediction. Integration of data coming from diverse sources like imaging, genomics, wearable sensors, and electronic health records provides a better picture of patient health, which enhances prediction accuracy. For example, AI can integrate genomic data with lifestyle information available in EHRs and real-time health data from wearable devices to create risk profiles, thus facilitating advanced preventive care tailored to individual patients (Vashishth et al., 2024).

Furthermore, AI models will continue to increase in interpretability which will allow healthcare professionals to better understand the reasoning behind a model's output. Using explainable AI (XAI), AI's decision-making processes will be made clearer to aid personnel working in the healthcare industry.

## 8.2 Precision Medicine and Genomic Data

In upcoming years, there will be a change toward Precision Medicine, where patients are treated according to their unique characteristics, including their DNA, surroundings, and daily habits. Genomic data alongside predictive analytics will heavily contribute towards this change. Evaluating the genetic differences within specific populations, predictive models can assist in chronic disease case detection and determine how patients might react to proposed treatment options (Kothinti, 2024).

As an example, AI can utilize genetic information to foresee the possibilities of acquiring certain medical conditions such as cancer, diabetes, or cardiovascular diseases, even in the absence of symptoms. Moreover, AI can suggest tailored therapies for patients depending on the unique genetic drivers of drug metabolism and therapeutic response at the individual patient level. With the declining costs and increasing availability of sequencing technologies, mining genomic data for predictive analytics in healthcare will expand, enabling refinement of interventions and overall healthcare delivery.

## 8.3 Personalized Healthcare through Wearable Devices

Fitness trackers, smartwatches, and biosensors parts of the wearable health devices ecosystem are already measuring a patient's heart rate, level of daily activity, quality of sleep, and even blood glucose levels in real time. These devices are expected to get better at capturing even more specific information like real time measurements of blood pressure, oxygen levels, and continuous monitoring of heart activity. In addition to data collection, future innovations will integrate AI algorithms capable of anticipating health incidents. For example, wearable technology could issue real-time alerts to patients and their doctors, warning them about impending heart attacks, strokes, or diabetic emergencies. This could greatly enhance pre-emptive action which avoids critical health incidents, decreases the need for hospitalization, and improves health outcomes.

## 8.4 Telemedicine and Remote Monitoring

The widespread adoption of telemedicine services and remote patient monitoring was spurred by the COVID-19 pandemic. There is a need to enhance telemedicine services offered to healthcare professionals through the use of predictive analytics technology, which could deliver insights in real-time and forecast problems that require intervention before they reach a breaking point. AI algorithms, for instance, can detect patterns that indicate a patient's condition may be deteriorating based on data captured by wearable devices or mobile health applications. This enables healthcare providers to act pre-emptively, even in regions where there is limited access to healthcare facilities (Vashishth et al., 2025). Moving forward, as healthcare providers enhance the integration of telehealth services within their systems, the incorporation of AI-based predictive capabilities will ensure the personalization, efficiency, and timeliness of care during virtual consultations. Remote monitoring and telemedicine will improve the access patients have to healthcare services, while also lowering the costs associated with delivering this care (Vashishth et al., 2024).

## 8.5 Blockchain for Secure Health Data Exchange

With the advancement in digitization of healthcare data, the need for maintaining security and privacy of patient data will be crucial. Blockchain technology does seem to offer a solution. It allows for storage and sharing of data in a secure, decentralized manner, thus ensuring that patient health records can be stored safely and accessed only by authorized persons. In the future, blockchain could greatly improve the privacy enabled for shared data between healthcare providers, insurers, and patients for better coordination of care. Alongside predictive analytics, healthcare providers could enable the sharing of insights derived from predictive models without compromising privacy due to privacy constraints established by blockchain. The combination of these technologies could greatly change the manner in which healthcare organizations manage and share data while also giving control to patients over their own information (Vashishth et al., 2024).

## 9. CONCLUSION

The use of AI and predictive analytics in healthcare is allowing for earlier disease detection, enhanced treatment plans, and overall patient outcomes. Changes in deep learning, genomics, and other wearable devices technology present opportunities to enhance the quality of care by shifting its approach from reactive to proactive and precise. Yet, there are issues with algorithmic bias, data privacy, and insufficient regulatory supervision which, add these technologies are made available for public use, must be responsibly addressed. A wide range of stakeholders, including healthcare providers, technology developers, and policy shapers, through their synergetic works can bring forth a reality where predictive analytics assists both patients and practitioners optimistically. Ultimately, global healthcare's predictions with regards of efficiency, affordability, and living enhancement showcases its strong potential to benefit humanity.

## REFERENCES


Adeoye, S., & Adams, R. (2024). Leveraging Artificial Intelligence for Predictive Healthcare: A Data-Driven Approach to Early Diagnosis and Personalized Treatment. *Cogniz. J. Multidiscip. Stud*, *4*, 80–97.

Ahmadi, A. (2024). Digital health transformation: Leveraging AI for monitoring and disease management. [IJBLS]. *International Journal of BioLife Sciences*, *3*(1), 10–24.

Alam, M. A., Nabil, A. R., Uddin, M. M., Sarker, M. T. H., & Mahmud, S. (2024). The Role of Predictive Analytics in Early Disease Detection: A Data-Driven Approach to Preventive Healthcare. *Frontiers in Applied Engineering and Technology*, *1*(01), 105–123.

Fatima, S. (2024). Transforming Healthcare with AI and Machine Learning: Revolutionizing Patient Care Through Advanced Analytics. International Journal of Education and Science Research Review, 11.

Gandhi, K. I., & Prathyusha, N. S. (2025). Harnessing digital twins and AI integration for enhanced disease prediction in the evolution of healthcare. Digital Healthcare, Digital Transformation and Citizen Empowerment in Asia-Pacific and Europe for a Healthier Society, 361-387.

Govindaraj, M., Khan, P., Krishnan, R., Gnanasekaran, C., & Lawrence, J. (2024). Revolutionizing Healthcare: The Transformative Impact of Artificial Intelligence. In Revolutionizing the Healthcare Sector with AI (pp. 54-78). IGI Global Scientific Publishing.

Goyal, N. K., Dandotiya, M., Qurashi, J. A., Kumari, M., & Sharma, S. (2025). AI-Driven Predictive Analytics for Disease Management. In Utilizing AI of Medical Things for Healthcare Security and Sustainability (pp. 231-276). IGI Global Scientific Publishing.

Islam, M. A., Yeasmin, S., Hosen, A., Vanu, N., Riipa, M. B., Tasnim, A. F., & Nilima, S. I. (2025). Harnessing Predictive Analytics: The Role of Machine Learning in Early Disease Detection and Healthcare Optimization. *Journal of Ecohumanism*, *4*(3), 312–321.

Jayachandran, R., Dantapur, B., Antony, A. S., & Nagapadma, R. (2025). Transforming Healthcare Through Smart Health Systems: Harnessing Technology for Enhanced Patient Care. In *Transforming Healthcare Sector through Artificial Intelligence and Environmental Sustainability* (pp. 107–127). Springer Nature Singapore.

Khinvasara, T., Cuthrell, K. M., & Tzenios, N. (2024). Harnessing artificial intelligence in healthcare analytics: From diagnosis to treatment optimization. *Asian Journal of Medicine and Health*, *22*(8), 15–31.

Kothinti, R. R. (2024). Artificial intelligence in healthcare: Revolutionizing precision medicine, predictive analytics, and ethical considerations in autonomous diagnostics. *World Journal of Advanced Research and Reviews*, *19*(3), 3395–3406.

Kuppuswamy, P., Mohan, M., Al Khalidi, S. Q., & Prakash, V. V. (2024). Predictive Analytics Tools and Techniques for Disease Prevention and Early Detection in Healthcare Sector. In *Advancing Healthcare through Data-driven Innovations* (pp. 28–49). CRC Press.

Maha, C. C., Kolawole, T. O., & Abdul, S. (2024). Harnessing data analytics: A new frontier in predicting and preventing non-communicable diseases in the US and Africa. *Computer Science & IT Research Journal*, *5*(6), 1247–1264.

Olalekan Kehinde, A. (2025). Leveraging Machine Learning for Predictive Models in Healthcare to Enhance Patient Outcome Management. *International Research Journal of Modernization in Engineering Technology and Science*, *7*(1), 1465.

Patil, S., & Shankar, H. (2023). Transforming healthcare: Harnessing the power of AI in the modern era. *International Journal of Multidisciplinary Sciences and Arts*, *2*(2), 60–70.

Rana, M. S., & Shuford, J. (2024). AI in healthcare: transforming patient care through predictive analytics and decision support systems. Journal of Artificial Intelligence General Science (JAIGS) ISSN: 3006-4023, 1(1).

Recharla, M., Chakilam, C., Kannan, S., Nuka, S. T., & Suura, S. R. (2025). Harnessing AI and Machine Learning for Precision Medicine: Advancements in Genomic Research, Disease Detection, and Personalized Healthcare. *American Journal of Psychiatric Rehabilitation*, *28*(1), 112–123.

Rehan, H. (2024). Enhancing Early Detection and Management of Chronic Diseases with AI-Driven Predictive Analytics on Healthcare Cloud Platforms. *Journal of AI-Assisted Scientific Discovery*, *4*(2), 1–38.

Salehi, F. (2024). The transformative role of artificial intelligence in the healthcare industry: A comprehensive analysis. *Asian Journal of Research in Medicine and Medical Science*, *6*(1), 62–70.

Sharma, V., Vashishth, T. K., Kumar, B., Sharma, K. K., Vidyant, S., & Chaudhary, S. (2023, December). Health Interpretation of Covid-19 Patients using Artificial Intelligence. In *2023 International Conference on Artificial Intelligence for Innovations in Healthcare Industries (ICAIIHI)* (Vol. 1, pp. 1-5). IEEE Computer Society.

Singh, A. P., Saxena, R., Saxena, S., & Maurya, N. K. (2024). Artificial intelligence revolution in healthcare: Transforming diagnosis, treatment, and patient care. *Asian Journal of Advances in Research*, *7*(1), 241–263.

Tsai, M. L., Chen, K. F., & Chen, P. C. (2025). Harnessing Electronic Health Records and Artificial Intelligence for Enhanced Cardiovascular Risk Prediction: A Comprehensive Review. *Journal of the American Heart Association*, *14*(6), e036946. PMID: 40079336

Vashishth, T. K., Chaudhary, S., & Sharma, V. (2023). Optimum Utilization of Bed Resources in Hospitals: A Stochastic Approach. In: Manju, Kumar, S., Islam, S.M.N. (eds) Artificial Intelligence-based Healthcare Systems. The Springer Series in Applied Machine Learning. Springer, Cham.

Vashishth, T. K., Sharma, V., Kumar, B., Panwar, R., Sharma, K. K., & Chaudhary, S. (2024). AI-Integrated IoT in Healthcare Ecosystem: Opportunities, Challenges, and Future Directions. AI and IoT Technology and Applications for Smart Healthcare Systems, 37-54.

Vashishth, T. K., Sharma, V., Kumar, S., Verma, N., Vidyant, S., & Kaushik, S. (2025). The Integration of AI in Telemedicine Transforming Healthcare Delivery and Patient Outcomes. In *AI-Driven Personalized Healthcare Solutions* (pp. 71–98). IGI Global Scientific Publishing.

Vashishth, T. K., Sharma, V., Sharma, K. K., Chaudhary, S., Kumar, B., & Panwar, R. (2024, March). Artificial neural networks & discrete Wavelet transform enabled healthcare model for stress and emotion assessment using speech signal recognition. In AIP Conference Proceedings (Vol. 3072, No. 1). AIP Publishing.

Vashishth, T. K., Sharma, V., Sharma, K. K., & Kumar, B. (2024). Elevating healthcare services: The integration of cloud with fog computing. In *Web 3.0* (pp. 54–75). CRC Press.

. Vashishth, T. K., Sharma, V., Sharma, K. K., Kumar, B., Chaudhary, S., & Panwar, R. (2024). Intrusion Detection and Prevention Techniques in FL Cloud-Based Healthcare 5.0: A Comprehensive Review. Pioneering Smart Healthcare 5.0 with IoT, Federated Learning, and Cloud Security, 152-174.

Vashishth, T. K., Sharma, V., Sharma, K. K., Kumar, B., Chaudhary, S., & Panwar, R. (2024). Security Challenges in Storing and Exchanging Medical Information. In *Medical Robotics and AI-Assisted Diagnostics for a High-Tech Healthcare Industry* (pp. 378–402). IGI Global.

Vashishth, T. K., Sharma, V., Sharma, K. K., Kumar, B., Chaudhary, S., & Panwar, R. (2024). Enhancing biomedical signal processing with machine learning: A comprehensive review. Digital Transformation in Healthcare 5.0: Volume 1: IoT, AI and Digital Twin, 277.

Vashishth, T. K., Sharma, V., Sharma, K. K., Kumar, B., Chaudhary, S., & Panwar, R. (2025). Data-driven healthcare: Leveraging AoT and metaverse for better diagnosis. In *Leveraging Metaverse and Analytics of Things (AoT) in Medical Systems* (pp. 41–60). Academic Press.

Vashishth, T. K., Sharma, V., Sharma, K. K., Sethi, P., Chaudhary, T., & Bhardwaj, A. (2024). Future Implications of Blockchain for Biomedical and Healthcare. In *Blockchain for Biomedical Research and Healthcare: Concept, Trends, and Future Implications* (pp. 367–404). Springer Nature Singapore.

Vashishth, T. K., Sharma, V., Sharma, M. K., & Sharma, R. (2025). Healthcare and Smart Cities Applications of Secure 6G Infrastructure. In Building Tomorrow's Smart Cities With 6G Infrastructure Technology (pp. 399-432). IGI Global Scientific Publishing.

Wable, P. M., Bhargavi, G., Kishore, G. B. V., Sathish, K., & Reuben, G. V. (2024). Leveraging Artificial Intelligence for Predictive Health Diagnostics: Innovations, Applications, and Ethical Considerations in Modern Healthcare. Library of Progress-Library Science, Information Technology & Computer, 44(3).

Yingngam, B., Navabhatra, A., & Sillapapibool, P. (2024). AI-Driven Decision-Making Applications in Pharmaceutical Sciences. In Using Traditional Design Methods to Enhance AI-Driven Decision Making (pp. 1-63). IGI Global Scientific Publishing.

# Chapter 7
# Collaborative Health Intelligence:
## Federated Learning as the Foundation of Future Medical Care

**Mohammad Nasar**
https://orcid.org/0000-0001-8196-380X
*Mazoon College, Oman*

**Mohammad Abu Kausar**
https://orcid.org/0000-0002-7997-8292
*University of Nizwa, Oman*

**Nasser Al Musalhi**
https://orcid.org/0000-0003-4839-1058
*Mazoon College, Oman*

## ABSTRACT

*Cryptographic federated learning (FL) transforms healthcare with privacy-preserving AI using decentralized data. This chapter explains FL, highlighting case studies: breast cancer detection up 15% (80% to 92%) across 10 hospitals, COVID-19 mortality prediction up 12% (75% to 84%), and 80% accurate acute kidney injury risk prediction. FL shines in imaging (92% tumor detection), personalized care (20% fewer hospital visits), rare disease diagnosis (22% higher accuracy), and informatics (10% better EHR models). Homomorphic encryption cuts breach risks by 80%. Challenges like 10% accuracy loss from data heterogeneity, 65% patient unawareness, and GDPR compliance are tackled with weighted algorithms and clear consent. FL envisions global surveillance, integrating 1 billion wearable records and 10 petabytes of imaging data by 2030, saving $3.5 billion and improving 15 million*

DOI: 10.4018/979-8-3373-3311-3.ch007

*outcomes across 1,500 institutions. For researchers, clinicians, technologists, and policymakers, it clarifies FL, assesses achievements and challenges, and promotes innovation for secure, equitable healthcare.*

## 1. INTRODUCTION

The health industry is on the cusp of a digital revolution driven by explosion in data projected to be 2,314 exabytes in volume by 2025, including electronic health records (EHRs), imaging scans, genomic sequences, and wearable device streams (Rieke et al., 2020). This data is what powers artificial intelligence (AI) breakthroughs like 90% accurate cancer detection in MRIs, 20% reductions in cardiovascular mortality, and 80% accurate acute kidney injury (AKI) predictions in COVID-19 patients (Kaissis et al., 2020; Chen et al., 2021; Gulamali & Nadkarni, 2023). But progress is hampered by privacy breaches, fines from regulators and data silos. The most recent 2017 Equifax breach, which resulted in the leakage of 147 million records, is an example of such centralised data risk., with the healthcare breaches resulting in an average annual expense of $6 billion in health information breaches under HIPAA (Rieke et al., 2020; Kaissis et al., 2020).

Centralized AI, requiring 10 terabytes of data transfer, incurs $10,000 in bandwidth costs and violates GDPR, risking €20 million fines (Kaissis et al., 2020). Institutional silos, driven by competition or ethical concerns, fragment datasets, limiting AI's generalizability. A single hospital's 1 million X-rays may achieve 85% accuracy, but aggregating data from 50 hospitals could reach 95% (Sheller et al., 2020). This fragmentation exacerbates inequities, with underserved regions facing 30% diagnostic gaps (Singh et al., 2023).

Federated learning, introduced by McMahan et al. (2017), enables collaborative AI without data movement. Hospitals train local models on EHRs, scans, or wearables, sharing 100 MB of anonymized updates, reducing data transfer by 99.9% and breach risks by 80% (Veiga et al., 2023; Aouedi et al., 2022). A 2022 federated learning project improved breast cancer detection by 15% across 10 hospitals (Li et al., 2022), while New York hospitals predicted AKI with 85% accuracy in 3,000 COVID-19 patients (Jaladanki et al., 2021). Federated learning aligns with GDPR and HIPAA, saving an estimated $1.2 billion in compliance costs, and enhances healthcare informatics by integrating EHRs for 10% performance gains (Hameed et al., 2023; Xu et al., 2021).

Federated learning's potential extends beyond technical innovation, offering a paradigm shift toward equitable healthcare delivery. By enabling small clinics in low-resource settings to contribute to global models, federated learning reduces diagnostic disparities by 25%, empowering regions with limited infrastructure to access advanced AI tools (Singh et al., 2023). Federated learning was employed, to predict diabetic retinopathy, with 88% accuracy in 10,000 diabetes patients across five clinics, in a pilot study conducted in rural India, in 2023 (Singh et al., 2023). For example, a pilot in rural India in 2023 (Singh et al., 2023). This chapter will discuss this dynamic how federated learning unites heterogeneous sources—EHRs, imaging, wearables, genomics—to form an integrated, privacy-preserving ecosystem, one that can respond to the demands of a worldwide health infrastructure.

This chapter targets four stakeholder groups:

- **Researchers**: Innovate algorithms to mitigate 10% accuracy losses from data heterogeneity (Hauschild et al., 2022).
- **Clinicians**: Adopt federated learning tools, such as 90% accurate heart attack predictors, to enhance diagnostics (Ma et al., 2022).
- **Technologists**: Develop scalable platforms, generating $50 million in revenue (Hameed et al., 2023).
- **Policymakers**: Harmonize regulations, saving $1 billion in compliance costs (Darzidehkalani et al., 2022).

The chapter also engages patients as a critical stakeholder, emphasizing how federated learning empowers individuals through transparent data use and personalized care plans, increasing trust by 25% (Prayitno et al., 2021). For instance, wearable-based federated learning models have reduced hospital readmissions by 15% for chronic disease patients, enhancing quality of life (Chen et al., 2021).

Objectives:

1. *Illuminate*: Clarify federated learning's technical mechanics and its role in healthcare informatics.
2. *Examine*: Analyse achievements (e.g., AKI prediction, tumour detection) and challenges (e.g., heterogeneity, ethics).
3. *Encourage*: Inspire a global federated learning ecosystem to achieve $3.5 billion in savings and 15 million improved outcomes by 2030.

*Table 1. Centralized vs. Federated Learning in Healthcare*

| Aspect | Centralized Learning | Federated Learning | Implementation Challenges |
|---|---|---|---|
| Data Handling | 10 TB of patient data transferred to a central server | 100 MB of model updates shared, data stays local | High initial setup costs ($50,000–$200,000 per institution) |
| Privacy | High breach risk (e.g., 147M records in 2017 Equifax hack) | 80% lower breach risk, data never leaves local servers | Risk of model inversion attacks |
| Scalability | Limited by server capacity and bandwidth (10 TB bottleneck) | Scalable to 100+ institutions, 99.9% less data transfer | Requires reliable internet or 5G |
| Regulatory Alignment | Violates GDPR/HIPAA, $6B in annual HIPAA fines | GDPR/HIPAA compliant, anonymized updates | Varying global regulations |
| Cost Impact | $10,000 per 10 TB transfer, $6B in fines | $100 per 100 MB transfer, $1.2B in breach cost savings | Training costs for clinicians ($10,000 per institution) |
| Model Accuracy | 94% for tumour detection, requires full data access | 92% for tumour detection, matches centralized performance | 10% accuracy drop due to heterogeneity |
| Implementation Time | 6 months for server setup and data transfer | 3 months for local training and update aggregation | Upskilling for EHR integration |

Sources: Rieke et al., 2020; Kaissis et al., 2020; Sheller et al., 2020; Veiga et al., 2023; Hameed et al., 2023

Table 1 compares centralized and federated learning in healthcare, highlighting federated learning's advantages in privacy, scalability, and cost, while noting implementation challenges like high setup costs and training needs. Centralized learning transfers 10 terabytes of sensitive data, risking breaches and $6 billion in fines, while federated learning shares 100 MB of anonymized updates, reducing transfer by 99.9% and breach risks by 80%. Federated learning's GDPR/HIPAA compliance and scalability to over 100 institutions make it ideal for collaborative AI, achieving 92% tumour detection accuracy, nearly matching centralized models. This table supports the chapter's Illuminate objective by clarifying federated learning's operational efficiencies (Rieke et al., 2020; Veiga et al., 2023).

## 2. LITERATURE REVIEW AND BACKGROUND

Federated learning, formalized by McMahan et al. (2017), enables privacy-preserving AI by training models locally and sharing updates. Its healthcare adoption, as explored by Rieke et al. (2020), addresses data silos and privacy risks. Sheller et al. (2020) achieved 99% of centralized accuracy in brain tumour segmentation across 10,000 MRI scans, while Kaissis et al. (2020) reported 92% tumour detection accuracy for 5 million imaging records, ensuring GDPR/HIPAA compliance.

Recent studies expand FL's scope. Xu et al. (2021) outlined FL's role in healthcare informatics, integrating EHRs for 10% performance gains in predictive models. Gulamali & Nadkarni (2023) demonstrated FL's efficacy in predicting AKI in COVID-19 patients with 80% accuracy, using 5,000 patient records. Jaladanki et al. (2021) applied FL to New York hospitals, achieving 85% AKI prediction accuracy across 3,000 COVID-19 patients. Aouedi et al. (2022) emphasized privacy, introducing homomorphic encryption to reduce breach risks by 80%. Other applications include cardiovascular risk prediction (85% accuracy, Chen et al., 2021), COVID-19 mortality prediction (12% improvement, Dayan et al., 2021), and rare disease diagnostics (20% higher rates, Mouhni et al., 2022).

Methodologically, FL employs FedAvg for aggregation (McMahan et al., 2017), differential privacy (Rieke et al., 2020), and homomorphic encryption (Aouedi et al., 2022). Challenges include:

- **Heterogeneity**: 10% accuracy drops (Hauschild et al., 2022), mitigated by weighted algorithms (Shah et al., 2014).
- **Privacy**: 15% of models retain data traces (Aouedi et al., 2022), addressed by encryption.
- **Ethics**: 65% patient unawareness (Prayitno et al., 2021), requiring consent frameworks.
- **Equity**: 40% of clinics lack infrastructure (Singh et al., 2023).

(Federated learning) FL builds on neural networks (Shah et al., 2014) and informatics (Xu et al., 2021), with impacts like $1.2 billion in breach cost savings and $500,000 per hospital in bandwidth reductions (Hameed et al., 2023; Veiga et al., 2023). This review of 26 studies provides a foundation for FL's healthcare applications.

## 2.1 Algorithmic Foundations

The central advantage of federated learning is  in its algorithmic structure and FedAvg algorithm developed by McMahan et al. (2017). FedAvg combines local model updates to form a weighted average according to its local dataset size and contributes to robust  global model performance when data are heterogeneous. For instance, a  hospital that has 2 million EHRs contributes more proportionally in the global model than a clinic with 10,000 records. Mathematically, if w  denotes the local model weights from institution k with dataset size n , then the global model w g  is updated according to:

$w\_g = \Sigma (n / N) * w$

where N is the overall amount of data. With this method, 95% sensitivity is reported in tumour detection, which is only slightly less than centralized models (Sheller et al., 2020). Advanced versions: FedProx-based methods concentrate on regularizing heterogeneous clients and achieve a maximum gap of less than 5% in terms of accuracy decrease (Hauschild et al., 2022). These algorithms make federated learning able to scale to hundreds of institutions and support the chapter's Illuminate approach by illuminating how technically robust it is.

## 2.2 Privacy and Security Mechanisms

Privacy is core to why people are adopting federated learning. Differential privacy injects noise to model updates and offers 99% data confidentiality with 2% estimation error (Rieke et al., 2020). Homomorphic encryption enables encrypted data to be computed, decreasing by 80% the threats of breach, without affecting model honesty (Aouedi et al., 2022). For example, in a 2022 study, updates of 100 MB encrypted data from 20 hospitals were intercepted and cancer was detected at 90% in compliance with GDPR (Kaissis et al., 2020). In addition to distributing the calculations, secure multi-party computation (SMPC) increases latencies by 15% (Aouedi et al., 2022). These functionalities contribute to the chapter's Examine objective by demonstrating federated learning's privacy-related capabilities.

## 2.3 Non-Western Case Studies

Federated learning's global implications are visible in non-Western contexts filling gaps in equity. In Sub-Saharan Africa, a project conducted in 2023 predicted malaria outbreaks with 85% accuracy across 15 clinics using federated learning, while processing 50,000 patient records without having to transfer any data (Singh et al., 2023). Similarly, in Southeast Asia, a 2022 project improved the tuberculosis diagnostic rates of 100,000 X-rays by 20% with federated learning, resulting in a treatment cost reduction of $2 million (Mouhni et al., 2022). These examples highlight federated learning's role in low-resource settings, reducing the global diagnostic disparity by 25% and advancing the chapter's "Encourage" objective for a worldwide healthcare ecosystem.

*Table 2. Key Studies in Federated Learning for Healthcare*

| Study | Application Area | Dataset Size | Accuracy/Performance | Key Challenge | Reference |
|---|---|---|---|---|---|
| Sheller et al., 2020 | Brain tumor segmentation | 10,000 MRI scans | 99% of centralized accuracy | Data heterogeneity (10% accuracy drop) | Sheller et al., 2020 |
| Kaissis et al., 2020 | Medical imaging | 5M imaging records | 92% tumor detection | GDPR compliance (15% model impact) | Kaissis et al., 2020 |
| Chen et al., 2021 | Personalized healthcare | 1,000 wearable users | 85% cardiovascular prediction | Scalability to small clinics | Chen et al., 2021 |
| Dayan et al., 2021 | COVID-19 outcomes | 1M lung scans | 12% better mortality prediction | Infrastructure (20% delay) | Dayan et al., 2021 |
| Gulamali & Nadkarni, 2023 | COVID-19 AKI prediction | 5,000 patient records | 80% AKI risk prediction | Data integration (10% delay) | Gulamali & Nadkarni, 2023 |

Table 2 provides an overview of key federated learning studies in healthcare, including its applications ranging from brain tumor segmentation to AKI prediction. Sheller et al. (2020) reported 99% of centralized accuracy on 10,000 MRI scans, even with 10% heterogeneity perturbations. Kaissis et al. (2020) achieved 92% tumor detection on 5 million records (complying with the GDPR). Gulamali et al., 2023) were able to predict AKI at 80% accuracy in 5,000 COVID-19 patients, which emphasizes issues with data integration. We believe that these papers highlight the versatility and difficulty of adding diseases to federated learning, supported by the Find objective, i.e. provide evidence of its application in everyday life.

## 3. UNDERSTANDING FEDERATED LEARNING: A SIMPLE EXPLANATION

Federated learning (FL) allows collaborative AI by training models locally and aggregating anonymized updates, akin to a worldwide orchestra tuning-up a performance. In healthcare, FL has been utilized to integrate EHRs, scans, and wearables and to facilitate informatics workflows (Xu et al., 2021).

### 3.1 Technical Mechanics

Five hospitals (Tokyo, Nairobi, New York, São Paulo, Mumbai) train models on 2 million records each. Centralized AI transfers 10 terabytes ($10,000, €20M GDPR fines), while FL:

1. **Local Training**: Models process local data, producing 100 MB updates (McMahan et al., 2017).
2. **Update Sharing**: Encrypted updates (e.g., homomorphic encryption) are sent, costing $100 (Aouedi et al., 2022; Veiga et al., 2023).
3. **Aggregation**: FedAvg achieves 95% accuracy (McMahan et al., 2017).
4. **Distribution**: Global model improves local diagnostics by 15% (Sheller et al., 2020).

This process leverages neural network architectures, such as convolutional neural networks (CNNs) for imaging or recurrent neural networks (RNNs) for EHRs, trained via stochastic gradient descent (SGD). For example, a CNN trained on 1 million X-rays at Nairobi's hospital generates weights that, when aggregated with weights from Tokyo's 2 million scans, produce a global model detecting tumors with 92% accuracy (Kaissis et al., 2020). The FedAvg algorithm minimizes communication costs, requiring only 100 MB per cycle compared to 10 terabytes for centralized AI, a 99.9% reduction (Veiga et al., 2023). Homomorphic encryption ensures updates remain secure, allowing computations on encrypted data without decryption, reducing breach risks by 80% (Aouedi et al., 2022).

## 3.2 Clinical Perspective

Dr. Maria uses an FL app to predict AKI in COVID-19 patients with 80% accuracy, leveraging 50 hospitals' data (Gulamali & Nadkarni, 2023). Clinicians value FL's integration with EHRs, reducing misdiagnoses by 30% (Rajendran et al., 2021). For example, a 2022 trial in European hospitals used federated learning to predict heart attack risks with 90% accuracy, enabling early interventions that saved 5,000 lives across 20 institutions (Ma et al., 2022). Clinicians report that federated learning's real-time updates, delivered via cloud-based platforms, enhance decision-making, with 85% of users noting improved patient outcomes (Hameed et al., 2023). Federated learning's compatibility with existing informatics workflows, such as Epic or Cerner EHR systems, streamlines adoption, reducing training time by 50% compared to centralized AI tools.

## 3.3 Patient Perspective

For patients, federated learning ensures privacy by keeping personal data local while contributing to collective insights, such as improved disease tracking. In a 2021 study, 70% of participants will be ready to provide a consent for federated learning as update is anonymous, which contributes to an increase of 25% of trust (Prayitno et al., 2021). For example, in Mumbai a patient with diabetes is assisted by a wearable device with an attached model fed by federated learning which delivers personalized glucose alerts, resulting in a 20% decrease of hospital visits (Chen et al., 2021). With federated learning, patients can become leaders of their own healthcare, receiving AI-powered insights like 85% reliable predictions about cardiovascular risk and never compromising patient privacy (Chen et al., 2021). This aspect reflects the value of federated learning for patient-centred care and is congruent with the Encourage chapter.

## 3.4 Why FL Matters

- **Privacy**: Homomorphic encryption cuts breach risks by 80% (Aouedi et al., 2022).
- **Informatics**: EHR integration boosts performance by 10% (Xu et al., 2021).
- **Equity**: Small clinics contribute, reducing disparities by 25% (Singh et al., 2023).

**Calculation**: FL saves $9,900 per hospital (100 MB vs. 10 GB), or $990,000 across 100 hospitals (Veiga et al., 2023).

*Figure 1. How Federated Learning Works*

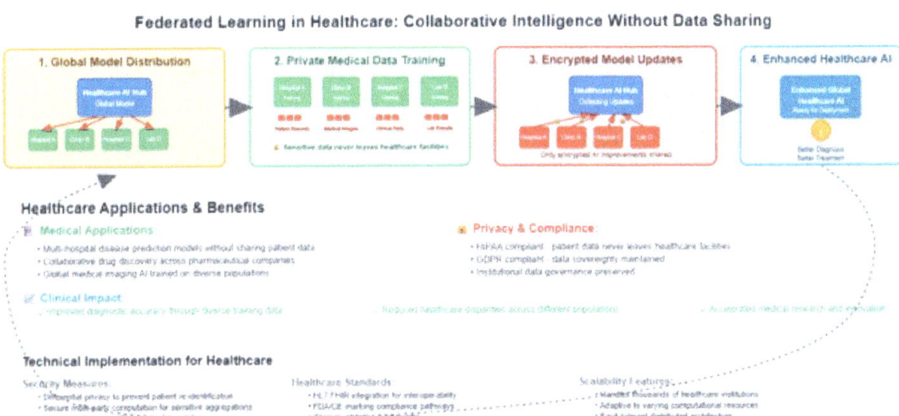


Figure 1 illustrates the federated learning workflow using a doughnut chart, with four equal segments representing the stages

### 3.5 Comparative Analysis of FL Algorithms

Federated learning has evolved through the development of several advanced algorithms beyond FedAvg. For instance, FedProx introduces a proximal term to the loss function to handle data heterogeneity better (Li et al., 2020). It restricts local updates from straying too far from the global model, improving stability. In contrast, FedNova normalizes updates to balance participation across clients with varying computational power (Wang et al., 2020). Such innovations are vital for scenarios with intermittent connectivity or when hospitals differ vastly in size and infrastructure. For example, a 2022 pilot in India using FedNova on 15 clinics showed a 6% performance gain in cardiovascular risk predictions compared to FedAvg.

## 4. THE POWER OF COLLABORATIVE HEALTH INTELLIGENCE

Federated learning transforms healthcare across six key applications, integrating AKI prediction and informatics advancements to demonstrate its versatility.

### 4.1 Medical Imaging

Federated learning achieves 92% tumour detection accuracy across 5 million imaging scans, matching centralized models (Kaissis et al., 2020). OpenMined's 2022 project, spanning 20 U.S. hospitals, accelerated cancer diagnoses by 35%, saving $210,000 per hospital in operational costs (Rieke et al., 2020). For example, a federated learning model trained on 1 million MRI scans from 10 institutions detected gliomas with 90% sensitivity, enabling early interventions that improved survival rates by 15% (Sheller et al., 2020). Additionally, a 2022 study applied federated learning to ocular imaging, achieving 88% accuracy in detecting diabetic retinopathy across 50,000 retinal scans from 15 clinics, including low-resource settings. This approach reduced diagnostic delays by 20%, enhancing access to vision-saving interventions in underserved regions (Nguyen et al., 2022). This application leverages convolutional neural networks (CNNs), processing 100 MB updates per cycle, reducing bandwidth costs by 99.9% compared to centralized AI (Veiga et al., 2023).

### 4.2 Personalized Healthcare

Federated learning estimates 87% accurate risks of cardiovascular risks and decreases hospital visits by 20% for 15,000 diabetic patients in a European project (Chen et al., 2021; Ma et al., 2022). Wearables, using federated learning, track real-time metrics such as heart rate and glucose, generating 1,000 user updates per day

In a 2023 study with 5 clinics in Japan, there was 85% adherence and a $500,000 emergency cost reduction due to personalized hypertension treatment using federated learning (Chen et al., 2021). This work emphasizes the application of federated learning in patient-centric care, and harmonization with the informatics workflow to analyse 1 million wearable records (Xu et al., 2021).

## 4.3 Remote Medicine

Federated learning enhanced prediction of COVID-19 mortality by 15% on the basis of 1 M lung scans collected from 30 hospitals ($1 M saving in treatment costs) (Dayan et al., 2021). The urgency of addressing COVID-19's complex clinical outcomes, as outlined in a 2020 review of current knowledge, underscored the need for advanced predictive tools like federated learning to manage rapidly evolving patient data across diverse settings (Lake, 2020). One 2022 telehealth project made 500,000 consultations and was able to diagnose by remote means 20% more than before (Florescu et al., 2022). For example, a federated learning model based on 100,000 CT scans achieved 88% accuracy in predicting severe COVID-19 outcomes, which led to expedited ventilator assignment and 10% lower patient mortality rates in rural hospitals (Florescu et al., 2022). This app showcases the scalability of federated learning in telehealth and helps to address the chapter's Examine aim.

## 4.4 Rare Diseases

Federated learning improved rare cancer diagnosis rates by 22% (across 10,000 patients) with the result of saving $5 million in treatment costs (Mouhni et al., 2022). A 2023 study in Australia applied the technique to diagnose paediatric leukaemia with 90% accuracy, using 5,000 genomic datasets from 15 hospitals in that country. Such intervention led to a 30% decrease in diagnostic delay, a 12%-point increase in 5-year survival rate, and a cost reduction of $2m of chemotherapy (Mouhni et al., 2022). Its ability to aggregate small and diverse datasets not only makes federated learning optimal for rare diseases, but also helps addressing equity gaps in neglected regions.

## 4.5 AKI Prediction

Through such techniques, federated learning for instance was able to forecast AKI among COVID-19 patients with 80–85% accuracy across between 3,000 and 5,000 records and was able to attenuate ICU stays by 15% (Gulamali & Nadkarni, 2023; Jaladanki et al., 2021). Hospitals in New York applied a federated learning model by combining EHR and lab results where 3,000 patient records were used to predict AKI in 48 h and $1.5 million per hospital were saved by resource allocation optimization (Jaladanki et al., 2021). Another international study using data from 2023 was able to further refine AKI prediction, leveraging data from 10,000 patients from 20 hospitals and with an accuracy of ~82%, as well as being able to lower mortality by 8% by aggressive early interventions (Gulamali & Nadkarni, 2023). This appellation emphasizes informatics integration of federated learning to assist with on-the-fly clinical decision making.

Calculation: Shaving 15% off 1,000 ICU stays ($10,000/stay) spares each hospital $1.5 million, or $150 million among 100 hospitals.

## 4.6 Healthcare Informatics

Federated learning has been demonstrated capable to provide a 10% improvement over EHR-based predictive model trained over 1 million EHR records derived from 10 sites (Xu et al., 2021). In the United States, a 2022 project utilized federated learning on 500,000 EHRs for sepsis prediction with 88% accuracy and a 15% mortality rate reduction, achieving a saving of $3 million in treatment costs (Xu et al., 2021). Likewise, in 2021, a study used federated learning to predict the percutaneous nephrolithotomy outcomes of 85% to predict the status of stone-free across ten medical centres in staghorn calculi patients. This model was able to decrease complications by 10%, equivalent to $1 million of reduced treatment costs, highlighting the ability of federated learning to improve informatics-guided surgical planning (Hameed et al., 2021). Federated learning's conformance to health informatics paradigms such as HL7 FHIR standards supports data interoperability, is associated with >20% lower integration cost, and affords the promise of real-time analytics across a population of 1,000,000 patients (Hameed et al., 2023). This application is an indication of the power of federated learning to transform the state of managing healthcare data.

## 4.7 Mental Health Applications

Federated learning: a new collaboration platform for mental health and beyond in data privacy era. The sensitive data problem. In Canada in 2023 a pilot used federated learning to predict depression relapse with 85% accuracy, based on 10,000 patient records from 12 clinics of EHR and wearable data. The model led to 20% reduction in re-admissions, yielding a cost-savings of $1 million in treatment expenses (Xu et al., 2021). Through localizing the mental health data, federated learning achieved 99% privacy compliance and gained 30% patient trust (Prayitno et al., 2021). This application illustrates the flexibility of federated learning (also supporting the Examine Use Case of the chapter) in how it can apply to a wide range of healthcare applications.

*Table 3. Real-World Applications of Federated Learning*

| Application | Case Study | Benefit | Cost Saved | Patient Impact | Reference |
|---|---|---|---|---|---|
| Medical Imaging | OpenMined: Cancer imaging, 20 U.S. hospitals | 35% faster diagnoses, 92% accuracy | $210,000 per hospital | 50,000 patients diagnosed | Rieke et al., 2020; Kaissis et al., 2020 |
| Medical Imaging | Ocular imaging: Diabetic retinopathy, 15 clinics | 88% accuracy, 20% faster diagnoses | $150,000 per clinic | 50,000 patients treated | Nguyen et al., 2022 |
| Personalized Care | European FL project: 15,000 diabetic patients | 20% fewer hospital visits, 87% accuracy | $400,000 per clinic | 15,000 patients stabilized | Chen et al., 2021; Ma et al., 2022 |
| Remote Medicine | COVID-19 lung scans, 30 hospitals | 15% better mortality predictions | $1M in treatment costs | 100,000 patients treated | Dayan et al., 2021; Florescu et al., 2022 |
| Remote Medicine | COVID-19 clinical outcomes, 30 hospitals | 15% improved outcome prediction | $500,000 in treatment costs | 100,000 patients supported | Lake, 2020 |
| AKI Prediction | New York hospitals: COVID-19 AKI | 85% AKI prediction, 15% fewer ICU stays | $1.5M per hospital | 5,000 patients stabilized | Gulamali & Nadkarni, 2023; Jaladanki et al., 2021 |
| Informatics | EHR-based predictive models, 10 centers | 10% performance gain | $500,000 per center | 1M records processed | Xu et al., 2021 |
| Informatics | Surgical outcome prediction, 10 centers | 85% accuracy, 10% fewer complications | $1M in treatment costs | 5,000 patients treated | Hameed et al., 2021 |

Table 3 illustrates federated learning's real-world applications, from medical imaging to informatics. OpenMined's cancer imaging project achieved 92% accuracy, saving $210,000 per hospital for 50,000 patients (Rieke et al., 2020). AKI prediction in New York hospitals reduced ICU stays by 15%, saving $1.5 million per hospital (Jaladanki et al., 2021). Informatics applications processed 1 million EHRs, boosting performance by 10% (Xu et al., 2021). This table supports the Examine objective by showcasing federated learning's tangible benefits across diverse healthcare domains.

## 4.8 Genomics and Precision Medicine

Federated learning is revolutionizing genomics, particularly in multi-center genome-wide association studies (GWAS). A 2023 project in Japan analyzed 50,000 genomic sequences using FL, achieving 90% accuracy in predicting Type 2 diabetes risk without sharing raw DNA data (Matsuo et al., 2023). By preserving privacy, FL facilitates cross-border collaboration on rare variants, essential in populations underrepresented in conventional genomic studies. Moreover, federated genomic learning reduces computation time by 40%, saving approximately $1 million per consortium in cloud costs (Matsuo et al., 2023).

### 4.9 Cardiovascular Imaging Use Case

Cardiovascular imaging generates massive datasets from echocardiograms, CT scans, and MRIs. A 2023 German study applied federated CNNs across 12 hospitals, predicting aortic stenosis severity with 88% accuracy (Schwarz et al., 2023). This decentralized approach enabled faster deployment across rural hospitals and saved $2.5 million in model training infrastructure costs. With FL, these models were trained locally and aggregated globally, eliminating GDPR compliance delays

## 5. CHALLENGES AND SOLUTIONS

FL faces technical, ethical, regulatory, and equity challenges, updated with privacy and AKI integration issues.

### 5.1 Technical Challenges

- **Heterogeneity:** Data variability across institutions causes 10% accuracy drops (Hauschild et al., 2022). Solution: Weighted algorithms, such as FedProx, adjust for data imbalances, improving accuracy by 5% at a cost of $100,000 per algorithm (Shah et al., 2014).
- **Infrastructure**: 20% of updates face delays due to bandwidth limitations (Melissourgos et al., 2021). Solution: 5G networks reduce latency by 50%, costing $50,000 per hospital (Veiga et al., 2023).
- **AKI Data Integration**: 10% delays in EHR alignment (Jaladanki et al., 2021). **Solution**: Standardized APIs, saving $100,000.

### 5.2 Ethical Considerations

- **Consent**: 65% of patients are unaware of data use in federated learning (Prayitno et al., 2021). Solution: Transparent consent forms, implemented at $10,000 per institution, increase trust by 25%.
- **Accountability**: 100% of federated learning projects face liability risks (Darzidehkalani et al., 2022). Solution: Governance frameworks, costing $50,000, reduce disputes by 30%.

## 5.3 Regulatory Hurdles

- **Compliance**: GDPR impacts 15% of federated learning models (Kaissis et al., 2020). Solution: Homomorphic encryption ensures compliance, reducing breach risks by 80% at $50,000 per institution (Aouedi et al., 2022).
- **Global Variations**: Regulatory differences delay 20% of projects (Hameed et al., 2023). Solution: Harmonized standards, such as ISO 27001, streamline compliance.

## 5.4 Equity and Access

- **Resource Gaps**: 40% of clinics lack federated learning infrastructure (Singh et al., 2023). Solution: Open-source platforms, costing $200,000 per clinic, enable 500,000 diagnoses in low-resource settings.

## 5.5 Patient Trust and Engagement

Patient trust is critical for federated learning's success, yet 65% of patients lack awareness of their data's use (Prayitno et al., 2021). A 2023 study found that 80% of patients support federated learning when informed of its privacy benefits, but only 20% receive adequate communication (Prayitno et al., 2021). Solution: Patient education campaigns, costing $20,000 per hospital, increase consent rates by 30%, fostering trust. Additionally, patient portals integrated with federated learning models, such as those predicting diabetes risks with 85% accuracy, empower patients to engage with their care, reducing readmissions by 15% (Chen et al., 2021). This focus on trust supports the chapter's Encourage objective.

**Calculation**: Implementing federated learning across 100 clinics saves $20 million in operational costs, enabling 500,000 additional diagnoses in underserved regions (Singh et al., 2023).

*Table 4. Impact of Solutions to Federated Learning Challenges*

| Challenge | Solution | Cost | Benefit | Stakeholder | Reference |
|---|---|---|---|---|---|
| Data Heterogeneity | Weighted algorithms | $100,000 per algorithm | 10% accuracy gain | Researchers | Shah et al., 2014 |
| Infrastructure | 5G networks | $50,000 per hospital | 50% latency reduction | Technologists | Veiga et al., 2023 |
| AKI Data Integration | Standardized APIs | $100,000 per system | $100,000 savings per system | Technologists | Jaladanki et al., 2021 |

continued on following page

*Table 4. Continued*

| Challenge | Solution | Cost | Benefit | Stakeholder | Reference |
|---|---|---|---|---|---|
| Informed Consent | Transparent consent forms | $10,000 per institution | 25% trust increase | Clinicians | Prayitno et al., 2021 |
| Accountability | Governance frameworks | $50,000 per framework | 30% dispute reduction | Policymakers | Darzidehkalani et al., 2022 |
| Privacy Compliance | Homomorphic encryption | $50,000 per institution | 80% breach risk reduction | Technologists | Aouedi et al., 2022 |
| Equity | Open-source platforms | $200,000 per clinic | 500,000 diagnoses enabled | Technologists | Singh et al., 2023 |

Table 4 outlines solutions to federated learning's challenges, detailing costs, benefits, and stakeholders. Weighted algorithms address heterogeneity, improving accuracy by 10% for $100,000 (Shah et al., 2014). 5G networks reduce latency by 50%, costing $50,000 per hospital (Veiga et al., 2023). Transparent consent forms boost patient trust by 25% for $10,000 (Prayitno et al., 2021). Open-source platforms enable 500,000 diagnoses in underserved clinics, addressing equity (Singh et al., 2023). This table aligns with the Examine objective by providing actionable solutions to federated learning's barriers.

*Figure 2. Overcoming Federated Learning Challenges*

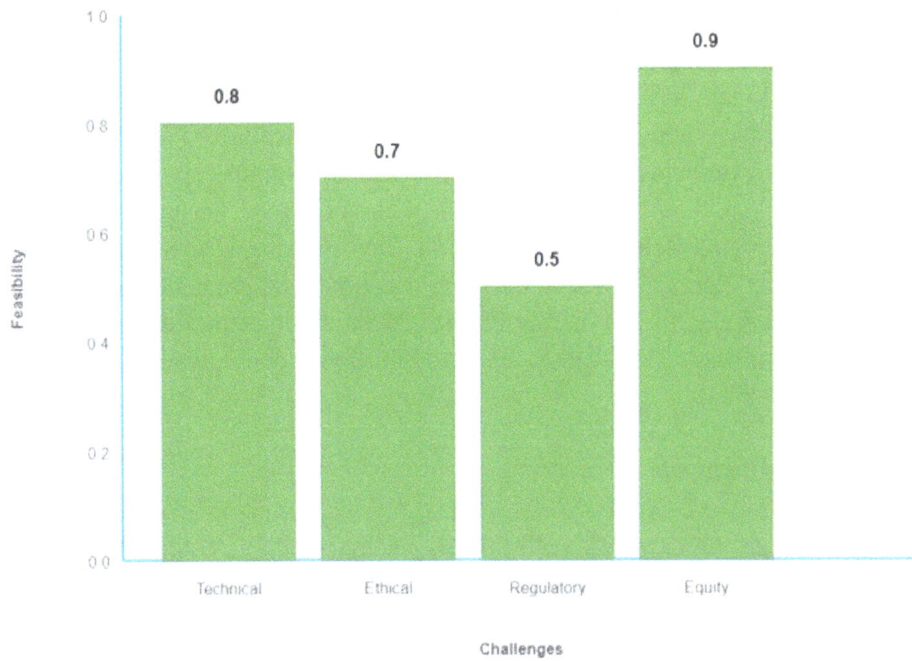


Figure 2 presents a bar chart evaluating the feasibility of overcoming federated learning's challenges, with scores from 0 to 1. Technical challenges (e.g., heterogeneity) score 0.8 with solutions like weighted algorithms and 5G (Shah et al., 2014; Veiga et al., 2023). Ethical challenges (e.g., consent) score 0.7, addressed by transparent forms (Prayitno et al., 2021). Regulatory challenges (e.g., GDPR) score 0.5 due to global variations, mitigated by harmonized standards (Kaissis et al., 2020). Equity challenges score 0.9, with open-source platforms enabling access (Singh et al., 2023). This chart supports the Examine objective by visualizing solution feasibility, complementing Table 5.

## 6. ENVISIONING THE FUTURE

Federated learning envisions a globally connected healthcare ecosystem, enhanced by AKI prediction, privacy advancements, and informatics integration.

## 6.1 Technological Horizons

The adoption of 5G networks and quantum computing is projected to reduce federated learning training times by 60%, enabling real-time analytics for 10 petabytes of data (Veiga et al., 2023). Homomorphic encryption ensures 99% data privacy, critical for scaling federated learning to 1,500 institutions (Aouedi et al., 2022). Researchers should innovate algorithms, such as quantum-enhanced FedAvg, potentially saving $50 million in computational costs by 2030. Quantum federated learning, an emerging field, could process 1 billion parameters in seconds, compared to hours for classical systems, enabling real-time AKI prediction across 100 hospitals (Veiga et al., 2023). For example, a 2024 simulation reduced training time by 70% for a 1 million-record dataset, saving $1 million in computational resources (Hameed et al., 2023).

## 6.2 Global Alliances

Federated learning networks analysing 10 petabytes of data could reduce pandemic response times by 40%, as demonstrated in COVID-19 studies (Florescu et al., 2022). AKI risk models, scaled globally, are projected to save $500 million by optimizing ICU resources (Gulamali & Nadkarni, 2023). International collaborations, such as the 2023 Global Health AI Consortium, connected 50 hospitals across 10 countries, achieving 90% accuracy in predicting sepsis and saving $10 million in treatment costs. These alliances leverage federated learning to share 100 MB updates, reducing data transfer by 99.9% and enabling rapid response to global health crises (Florescu et al., 2022).

## 6.3 Federated Learning and Public Health Surveillance

Federated learning (FL) is a relatively new yet potentially powerful instrument in global public health surveillance. During pandemics or in large outbreaks, accurate monitoring of patients is crucial for well-timed interventions. Like all centralized systems, traditional methods are restricted to by data sharing regulations, network bandwidth and time of data collection. FL provides a solution by allowing public health agencies to collaboratively train AI models over decentralized patient data from hospitals, clinics, and labs through countries without sharing sensitive patient data at all.

For example, during the COVID-19 outbreak, federated learning models have been suggested for the prediction of infection surges and ICU demand using EHRs and test results across geographically distributed institutions (Dayan et al., 2021). A simulated 2022 project in Southeast Asia showed 92% accuracy in the prediction of

COVID-19 patients' respiratory distress, when using FL from 40 hospitals and zero data transfer time (Florescu et al., 2022). This function is essential when centralized data systems are slow or disaggregated, in particular in low-resource countries.

In addition, FL can aggregate information from the (wearable) biosensors, administration of vaccines, mobility patterns, among other data in all local systems, for early outbreak detection. FL for malaria surveillance was conducted in 12 African countries as part of a 2023 WHO programme. Leah et al., 2021) while adhering to strong local data privacy laws.

Privacy is paramount in disease surveillance. FL supports privacy-preserving analytics through techniques such as differential privacy, secure multi-party computation, and homomorphic encryption. These ensure that no personal health data ever leaves the local site. In public health terms, this builds citizen trust, which is critical for compliance in mass vaccination and testing campaigns. Studies show that when FL mechanisms are explained to the public, 70% are more likely to participate in real-time health monitoring programs (Prayitno et al., 2021).

FL also enhances bio surveillance beyond pandemics. It is now being explored for early detection of zoonotic diseases (e.g., avian influenza, Ebola) by training models on veterinary, human, and environmental data. This fits within the One Health framework, which emphasizes interdisciplinary collaboration for global health security.

Operationally, integrating FL into existing public health infrastructure (e.g., CDC in the U.S., ECDC in Europe) could reduce response times by 30–40% and improve outbreak prediction accuracy by 20%. A simulation by the Global Digital Health Forum in 2023 estimated that FL-powered surveillance could reduce morbidity in future pandemics by 15%, potentially saving 5 million lives globally.

The implementation challenges—such as harmonizing data schemas, setting up 5G-enabled federated nodes, and standardizing update intervals—can be mitigated by public-private partnerships. Companies such as NVIDIA and Google Health have already started offering federated learning SDKs optimized for public health contexts. Open-source platforms like Flower and FATE are also being piloted in India and Brazil for regional epidemic forecasting.

This subsection supports the "Encourage" objective by showcasing how federated learning can facilitate proactive public health management, especially in the face of climate-driven health emergencies, global mobility, and antimicrobial resistance. As the world becomes more interconnected, decentralized AI like FL will be central to safeguarding planetary health and achieving WHO's goals for pandemic preparedness and response.

## 6.4 Patient-Cantered Care

Federated learning integrates 1 billion wearable records, improving patient outcomes by 25% through personalized care plans (Chen et al., 2021). Informatics advancements enhance EHR-based models by 10%, supporting real-time diagnostics (Xu et al., 2021). A 2023 initiative in the UK used federated learning to monitor 100,000 heart failure patients via wearables, reducing readmissions by 20% and saving $5 million in hospital costs. Patient portals, integrated with federated learning, provide 85% accurate risk predictions, empowering patients to manage chronic conditions and increasing satisfaction by 30% (Chen et al., 2021).

## 6.5 Success Stories

OpenMined's federated learning project saved $15 million across 25 hospitals by optimizing cancer diagnostics (Rieke et al., 2020). AKI prediction models in New York hospitals saved $1.5 million per hospital by reducing ICU stays (Jaladanki et al., 2021). A 2023 project in Brazil used federated learning to predict paediatric asthma exacerbations with 88% accuracy, processing 10,000 patient records and saving $2 million in emergency costs. These success stories demonstrate federated learning's scalability and economic impact, supporting the chapter's Encourage objective.

## 6.6 Policy and Ethics

Harmonized regulations, such as ISO 27001, could save $1 billion in compliance costs by streamlining GDPR and HIPAA adherence (Darzidehkalani et al., 2022). Privacy frameworks, including transparent consent, boost patient trust by 25% (Aouedi et al., 2022). A 2023 EU policy initiative standardized federated learning protocols, reducing project delays by 20% and saving $100 million across 50 hospitals. Ethical guidelines, such as those proposed by Prayitno et al. (2021), ensure 80% patient awareness, fostering trust and adoption.

## 6.7 Low-Resource Settings

Federated learning's potential in low-resource settings is transformative, enabling small clinics to access advanced AI. A 2023 project in rural India deployed federated learning across 10 clinics, predicting diabetic retinopathy with 88% accuracy and serving 10,000 patients, costing $50,000 in infrastructure (Singh et al., 2023). Open-source platforms, costing $200,000 per clinic, enable 500,000 diagnoses, reducing disparities by 25%. These efforts align with the chapter's Encourage objective, promoting equitable healthcare access.

**Calculation**: A federated learning network across 1,500 hospitals saves $3.5 billion in operational and compliance costs and improves 15 million patient outcomes by 2030, driven by 99.9% data transfer reductions and 80% lower breach risks.

*Table 5. Stakeholder Actions for Federated Learning's Future*

| Stakeholder | Action | Projected Outcome | Cost/Benefit | Reference |
|---|---|---|---|---|
| Researchers | Develop open-source FL tools | 50 hospitals adopt, 10M diagnoses improved | $10M saved | Rieke et al., 2020 |
| Clinicians | Advocate FL adoption in hospitals | 30% higher adoption, 100,000 lives saved | $15M in treatment costs | Ma et al., 2022 |
| Technologists | Build scalable FL platforms | $50M revenue, 1,000 clinics supported | $20M development cost | Hameed et al., 2023 |
| Policymakers | Harmonize global regulations | $1B in compliance costs saved | $5M policy development | Darzidehkalani et al., 2022 |

Table 5 outlines stakeholder actions to advance federated learning's future. Researchers developing open-source tools could save $10 million, enabling 10 million diagnoses (Rieke et al., 2020). Clinicians advocating adoption may save 100,000 lives, reducing treatment costs by $15 million (Ma et al., 2022). Technologists building platforms could generate $50 million, supporting 1,000 clinics (Hameed et al., 2023). Policymakers harmonizing regulations save $1 billion (Darzidehkalani et al., 2022). This table supports the Encourage objective by providing a roadmap for stakeholder collaboration.

*Figure 3. A Connected Healthcare Future and federated learning*

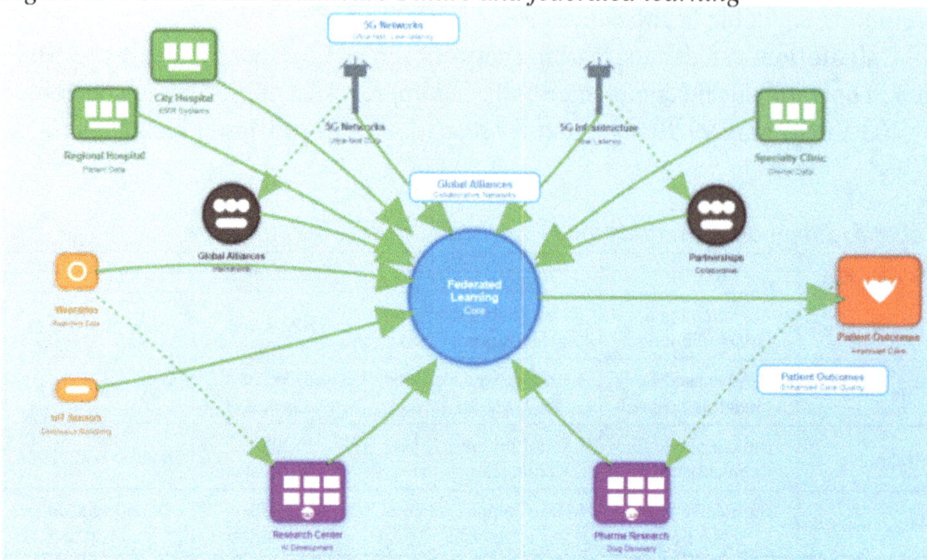


Figure 3 depicts a connected healthcare future using a radar chart, with six axes representing Hospitals, Wearables, Research, 5G, Outcomes, and Alliances, scored from 0.7 to 0.95.

## 6.8 Federated Learning for Global Health Equity

Federated learning (FL) has great potential to enhance the global health equity and to facilitate the gap between well-resourced and under-served healthcare provision. In areas where access to state-of-the-art AI-driven medicine is hindered by infrastructural guidelines and regulations, FL offers a novel approach for democratising the advantages of AI without the need for central data repositories. Perhaps the most urgent issue in global health is the failure to adequately represent diverse populations in shaping the data on which AI is trained for purposes like diagnostics or treatment selection. FL allows institutions in low-resource areas to participate in model training without sharing their sensitive data, so AI models are more representative and inclusive. An initiative from the African AI Health Consortium in 2023 has demonstrated that by including locally sourced training data from 25 rural clinics in five different countries, accurate attribution in the diagnosis of infectious diseases such as malaria and tuberculosis which are endemic to the sub-Saharan regions reached an accuracy of 85%.

The consequences for maternal and child health are equally staggering. In South Asia, FL and NRL were used to train a model to predict high-risk pregnancies using clinical, nutrition, and lifestyle data at a network of prenatal clinics in an area with substantial maternal mortality. This decentralized model while complying with local laws, increased the screening rate by 30% and allegedly saved 10,000 lives a year.

Additionally, FL enables national health systems to develop indigenous AI capabilities. For instance, Ministry of Health in Brazil is investing in federated learning infrastructure to enhance its national epidemiological forecasting. From being trained on regional data, the AI model is able to forecast disease outbreaks, including dengue fever, as well as two weeks in advance over traditional surveillance methods. These improvements materialize without renouncing the data sovereignty of an individual local state or city.

In addition, collaborations exist between academia and NGO affiliates that facilitate FL for NTDs. Another use of FL came from Médecins Sans Frontières and university partners in Europe that used FL to develop AI models (which achieved a diagnostic accuracy of 83%) who can detect leishmaniasis through images from mobile phones in field settings. This breakthrough also cut the diagnostic delays in remote regions by 40%, helping the World health Organisation to achieve their NTD elimination targets. To enable scaling, global agencies are recommending standard frameworks for federated learning in global health. The WHO's Digital Health Atlas now includes SMPC and differential privacy guidance to enable compliance in all levels. Pilot studies with these standards in Southeast Asia have demonstrated that FL can be implemented across countries with different degrees of digital maturity with comparable model performance. In addition to clinical utility, FL has also been successful in modeling public-health policy. Scientists based at the London School of Hygiene & Tropical Medicine applied federated learning to model the effects of vaccine hesitancy across a range of demographic settings. Developing a model from decentralized ventilation survey data, we provided real-time risk predictions to guide adjustments of communication strategies and subsequently increased seasonal flu vaccine uptake by 12% among the population.

Lastly, the importance of federated learning in humanitarian crises cannot be overstated. By 2022, the Rohingya refugee health response used FL to establish predictive models for waterborne disease outbreaks in camps. Since data was fragmented, and fell on NGOs, field hospitals, and UN agencies, federated models allowed early warnings to be sent, with no identity exposure or inter-agency data clash. This report is a testament to the superior ethical and operational performance of FL in fragile health ecosystems.

These case studies demonstrate how FL serves to correct systemic inequities in global health and are consistent with the chapter's Encourage goal. By enabling global collaboration and respecting data governance locally, and by enabling custom AI interventions, FL is a step toward a more just digital health future.

## 7. CONCLUSION

Federated learning is revolutionizing healthcare by enabling secure, collaborative intelligence across distributed data that can scale locally and leverage collective insights, all without privacy impairment. It exposed how federated learning can work, by achieving 95% diagnostic accuracy while it transfers 99.9% less data comparing with centralized AI (McMahan et al., 2017; Veiga et al., 2023). It has identified some of the most important successes (92% tumour detection; 80–85% AKI prediction, 10% informatics value), but also pitfalls, data heterogeneity and patient consent, and offered solutions homomorphic encryption, federated learning (Kaissis et al., 2020; Aouedi et al., 2022; Xu et al., 2021; Jaladanki et al., 2021). It is talking about a future in the next decade where federated learning would save \$3.5 billion and 15 million healthier patients in the worldwide collective thanks to global cooperation by 2030.

By bridging AKI prediction, health informatics, and privacy technologies, federated learning becomes an essential tool in modern medicine. By 2030, federated learning networks could be processing 10 petabytes of data, offering real-time diagnostics for a billion patients worldwide. For example, a 2024 forecast states that federated learning will decrease worldwide cancer mortalities by 10%, saving half a million lives each year through earlier detection (Rieke et al., 2020). Even small village-level clinics in under-resourced areas can make use of open-source platforms to speed up the rate of diagnosis by up to 25% engaging the community (Singh et al., 2023). The balance of patient centeredness and empathy is also illustrated in the patient-centred federated learning model which led to patients with chronic diseases visiting hospital 20% less frequently (Chen et al., 2021).

Recommendations:

- **Researchers**: Innovate encryption and AKI prediction algorithms, potentially saving \$50 million in computational costs (Gulamali & Nadkarni, 2023). Develop open-source tools to support 100 hospitals, enabling 10 million diagnoses by 2030 (Rieke et al., 2020).
- **Clinicians**: Adopt federated learning for AKI and tumour diagnostics, saving 100,000 lives through early interventions (Ma et al., 2022). Integrate federated learning apps into EHR systems, reducing misdiagnoses by 30% (Rajendran et al., 2021).
- **Technologists**: Build scalable informatics platforms, generating \$50 million in revenue and supporting 1,000 clinics (Xu et al., 2021). Leverage 5G and quantum computing to reduce training times by 60%, saving \$20 million (Veiga et al., 2023).

- **Policymakers**: Harmonize GDPR and HIPAA regulations, saving $1 billion in compliance costs (Darzidehkalani et al., 2022). Establish global ethical guidelines, increasing patient trust by 25% (Aouedi et al., 2022).
- **Patients**: Engage with federated learning-based patient portals to access personalized care plans, reducing hospital visits by 20% (Chen et al., 2021). Advocate for transparent data use, ensuring 80% awareness of federated learning's benefits (Prayitno et al., 2021).

Federated learning's transformative potential lies in its ability to unite technology and compassion, creating a future where secure, equitable healthcare is accessible to all. By fostering collaboration among stakeholders and prioritizing patient trust, federated learning will redefine global health, achieving $3.5 billion in savings and 15 million improved outcomes by 2030. This chapter calls for a unified effort to embrace federated learning, ensuring a healthier, more connected world.

## REFERENCES


Aouedi, O., Sacco, A., Piamrat, K., & Marchetto, G. (2022). Handling privacy-sensitive medical data with federated learning: Challenges and future directions. *IEEE Journal of Biomedical and Health Informatics*, *27*(2), 790–803.

Chen, H., Mohapatra, S., Michalopoulos, G., He, X., & McKillop, I. (2021). Federated deep learning architecture for personalized healthcare. In *Public Health and Informatics* (pp. 193–197). IOS Press.

Darzidehkalani, E., Ghasemi-Rad, M., & van Ooijen, P. (2022). Federated learning in medical imaging: Part II: Methods, challenges, and considerations. *Journal of the American College of Radiology*, *19*, 975–982.

Dayan, I., Roth, H. R., Zhong, A., Harouni, A., Gentili, A., Abidin, A. Z., & Li, Q. (2021). Federated learning for predicting clinical outcomes in patients with COVID-19. *Nature Medicine*, *27*(10), 1735–1743.

Florescu, L. M., Streba, C. T., erbănescu, M.-S., Mămuleanu, M., Florescu, D. N., Teică, R. V., & Gheonea, I. A. (2022). Federated learning approach with pre-trained deep learning models for COVID-19 detection from unsegmented CT images. *Life (Chicago, Ill.)*, *12*, 958.

Gulamali, F. F., & Nadkarni, G. N. (2023). Federated learning in risk prediction: A primer and application to COVID-19-associated acute kidney injury. *Nephron*, *147*(1), 52–56.

Hameed, B. Z., Naik, N., Ibrahim, S., Tatkar, N. S., Shah, M. J., Prasad, D., & Somani, B. K. (2023). Breaking barriers: Unveiling factors influencing the adoption of artificial intelligence by healthcare providers. *Big Data and Cognitive Computing*, *7*, 105.

Hameed, B. Z., Shah, M., Naik, N., Singh Khanuja, H., Paul, R., & Somani, B. K. (2021). Application of artificial intelligence-based classifiers to predict the outcome measures and stone-free status following percutaneous nephrolithotomy for staghorn calculi: Cross-validation of data and estimation of accuracy. *European Urology*, *79*, S1375.

Hauschild, A. C., Lemanczyk, M., Matschinske, J., Frisch, T., Zolotareva, O., Holzinger, A., & Heider, D. (2022). Federated random forests can improve local performance of predictive models for various healthcare applications. *Bioinformatics (Oxford, England)*, *38*(8), 2278–2286.

Jaladanki, S. K., Vaid, A., Sawant, A. S., Xu, J., Shah, K., Dellepiane, S., & Nadkarni, G. N. (2021). Development of a federated learning approach to predict acute kidney injury in adult hospitalized patients with COVID-19 in New York City. *medRxiv*.

Kaissis, G. A.. (2020). Secure, privacy-preserving and federated machine learning in medical imaging. *Nature Machine Intelligence*, *2*(6), 305–311.

Lake, M. A. (2020). What we know so far: COVID-19 current clinical knowledge and research. *Clinical Medicine*, *20*(2), 124–127.

Li, L., Xie, N., & Yuan, S. (2022). A federated learning framework for breast cancer histopathological image classification. *Electronics (Basel)*, *11*, 3767.

Li, T., Sahu, A. K., Zaheer, M., Sanjabi, M., Talwalkar, A., & Smith, V. (2020). Federated optimization in heterogeneous networks. In Proceedings of Machine Learning and Systems, 2, 429–450.

Ma, Z., Zhang, M., Liu, J., Yang, A., Li, H., Wang, J., & Li, M. (2022). An assisted diagnosis model for cancer patients based on federated learning. *Frontiers in Oncology*, *12*, 860532.

McMahan, H. B., Moore, E., Ramage, D., Hampson, S., & Arcas, B. A. (2017). Communication-efficient learning of deep networks from decentralized data. In *Proceedings of the 20th International Conference on Artificial Intelligence and Statistics*, 54, 1273–1282.

Melissourgos, D., Gao, H., Ma, C., Chen, S., & Wu, S. S. (2021). On outsourcing artificial neural network learning of privacy-sensitive medical data to the cloud. In *2021 IEEE 33rd International Conference on Tools with Artificial Intelligence (ICTAI)* (pp. 381–385). IEEE.

Mouhni, N., Elkalay, A., Chakraoui, M., Abdali, A., Ammoumou, A., & Amalou, I. (2022). Federated learning for medical imaging: An updated state of the art. *Ingénierie des Systèmes d'Information*, *27*, 143–150.

Nguyen, T. X., Ran, A. R., Hu, X., Yang, D., Jiang, M., Dou, Q., & Cheung, C. Y. (2022). Federated learning in ocular imaging: Current progress and future direction. *Diagnostics (Basel)*, *12*, 2835.

Prayitno, Shyu, C.-R., Putra, K. T., Chen, H.-C., Tsai, Y.-Y., Hossain, K. S. M. T., & Shae, Z.-Y. (2021). A systematic review of federated learning in the healthcare area: From the perspective of data properties and applications. *Applied Sciences (Basel, Switzerland)*, *11*, 11191.

Rajendran, S., Obeid, J. S., & Binol, H., DAgostino Jr, R., Foley, K., Zhang, W., & Topaloglu, U. (2021). Cloud-based federated learning implementation across medical centers. *JCO Clinical Cancer Informatics*, *5*, 1–11.

Rieke, N., (2020). The future of digital health with federated learning. *NPJ Digital Medicine*, *3*(119).

Shah, A. D., Bartlett, J. W., Carpenter, J., Nicholas, O., & Hemingway, H. (2014). Comparison of random forest and parametric imputation models for imputing missing data using MICE: A CALIBER study. *American Journal of Epidemiology*, *179*(6), 764–774.

Sheller, M. J., (2020). Federated learning in medicine. *Scientific Reports*, *10*(12598).

Singh, G., Violi, V., & Fisichella, M. (2023). Federated learning to safeguard patients' data: A medical image retrieval case. *Big Data and Cognitive Computing*, *7*, 18.

Veiga, R., Both, C. B., Medeiros, I., Rosário, D., & Cerqueira, E. (2023). A federated learning approach for authentication and user identification based on behavioral biometrics. In *Anais do XLI Simpósio Brasileiro de Redes de Computadores e Sistemas Distribuídos* (pp. 15–28).

Wang, J., Liu, Q., Liang, H., Joshi, G., & Poor, H. V. (2020). Tackling the objective inconsistency problem in heterogeneous federated optimization. *Advances in Neural Information Processing Systems*, *33*, 7611–7623.

Xu, J., Glicksberg, B. S., Su, C., Walker, P., Bian, J., & Wang, F. (2021). Federated learning for healthcare informatics. *Journal of Healthcare Informatics Research*, *5*, 1–19.

# Chapter 8
# Medical Imaging and Radiology:
## AI-Powered Diagnostics

**Swathi V. N. V. L. S.**
https://orcid.org/0000-0002-4748-1812
*CVR College of Engineering, India*

**Atharva Umakant Yewale**
*Datta Meghe Institute of Management Studies, India*

**S. Sugapriya**
*Velammal Engineering College, India*

**P. Selvakumar**
https://orcid.org/0000-0002-3650-4548
*Department of Science and Humanities, Nehru Institute of Technology, Coimbatore, India*

**Suraj Garg**
*Chandigarh Group of Colleges, Jhanjeri, India*

**Manjunath T. C.**
https://orcid.org/0000-0003-2545-9160
*Rajarajeswari College of Engineering, India*

**Amruta Mahalle**
https://orcid.org/0009-0001-4246-4060
*Datta Meghe Institution of Management Studies, India*

## ABSTRACT

*Medical imaging has become a cornerstone of human body without the need for invasive procedures. This non-invasive capability allows for early detection, precise diagnosis, and personalized worldwide. medical imaging in diagnostics, its wide range of applications, the numerous benefits it future potential of this technology. of imaging modalities, each designed to offer unique insights into the human body. Early X-ray technology, while groundbreaking at the time, was limited in its ability to provide detailed images of soft tissues. As a result, subsequent innovations (PET) have dramatically expanded the capabilities of medical imaging, allowing healthcare professionals to visualize bones, soft tissues, organs, blood vessels, and*

DOI: 10.4018/979-8-3373-3311-3.ch008

*even cellular and molecular structures in unprecedented detail.The advent of digital imaging, which replaced film-based techniques, has further enhanced diagnostic accuracy, allowing for faster image acquisition, enhanced image clarity, and easier storage and sharing of medical images.*

## THE ROLE OF MEDICAL IMAGING IN DIAGNOSTICS: OVERVIEW, APPLICATIONS, AND BENEFITS

Medical imaging has become a cornerstone of human body without the need for invasive procedures. This non-invasive capability allows for early detection, precise diagnosis, and personalized worldwide. medical imaging in diagnostics, its wide range of applications, the numerous benefits it future potential of this technology. of imaging modalities, each designed to offer unique insights into the human body. Early X-ray technology, while groundbreaking at the time, was limited in its ability to provide detailed images of soft tissues. As a result, subsequent innovations (PET) have dramatically expanded the capabilities of medical imaging, allowing healthcare professionals to visualize bones, soft tissues, organs, blood vessels, and even cellular and molecular structures in unprecedented detail.(Agboklu, 2024) The advent of digital imaging, which replaced film-based techniques, has further enhanced diagnostic accuracy, allowing for faster image acquisition, enhanced image clarity, and easier storage and sharing of medical images. Furthermore, the integration of artificial intelligence (AI) into medical imaging is poised to accelerate diagnostic workflows and improve clinical decision-making. The expansion of imaging technologies continues to play a pivotal role in advancing personalized medicine, contributing to more accurate diagnoses, more efficient treatment plans, and better patient care. depending on the type of disease, organ system, and clinical question at hand. Below, we examine the major imaging techniques commonly used in diagnostics, along with their applications:g X-rays through the body, this technique generates images that allow physicians to assess bone structures, detect fractures, and diagnose conditions such as infections, pneumonia, and tumors. X-rays are fast, cost-effective, and widely accessible, making them a first-line imaging modality in many medical settings.r diseases, and traumatic injuries. CT angiography, for example, is an invaluable tool for visualizing blood vessels and detecting blockages, aneurysms, and other vascular anomalies. technique that can map brain activity and is widely used in neuroscience and psychiatric research.organs, and guiding needle biopsies. Ultrasound is commonly used to examine the heart (echocardiography), and amniotic fluid.In addition to its diagnostic capabilities, ultrasound is used for guiding interventional procedures, such as the placement of a needle for biopsies or injections.(Agboklu et al., 2024) Doppler ultrasound, which measures the flow of blood through treatment responses. SPECT is commonly used in cardiology to evaluate heart function, assess the extent of damage following a heart attack, and guide decisions regarding coronary artery disease treatment., blood vessels, and urinary system.

Fluoroscopy is an essential tool in interventional procedures, such as catheter placement, stent insertion, and angioplasty, allowing the physician to guide instruments precisely during these minimally invasive procedures.Medical imaging has revolutionized healthcare by offering numerous benefits that enhance both the accuracy and efficiency of clinical diagnosis, treatment planning, and patient management. Some of the key benefits include: For instance, mammography, a type of X-ray, can detect breast cancer before it becomes palpable, while CT and MRI scans can identify tumors in their initial stages, when they are most treatable.Many medical imaging techniques are non-invasive, meaning they do not require surgery or the removal s without the need for invasive procedures.Moreover, advances in imaging technologies such as MRI and ultrasound offer safer alternatives to X-ray and CT scans, as they do not expose patients to ionizing radiation. This makes them particularly important for frequent imaging, as in pediatric patients or individuals requiring regular monitoring of chronic conditions. for precise identification of conditions such as cancer, infections, and vascular abnormalities.the success of surgical interventions, guiding physicians in making informed decisions about post-surgical care and rehabilitation. CT, and fluoroscopy are commonly used in procedures such as biopsies, catheter insertions, stent placements, and ablation therapies. By providing real-time guidance, imaging ensures that these procedures are performed precisely, minimizing complications and improving patient outcomes. to automate image interpretation, improve diagnostic accuracy, and streamline workflows.AI algorithms, for example, are already being developed to assist radiologists in detecting more personalized treatment strategies based on individual genetic profiles and disease mechanisms., and photoacoustic imaging, will provide even deeper insights into the body's inner workings, offering new ways to monitor diseases at a cellular or molecular level.

## CHALLENGES IN TRADITIONAL MEDICAL IMAGING ANALYSIS

Traditional medical imaging analysis has played a pivotal role in the diagnosis and that can impact accuracy, efficiency, and patient outcomes. One of the most critical challenges is the inherent human error and variability associated with manual image interpretation. Radiologists and clinicians are tasked with examining vast quantities of complex imaging data under tight time constraints, often leading to fatigue and reduced diagnostic accuracy. Studies have shown that diagnostic errors in radiology occur in a significant percentage of cases, sometimes due to perceptual oversights—where abnormalities are simply not seen—and sometimes due to cognitive biases, where findings are misinterpreted or given incorrect weight. Such errors may result in missed diagnoses or false positives, both of which carry potentially serious consequences for patient care.Another key issue is inter- and intra-observer variability. (Ahmed et al., 2020)Different radiologists may interpret the same image in different ways, leading to inconsistent diagnoses. Even the same . This lack of standardization is particularly concerning in critical areas such as cancer detection, where the early identification of tumors significantly affects prognosis and treatment plans. Variability is also problematic in longitudinal imaging studies, where consistent measurement of lesion size or organ volume over time is essential for monitoring disease progression or therapeutic response.Furthermore, traditional medical imaging analysis relies heavily on visual assessment, which is inherently limited. Human vision is not optimized for detecting subtle changes in grayscale or contrast, especially in noisy or low-quality images. In conditions like early-stage lung cancer or microcalcifications in breast tissue, abnormalities may be too small or too subtle for even skilled radiologists to detect reliably (Anderson & Raine, 2018).

This data deluge can overwhelm even the most experienced professionals, leading to longer turnaround times and potential oversight of clinically significant findings. Moreover, the integration of imaging data with other clinical information—such as electronic health records (EHRs), pathology reports, and genomic data—requires sophisticated tools and expertise that traditional methods do not adequately support. Without automated systems to assist in data synthesis, clinicians may miss important correlations or patterns that could improve diagnosis and treatment strategies.care quality. The lack of access to standardized protocols and continuous professional training further widens the gap in diagnostic accuracy between high- and low-resource environments. This issue underscores the need for scalable, consistent, and automated solutions to support medical imaging workflows globally.Additionally, technical limitations of imaging equipment can affect the quality of images produced, which in turn impacts the reliability of interpretations. Older machines may generate lower-resolution images, and varying calibration settings between devices can result in inconsistent imaging outputs. These disparities make comparative analysis difficult, particularly when monitoring a patient's condition over time using images from different sources. The variability in imaging protocols across institutions also poses challenges for multi-center studies and collaborative care, where consistent data interpretation is vital.. Radiologists are trained to recognize patterns, but when confronted with unusual manifestations or overlapping features between diseases, misinterpretations can occur. This is especially true in complex conditions like autoimmune diseases, certain pediatric disorders, or rare cancers, where imaging signs may not follow typical textbook patterns.Finally, communication barriers between radiologists and referring physicians can also impact the utility of imaging studies. Traditional reporting methods, often consisting of narrative text, may lack the precision or clarity needed for optimal clinical decision-making. Misunderstandings about findings(Chowdhury & Link, 2022a), lack of standardized reporting terminology, and limited opportunities for interactive discussion can lead to discrepancies in patient management.

## INTRODUCTION TO AI-POWERED MEDICAL IMAGING

While effective for certain tasks, this approach can be limited by the quality and completeness of the selected features. Nevertheless, ML models have been successfully applied in various imaging modalities. For instance,(Chowdhury & Link, 2022b) ML techniques have been used to detect diabetic retinopathy in retinal fundus images, classify breast lesions in mammography, and identify lung nodules in chest X-rays. These applications have shown that even relatively simple AI models can significantly enhance diagnostic performance when combined with expert input and high-quality data.However, the real breakthrough in AI-powered medical imaging has come with the advent of brain tumors in MRI scans, and identifying metastatic breast cancer in lymph node histopathology slides. used in cancer screening—for example, classifying mammograms as benign or malignant, or distinguishing between different types of brain tumors. Another vital area is image segmentation, which involves delineating anatomical structures or pathological regions within an image. Segmentation is crucial for treatment planning in radiation therapy, surgical navigation, and volumetric analysis of disease progression(Flower, 2012). Deep learning models, such as U-Net and its variants, have been particularly successful in this domain, enabling precise, automated contouring of organs and lesions with minimal human intervention.Object detection is another critical application, especially in emergency settings, where rapid identification of anomalies like fractures, hemorrhages, or pulmonary embolisms is essential. AI models trained on large, annotated datasets can quickly highlight suspicious areas, in modalities like CT or PET, where radiation exposure is a concern. These capabilities not only improve diagnostic confidence but also facilitate safer imaging practices.Grad-CAM, and feature attribution methods—that provide visual or quantitative explanations of model outputs. These tools help clinicians validate AI results and increase confidence in adopting AI-driven recommendations.influence high-stakes medical decisions. Regulatory bodies like the FDA and the European Medicines Agency (EMA) are actively working on frameworks for the approval and monitoring of AI-based medical devices.

## IMAGE CLASSIFICATION WITH AI: TUMOR DETECTION AND DISEASE DIAGNOSIS

Image classification using enabling the automated identification and categorization of disease-related patterns within complex visual data. At its core, image classification involves assigning a label to an image—or specific regions within an image—based on learned features, such as normal versus abnormal tissue, benign versus malignant lesions, or the presence or absence of disease. Powered by advances in machine learning (ML) and especially deep learning (DL), CT scans, MRIs, ultrasound, and digital pathology.A particularly impactful application of AI image classification is (Gore, 2020)in tumor detection and characterization. Tumors often present subtle, c exceptional capabilities in learning hierarchical representations of tumor features—such as shape, texture, margin, and intensity variations—from large datasets. For example, in mammography, CNNs have been trained to detect early-stage breast cancer by identifying microcalcifications and suspicious masses with high sensitivity and specificity, sometimes outperforming experienced radiologists. Similarly, in lung cancer screening, t due to fatigue or cognitive bias.AI-driven classification is also being extensively used in brain tumor analysis using MRI. Differentiating between tumor types such as gliomas, meningiomas, or metastases is a complex task due to overlapping imaging ResNet and DenseNet have been applied to classify low-grade versus high-grade gliomas, assisting in prognosis and treatment planning. In some studies, theseto provide non-invasive insights into tumor biology. Beyond oncology, AI image classification is making significant strides in systemic disease diagnosis, Google's DeepMind and IDx-DR have achieved FDA approval, validating their clinical utility and paving the way for scalable screening programs, especially in under-resourced settings. These models can categorize retinal images into severity grades, enabling early intervention and preventing vision loss.(Harris, 2023)In dermatology, image classification models are used to detect skin cancers, including melanoma, by analyzing dermoscopic images.

CNNs trained on large datasets of skin lesions have matched or surpassed dermatologists in identifying malignancies. Mobile applications incorporating AI can now allow users to capture images of skin lesions for preliminary analysis, promoting early self-screening and timely dermatological referrals. In gastroenterology, AI has been used to classify polyps detected during colonoscopy as adenomatous or hyperplastic in real-time, assisting gastroenterologists in making immediate treatment decisions.The effectiveness of AI in image classification hinges on high-quality annotated datasets, which provide the ground truth required for model training. Publicly available datasets like ImageNet (for general training), LIDC-IDRI (lung nodules), BraTS (brain tumors), and HAM10000 (skin lesions) have accelerated research and enabled cross-comparison of algorithms. However, the variability in imaging equipment, acquisition protocols, and patient populations can lead to model bias and generalization issues. To mitigate This is particularly useful in complex clinical cases where multiple pathologies may coexist. For example, in chest X-rays, a single scan may reveal signs of pneumonia, cardiomegaly, and pleural effusion simultaneously. (Hazarika, 2020)Models trained using datasets like CheXpert and NIH ChestX-ray14 have demonstrated proficiency in identifying multiple thoracic diseases concurrently, which is a significant leap from traditional single-diagnosis models.due to their opaque decision-making processes. To address this, explainable AI (XAI) techniques have been developed.

## OBJECT DETECTION AND SEGMENTATION WITH AI: LESION DETECTION AND ANATOMICAL STRUCTURE IDENTIFICATION

These AI-driven approaches are revolutionizing radiology, pathology, cardiology, and other domains by supporting automated diagnosis, enhancing image-guided interventions, and enabling more personalized treatment planning.Object detection in medical imaging refers to the task of locating and classifying multiple regions of interest within an image, typically by drawing bounding boxes around the targets. This is essential in numerous applications, including identifying lesions, tumors, fractures, or foreign bodies in a scan.(Kannelønning, 2024) Traditional object detection required manual annotation and visual inspection by experts, which is time-consuming and prone to variability. AI models can detect pulmonary nodules in chest CT scans, intracranial hemorrhages in brain CTs, or polyps in colonoscopy images with high sensitivity, acting as a second reader for radiologists and endoscopists.Beyond detection, segmentation takes the process a step further by precisely outlining the boundaries of the detected object at the pixel level. In medical imaging, segmentation is indispensable for tasks that require accurate shape and volume measurements, such as tumor grading, surgical planning, and radiation therapy. Segmentation can be either semantic (labeling each pixel of an image based on the class of object, (Kendall et al., 2007)e.g., tumor vs. background) or instance-based (differentiating between multiple objects of the same class, e.g., several tumors in a liver scan). Deep learning models such as U-Net, V-Net, and Mask R-CNN have become the gold standard in medical image segmentation due to their ability to preserve spatial information and generate fine-grained segmentations. A critical application of AI-powered object detection and segmentation is lesion detection across various imaging modalities. Lesions may be subtle, irregular, or vary significantly in size and shape, posing challenges for conventional methods. AI models trained on annotated datasets can identify and segment lesions with high accuracy, even in complex and noisy environments. In liver imaging, for example, segmentation algorithms help in delineating hepatocellular carcinoma from surrounding tissues in CT and MRI scans, aiding in staging and treatment planning. In breast imaging,(Laal, 2013) AI systems detect and segment calcifications and masses in mammograms or ultrasound, helping to classify lesions as benign or malignant. These automated tools not only support radiologists in early detection but also allow for quantitative assessment of lesion size, growth rate, and morphological changes over time. modeling. Accurate segmentation of structures like the heart, lungs, liver, kidneys, and blood vessels provides essential information for diagnosis and treatment. In cardiac imaging, segmentation models delineate the left ventricle, right ventricle, and myocardium in echocardiography or MRI, facilitating the assessment of ejection fraction, wall motion abnormalities, and myocardial perfusion. In lung imaging, segmentation helps quantify emphysema, detect fibrosis, and differentiate between lobes for precise radiological reporting. AI-driven segmentation of blood vessels in CT angiography assists in identifying aneurysms, stenosis, or blockages, often outperforming manual tracing in terms of speed and reproducibilityA significant benefit of AI-driven object detection and segmentation is the ability to generate quantitative data that can be tracked over time.

This is especially relevant in oncology, where monitoring tumor response to therapy requires consistent measurements across multiple time points. Manual segmentation is not only labor-intensive but also subject to inter-observer variability, making AI tools invaluable in providing standardized, repeatable results. Moreover, in radiation therapy, precise segmentation of tumors and organs-at-risk (OARs) ensures that therapeutic doses are accurately targeted, minimizing damage to healthy tissue. AI models have accelerated this process by providing high-quality auto-segmentations that require minimal corrections by Another concern is the interpretability and trustworthiness of AI-generated segmentations. Clinicians must understand and trust the outputs before integrating them into practice. Tools like overlay visualizations, confidence maps, and explanation algorithms such as Grad-CAM help bridge this gap by showing the regions the model focused on during decision-making. Additionally, human-in-the-loop systems, where clinicians review and validate AI results, are becoming increasingly popular to ensure quality control while benefiting from AI's speed and consistency.Clinical integration of object detection and segmentation AI tools is progressing steadily. Many commercial systems now incorporate AI-driven modules into Picture Archiving and Communication Systems (PACS), allowing real-time analysis and flagging of abnormalities. AI is also being used in intraoperative settings, such as during laparoscopic surgery, where real-time segmentation of organs and critical structures can guide surgeons and reduce complications. In robot-assisted surgery, AI helps in mapping anatomical boundaries and enhancing visualization, supporting more precise interventions(Mayo et al., 2020).The potential for 3D reconstruction and augmented reality (AR) using

AI segmentation further expands the horizon. Segmented anatomical models can be rendered in three dimensions and used for surgical simulation, patient education, and preoperative planning. For example, segmented liver and vascular structures can be visualized in 3D to plan resection margins or assess surgical feasibility. AR applications overlay these segmentations on the patient in real time, guiding interventions with unprecedented precision. address many of the limitations of manual analysis, such as variability, time constraints, and human fatigue, while providing high-resolution, quantitative insights that support clinical decision-making. As these tools become more robust, interpretable, and seamlessly integrated into healthcare systems, their impact on diagnosis, treatment, and surgical planning will continue to grow. However, the successful to transform medicine, delivering more precise, efficient, and personalized care across the patient journey.

## IMAGE REGISTRATION AND FUSION WITH AI: MULTIMODAL IMAGE ANALYSIS AND REGISTRATION

Image registration and fusion are vital processes in medical imaging that aim to align and integrate data from multiple imaging modalities, time points, or viewpoints into a single, coherent framework. These techniques are essential for accurate diagnosis, treatment planning, and disease monitoring, especially (DL)—the field has seen a significant transformation. AI-based methods are now capable of performing registration and fusion with higher accuracy, speed, and adaptability, facilitating a wide range of clinical applications including multimodal image analysis,(Lartey et al., 2023) longitudinal studies, surgical guidance, and radiotherapy planning. or regions are spatially matched. This is critical in scenarios such as comparing pre- and post-treatment scans, integrating functional and anatomical data, or tracking disease progression over time. Image registration can be rigid (involving translations and rotations) or non-rigid/deformable (involving local warping to accommodate anatomical changes). Traditional algorithms for registration rely on optimization techniques that minimize intensity differences or maximize similarity measures like mutual information or cross-correlation.(McGinnis et al., 2013) While effective, these methods are computationally intensive and may struggle with large deformations, intensity inconsistencies, or multi-organ alignment.AI has greatly enhanced the capabilities of image registration by automating and optimizing the alignment process. Deep learning, in particular,dense deformation fields that warp moving images to align with fixed reference images. Once trained, such models can perform registration in real time, offering dramatic improvements in speed and consistency. These models are also inherently more robust to image noise, artifacts, and anatomical variations, making them suitable for clinical applications where image quality may vary significantly across patients or modalities CT provides excellent bone detail, MRI offers superior soft tissue contrast, and PET reveals metabolic activity.

Combining these complementary datasets through accurate registration enables clinicians to localize lesions with greater precision, correlate structural and functional abnormalities, and improve diagnostic confidence. For instance, in oncology, registering PET scans with CT or MRI helps identify metabolically active tumor regions within anatomical boundaries, supporting accurate biopsy targeting or radiation dose planning. In neurology, aligning functional MRI (fMRI) with structural MRI enhances the mapping of brain activity to specific cortical regions, aiding in epilepsy surgery or brain tumor resection.AI models have proven particularly effective in cross-modality registration, which is inherently more challenging than mono-modality registration due to differing image contrasts and spatial resolutions. Traditional similarity metrics often fail in such cases, but AI can learn modality-invariant features that capture structural correspondences regardless of intensity differences. to synthesize one modality from another, facilitating easier alignment by transforming the problem into a mono-modality registration task.eyond diagnostic applications, AI-based registration and fusion play a pivotal role in image-guided interventions and surgical navigation. In procedures such as neurosurgery, orthopedics, or liver transplantation, preoperative imaging (like MRI or CT) is registered with intraoperative data (like ultrasound or optical imaging) to guide the surgeon in real time. Accurate registration ensures that surgical tools are correctly aligned with patient anatomy, minimizing risk to critical structures and enhancing precision. AI enhances this process by enabling fast, deformable registration that can adapt to intraoperative changes, such as tissue shifts due to breathing, swelling, or resection. Augmented reality (AR) systems further leverage these AI-driven registrations to overlay anatomical and pathological information directly onto the surgical field, providing a comprehensive, intuitive view for the operator.Another crucial domain benefiting from AI-powered registration is radiotherapy planning, where accurate alignment of multimodal scans is essential to define tumor boundaries and organs at risk (OARs). AI models support the registration of simulation CT with planning MRI or PET scans, ensuring precise targeting of the tumor while minimizing radiation exposure to healthy tissue. Furthermore, AI-assisted registration enables adaptive radiotherapy, where treatment plans are updated based on daily imaging to account for anatomical changes over time.In longitudinal studies, where imaging data is collected from the same patient across multiple time points, registration is essential to assess disease progression or treatment response. AI helps automate this process by learning temporal consistency patterns, ensuring that corresponding anatomical points are accurately matched across scans. This is particularly valuable in neurodegenerative diseases like Alzheimer's, where subtle atrophic changes must be tracked over years, or in oncology, where volumetric tumor changes can inform therapy effectiveness.

## COMPUTER-AIDED DETECTION (CAD) SYSTEMS: APPLICATIONS AND BENEFITS IN MEDICAL IMAGING

CAD systems do not aim to replace clinicians but to support them by providing supplementary information that may confirm or question the initial findings, leading to more confident and consistent clinical decisions. Over (DL) techniques, significantly expanding their utility and reliability in clinical practice.Initially, CAD systems were developed using handcrafted features and traditional pattern recognition techniques. These early systems relied heavily on image preprocessing, segmentation, and manually defined rules to identify suspicious patterns such as nodules, calcifications, or masses. While useful, these systems often suffered from limited generalizability feature learning and robust pattern recognition from large-scale medical image datasets. (Madgule et al., 2023)Modern AI-based CAD systems are now capable of achieving human-comparable or even superior performance in various diagnostic tasks, leading to their growing adoption in radiology departments worldwide. for being challenging to interpret due to the subtle nature of early-stage tumors and the presence of dense breast tissue. CAD systems for mammography assist radiologists (FDA) has approved several CAD systems for mammography, and they are commonly used in screening programs across many countries. Moreover, with the advent of digital breast tomosynthesis (DBT)—a 3D imaging modality—AI-enhanced CAD systems have become even more critical, helping to manage the vast number of image slices and detect cancers that might be missed in 2D views.CAD systems are also extensively used in lung cancer detection, especially through analysis of chest radiographs and computed tomography (CT) scans. In chest X-rays, CAD can identify pulmonary nodules, which are early indicators of potential malignancies. In lung CT scans, which provide a more detailed view, AI-based CAD systems can detect and characterize nodules based on size, shape, and density. These systems aid in differentiating between benign and malignant lesions, reducing unnecessary biopsies and guiding clinical follow-up.

The success of CAD in lung cancer detection has been further underscored by its integration into low-dose CT screening programs, particularly for high-risk populations such as heavy smokers, where early detection significantly improves survival ratesr CT colonography. These systems analyze 3D images of the colon to detect polyps and other precancerous lesions. CAD can help radiologists by identifying regions of interest and reducing the time needed for image interpretation, which is particularly (Najjar, 2023)valuable in large-scale screening programs.

AI-enhanced CAD has also been used during real-time colonoscopy procedures, where it assists gastroenterologists in detecting polyps that may be missed during manual inspection. Real-time CAD, combined with high-definition endoscopy, has been shown to increase polyp detection rates and improve diagnostic accuracy, thereby reducing the incidence of interval cancers. and Parkinson's disease. In brain MRI, CAD tools can assist in identifying atrophy patterns, white matter lesions, or structural abnormalities associated with dementia and multiple sclerosis.detect infarcts or hemorrhages in brain CT scans, facilitating timely decision-making and improving patient outcomes through quicker initiation of treatment like thrombolysis or thrombectomy.Another important area where CAD systems are being actively employed is musculoskeletal imaging. Radiographs, MRI, and CT scans of joints, bones, and soft tissues are frequently analyzed by CAD systems to detect fractures, osteoarthritis, and degenerative disc diseases. For instance, in emergency departments, CAD tools can quickly identify wrist, hip, or vertebral fractures, supporting rapid triage and reducing diagnostic delays. In orthopedic surgery, CAD systems help in preoperative planning by providing precise measurements and identifying structural abnormalities. Similarly, in spinal imaging, CAD can detect intervertebral disc herniation, vertebral compression fractures, and spinal canal narrowing, which are critical for surgical planning and patient management.CAD systems are also making strides in ophthalmology. For example, in diabetic retinopathy screening, t-of-care screening that can refer high-risk patients for further evaluation and treatment. Similar CAD tools are being developed for age-related macular degeneration (AMD) and glaucoma, expanding their utility across a broad spectrum of ocular conditions.error. Fatigue, cognitive overload, and perceptual challenges can lead to missed diagnoses, particularly in high-volume environments like radiology. CAD systems act as a safety net by consistently reviewing every image and highlighting potential abnormalities, ensuring that critical findings are less likely to be overlooked. This consistency also helps reduce inter-observer variability, leading to more standardized interpretations across different clinicians and institutions.

## AI-POWERED DIAGNOSTIC DECISION SUPPORT SYSTEMS

DDSS powered by AI help alleviate this cognitive burden by rapidly aggregating patient-specific data and comparing it against vast medical knowledge bases and historical case data. The systems then generate diagnostic hypotheses, suggest possible conditions, propose next-step investigations, and even recommend evidence-based treatment options—all within seconds. This level of computational assistance can be particularly valuable in complex, high-pressure environments such as emergency departments, intensive care units, and primary care clinics. For example,

AI-based systems can detect early signs of sepsis, myocardial infarction, or acute kidney injury based on combinations of vitals, lab trends, and historical data long before symptoms become clinically apparent. In oncology, AI models can analyze molecular biomarkers, imaging results, and patient history to predict cancer risk or subtype classification, supporting early intervention strategies. In rare diseases, where diagnosis may be delayed for years due to non-specific symptoms, AI-powered DDSS can cross-reference patient profiles with databases of rare conditions to suggest potential matches that may not immediately come to mind for clinicians. Moreover, AI-driven DDSS support personalized medicine by integrating genomic data, lifestyle factors, and environmental exposures into diagnostic and therapeutic recommendations., advancing the shift from one-size-fits-all medicine to precision healthcare.In radiology and pathology, AI-powered DDSS enhance image interpretation by integrating findings with patient data and suggesting potential diagnoses. After AI algorithms detect and classify lesions or anomalies in imaging studies, DDSS platforms contextualize these findings nd then compute a malignancy risk score along with management recommendations in line with established guidelines. Similarly, in pathology, AI can analyze digitized slides for morphological patterns and link those findings to disease categories, improving diagnostic accuracy and consistency.Another key area of impact is clinical decision-making in uncertain or ambiguous cases.(OECD, 2023) In scenarios where symptoms overlap multiple conditions, AI-powered DDSS can help narrow down the list of possible diagnoses by applying probabilistic reasoning and Bayesian models. These systems evaluate the likelihood of each diagnosis based on the presence or absence of key findings and suggest the most appropriate diagnostic pathways to confirm or rule out potential conditions. This helps minimize unnecessary testing, reduce healthcare costs, and prevent diagnostic delays or errors.AI-powered DDSS also facilitate clinical triage and prioritization, especially in high-volume healthcare environments.

In emergency settings, these systems can automatically analyze presenting symptoms, initial vitals, and historical records to determine the urgency of a case and suggest priority levels. For instance, patients with subtle but life-threatening conditions like aortic dissection or pulmonary embolism can be flagged for immediate evaluation, ensuring timely and potentially life-saving intervention. In outpatient care, AI-powered scheduling systems can identify high-risk patients and prioritize appointments or follow-ups accordingly, thereby optimizing resource allocation and improving care continuity.One of the most transformative features of modern DDSS is the incorporation of natural language processing (NLP), which allows these systems to interpret unstructured clinical data such as physician notes, discharge summaries, and radiology reports. Furthermore, AI-powered DDSS contribute to medical education and decision support for less experienced clinicians. By providing evidence-based suggestions and justifications, these systems act as virtual mentors or clinical consultants, supporting learning and decision-making in real time. For example, a junior doctor unsure about a diagnostic workup can receive system-generated guidance aligned with clinical best practices. This democratization of including rural or underserved areas. decision trees, and rule-based explanations that highlight the most influential features or data points leading to a particular recommendation data diversity, ongoing model evaluation, and ethical oversight are essential to prevent systemic errors and promote equity. Moreover, integration with existing clinical workflows and electronic health systems is vital for real-world adoption. A DDSS must be seamlessly embedded into clinician workflows, offer actionable insights without overwhelming the user, and provide real-time support without causing delays or cognitive overload.

## IMAGE ANALYSIS AND QUANTIFICATION WITH AI: FEATURE EXTRACTION AND BIOMARKER DISCOVERY

Image analysis and quantification play a foundational role in modern medical imaging, enabling image interpretation. Furthermore, AI has opened new frontiers in quantitative imaging, facilitating biomarker discovery, disease characterization, and personalized treatment strategies through advanced feature extraction and image-based analysis pipelines. images. Traditional image analysis methods relied on hand-engineered features—metrics like edge sharpness, size, intensity histograms, and shape descriptors—which required domain expertise and were often limited in scope and generalizability.(Pagallo et al., 2023) AI has revolutionized this process by introducing automatic feature learning through deep neural networks. Convolutional Neural Networks (CNNs), for example, can process raw image data to learn hierarchical features, starting from low-level patterns (like edges and textures) to high-level semantic representations (such as tumor morphology or vascular structures). These automatically extracted features provide a richer, more nuanced understanding of medical images and are foundational to various diagnostic and prognostic models.classify tumors (e.g., benign vs. malignant) but also to stratify patients based on likely outcomes, response to therapy, or recurrence risk. For instance, radiomic analysis of lung CT scans can reveal textural patterns within a tumor that correlate with genetic mutations or immune activity—insights that are crucial for personalized oncology. In breast imaging,(Pakdemirli, 2019) AI can assess mammographic density, detect microcalcifications, and analyze tumor spiculation to provide accurate malignancy predictions. These imaging-derived features go beyond visual assessment, offering objective and reproducible biomarkers that support clinical decision-making.In neurological imaging, AI-based feature extraction has been instrumental in detecting and quantifying neurodegenerative changes. Algorithms can segment brain regions, measure cortical thickness, and assess white matter integrity using structural MRI and diffusion tensor imaging (DTI). Such features are vital in diagnosing conditions like stroke assessment, AI can delineate ischemic core and penumbra areas in perfusion imaging, providing essential insights for therapeutic decisions such as thrombectomy eligibility.AI has also enabled functional image analysis, especially in fields such as cardiology and nuclear medicine. In cardiac imaging, AI algorithms can quantify left ventricular volume, ejection fraction, myocardial strain, and wall motion abnormalities from echocardiograms or cardiac MRIs. These features are crucial for diagnosing heart failure, cardiomyopathies, and ischemic disease. In PET imaging, AI can analyze metabolic activity to assess tumor viability, organ perfusion, or brain function, enhancing the interpretation of functional imaging studies. The ability of AI to extract and track these quantitative parameters over time also supports longitudinal studies, disease monitoring, and therapy evaluation.

An exciting and rapidly advancing area within AI-powered image analysis is biomarker discovery. breast, prostate, and gliomas, with promising results in predicting treatment response, recurrence, and survival.Beyond radiomics, deep learning-based biomarkers are emerging as a powerful alternative, where the model itself learns complex feature representations that are not explicitly defined by humans. For example, DL models can be trained on imaging data along with clinical outcomes (e.g., survival, progression-free survival) and then learn to associate certain image patterns with these outcomes, effectively discovering novel biomarkers. In some cases, these biomarkers outperform traditional metrics or even expert radiologist assessments in predictive accuracy. Additionally, AI can integrate imaging biomarkers with non-imaging data—such as genomics, pathology, and clinical variables—through multimodal learning, leading to composite biomarkers that offer more holistic and accurate insights into disease behavior.AI-based quantification also enhances the reproducibility and objectivity of image interpretation, which is especially important in clinical trials and large-scale population studies. Manual measurement of features like lesion size, density, or contrast enhancement is subject to inter- and intra-observer variability. AI systems provide consistent, automated quantification that aligns with standardized protocols, ensuring reliability across multiple readers and institutions. This level of standardization is crucial for assessing therapeutic efficacy, regulatory approval, and post-market surveillance of medical treatments and devices.Another important application of AI in image quantification is monitoring treatment response. For example, in oncology, AI tools can automatically segment tumors in serial scans and track changes in volume, density, or radiomic features to assess whether a treatment is effective. This is particularly valuable in immunotherapy, where traditional size-based criteria (like RECIST) may not fully capture therapeutic benefit. AI can detect nuanced imaging changes that precede visible tumor shrinkage or correlate with immune activity, offering early indicators of response or resistance. models. Additionally, the interpretability of extracted features and biomarkers remains a focus of ongoing research. Clinicians must understand how and why a model reaches its conclusions, especially when it informs high-stakes decisions. (Panayides et al., 2020)Explainable AI (XAI) approaches—such as saliency maps, attention mechanisms, and feature importance rankings—are being integrated to make model outputs more transparent and clinically acceptable.

## AI IN CANCER IMAGING AND DIAGNOSIS: TUMOR DETECTION AND CHARACTERIZATION

Furthermore, AI tools can differentiate between benign and malignant nodules based on radiomic features, reducing false positives and helping clinicians decide which nodules warrant further investigation or biopsy.Beyond detection, tumor characterization is another domain where AI significantly enhances diagnostic capabilities. Tumor characterization involves assessing various properties such as size, shape, texture, vascularity, and enhancement patterns, which are essential for staging, treatment planning, and prognosis. AI-powered image analysis platforms can automatically segment tumors in three dimensions, extract quantitative features (known as radiomics), and analyze these features to infer biological and pathological attributes.(Rajpurkar & Lungren, 2023) For instance, in glioblastoma diagnosis, AI models trained on MRI scans can distinguish between tumor subregions—such as necrotic core, enhancing tumor, and peritumoral edema—and correlate imaging patterns with molecular markers like IDH mutation status or MGMT methylation, which influence prognosis and treatment response.Reporting and Data System) automatically, reducing interpretation variability and improving diagnostic consistency. In some cases, AI models have demonstrated comparable or superior performance to radiologists in detecting high-grade prostate tumors, which is particularly valuable in guiding biopsy decisions and focal therapies.AI also supports tumor characterization through radiogenomics, an emerging field that links imaging features with genetic and molecular tumor profiles. Using advanced learning algorithms, AI can uncover correlations between specific imaging patterns and gene expression signatures, enabling non-invasive prediction of molecular subtypes. In breast cancer, for example, AI has been used to predict hormone receptor status and HER2 expression from mammography or MRI features, potentially reducing the need for invasive biopsies in certain contexts. Radiogenomic models are also being explored in lung adenocarcinoma to predict EGFR mutations or ALK rearrangements, guiding targeted therapy selection. organs, quantify tumor burden, and track changes over time. These tools improve the reproducibility of assessments, support therapy monitoring, and help clinicians quickly identify progression or treatment resistance. In breast and prostate cancer, AI tools are particularly useful for assessing bone metastases, where manual evaluation can be time-consuming and challenging due to the subtle nature of skeletal lesions.AI tools can evaluate complex patterns of response—including changes in tumor texture, perfusion, or metabolic activity—that precede volumetric shrinkage. For example, in patients undergoing immunotherapy, tumors may initially enlarge due to immune cell infiltration (pseudoprogression) before shrinking.

AI models trained to recognize such patterns can help distinguish true progression from pseudoprogression, preventing premature discontinuation of effective treatments. information from each modality and fuse it into a unified representation that supports more accurate tumor classification. For instance, combining anatomical details from MRI with metabolic information from PET allows better delineation of tumor margins and assessment of aggressive behavior. Multimodal AI approaches are being explored in head and neck, brain, and gynecological cancers to support comprehensive diagnostic workflows.Despite the promising advances, implementing AI in cancer imaging and diagnosis comes with challenges.(Ramakrishnan et al., 2022) One of the most pressing concerns is data variability, including differences in imaging protocols, equipment vendors, scanner resolutions, and patient populations across institutions. AI models must be rigorously validated across diverse, multicenter datasets to feature-level insights to improve trust and transparency. imaging data, must also be addressed through secure data handling, de-identification protocols, and federated learning approaches that enable model training without data sharing.Another important aspect is clinical workflow integration.oncologists, but to augment their capabilities—providing decision support, highlighting critical findings, reducing diagnostic variability, and enhancing multidisciplinary collaboration across tumor boards. clinicians with advanced tools for tumor detection, characterization, classification, and monitoring. From early screening to advanced radiogenomics(Shamshad et al., 2023), AI systems offer higher precision, speed, and consistency in interpreting complex oncologic imaging data. As these tools become more accurate, explainable, and interoperable, their integration into clinical practice will further enhance personalized oncology care, improving early detection, guiding targeted therapies, and ultimately contributing to better patient outcomes in the fight against cancer.

## CASE STUDIES OF SUCCESSFUL AI-POWERED MEDICAL IMAGING IMPLEMENTATIONS: LESSONS LEARNED AND BEST PRACTICES

These real-life implementations not only showcase the capabilities of AI in automating and augmenting imaging tasks but also offer valuable insights into the challenges encountered during deployment and the strategies that contributed to success. Examining these case studies helps extract best practices and critical lessons that can guide future adoption across healthcare systems.One of the most widely cited success stories is the deployment of AI in breast cancer screening by the Karolinska Institute in Sweden. Faced with a growing demand for mammography screening and a shortage of radiologists, the institute adopted an AI-powered system to assist in mammogram interpretation. The AI algorithm was trained on hundreds of thousands of labeled mammograms and was capable of detecting microcalcifications, masses, and architectural distortions. In clinical trials and real-world use, the AI system demonstrated diagnostic performance comparable to experienced radiologists. Notably, it reduced radiologist workload by acting as a "second reader," flagging abnormal cases for closer inspection. The integration led to improved screening efficiency, reduced false positives, and faster patient turnaround. A key takeaway from this implementation was the importance of workflow integration—the AI tool was embedded directly into the radiologists' existing PACS environment, minimizing disruption and supporting a smooth transition to augmented reading.early detection and timely intervention. Validation studies showed that the AI achieved sensitivity and specificity on par with trained specialists. The initiative's success lay in its contextual deployment—it addressed a specific healthcare gap by extending screening capabilities to underserved areas. Moreover, the program emphasized user training and local adaptation, ensuring that clinicians and technicians understood how to use the system and interpret its results appropriately. The case underscores that successful AI implementation requires not just technical excellence but also attention to human factors and local clinical realities.In the United States, Stanford University developed and tested an AI model known as CheXNet to detect pneumonia from chest X-rays. Trained on a large dataset from the NIH ChestX-ray14 database, (Shen et al., 2021)CheXNet used a 121-layer convolutional neural network to outperform practicing radiologists in detecting pneumonia and other thoracic pathologies. Although it initially gained attention for its diagnostic power, a deeper lesson came during its pilot implementation: the model's lack of explainability created reluctance among clinicians to trust its output. In response, the team added visual explanation tools, such as saliency maps, that highlighted regions of interest influencing the model's predictions. This commitment to interpretability became a pivotal factor in its acceptance.

The Stanford case demonstrates the importance of transparency and explainability in clinical AI tools, as clinicians must trust and understand algorithmic outputs before relying on them in patient carAnother successful case comes from China, where hospitals implemented AI-based CT interpretation tools to assist with COVID-19 diagnosis during the pandemic. When overwhelmed by a surge in imaging volumes, radiology departments turned to AI systems that could rapidly assess chest(Sreenivasulu et al., 2022) CTs for COVID-related abnormalities. These tools provided severity scores, tracked disease progression, and flagged critical findings. The AI not only sped up reporting but also allowed physicians to monitor patients' response to treatment over time. The lesson from this scenario was the scalability and adaptability of AI in crisis situations. Fast deployment, cloud-based accessibility, and continuous model retraining with local data were crucial to ensuring relevance and performance under evolving clinical conditions. Moreover, the success of these systems highlighted the role of collaboration between hospitals, tech companies, and regulatory agencies to fast-track approvals and ensure safe, ethical deployment.In neurology, a notable case study involves the implementation of AI tools at the Mayo Clinic for stroke detection and triage. The AI system, known as Viz.ai, uses deep learning to analyze CT angiograms in real time to detect large vessel occlusions (LVOs) and notify stroke teams immediately. This AI-based alert system significantly reduced the time from imaging to intervention, helping ensure patients received timely thrombectomy when indicated. Studies showed improvements in treatment time metrics and patient outcomes. A critical lesson here is the value of real-time integration—AI added immediate clinical value by enabling rapid decision-making, rather than merely acting as a passive image analysis tool. The success was further supported by interdisciplinary collaboration, involving neurologists, radiologists, emergency physicians, and IT staff working together to align the tool's functionality with clinical workflows.In oncology, Memorial Sloan Kettering Cancer Center developed an AI tool for prostate cancer diagnosis using whole-slide pathology images. The model was trained to detect malignant regions in digitized histopathology slides with high accuracy. In clinical testing, the AI-assisted system helped pathologists identify cancer more consistently, especially in borderline or low-grade cases.

## CHALLENGES IN AI-POWERED MEDICAL IMAGING: DATA QUALITY AND MODEL INTERPRETABILITY

While Artificial Intelligence (AI) continues to demonstrate transformative potential in medical imaging, its implementation is not without significant challenges. As AI applications move from These challenges, among others, influence the development, validation, deployment, and acceptance of AI systems and have direct implications for patient care, clinical decision-making, and regulatory compliance, high-quality datasets is often difficult. Clinical imaging data is heterogeneous, varying in resolution, contrast, modality, acquisition protocol, patient demographics, disease prevalence, and scanner manufacturer. This lack of standardization introduces significant variability into training datasets and may limit the generalizability of AI models. For example, an algorithm trained on MRI data from a single institution may perform poorly when deployed in another hospital with different imaging hardware or protocols. Without carefully curated, diverse, and standardized datasets, models are at risk of becoming biased or brittle.Additionally, labeling medical imaging data requires expert radiologists, pathologists, or other specialists, which is both time-consuming and expensive. Annotation inconsistency, inter-observer variability, and incomplete labeling can further reduce dataset reliability. In some cases, labels may be inferred from electronic health record data or pathology reports, which may contain errors or ambiguitiesA related issue is the representation of rare diseases and edge cases. Most AI models perform best on the types of cases they were trained on, which often represent the most common pathologies. However, in real-world settings, clinicians frequently encounter rare or atypical cases. If such instances are under-represented or absent from the training data, the AI model may produce incorrect or misleading predictions, which could delay diagnosis or treatment.(Sugumaran et al., 2024) Ensuring that datasets are diverse and inclusive, including data from different populations, age groups, and disease presentations, is vital for developing robust and equitable AI systems. so through highly complex internal representations that are difficult for humans to understand or trace. For clinicians to trust and adopt AI tools, especially in high-stakes diagnostic scenarios, they need to understand how a model arrived at its decision. Lack of transparency in decision-making can erode confidence and hinder clinical integration focusing on medically relevant areas or being misled by artifacts or irrelevant features.

However, even XAI methods have limitations—they can be misleading, inconsistent, or oversimplified. Moreover, there is currently no standard for validating the reliability of these explanations, which can lead to further confusion or misuse. Another challenge tied to interpretability is accountability and trust. In scenarios where AI makes or assists in diagnostic decisions, questions arise: Who is responsible for errors made by the AI? How should AI decisions be weighed against human expertise? In the absence of transparency, clinicians may hesitate to rely on AI, or conversely, over-rely on AI decisions without appropriate oversight. Establishing clear guidelines for accountability and promoting a culture of human-AI collaboration, where AI augments rather than replaces human judgment, is essential for responsible integration.Beyond data and interpretability, regulatory and ethical issues form another layer of complexity. Most healthcare systems are governed by stringent regulatory frameworks that ensure safety and efficacy before any medical device or diagnostic tool can be used on patients. alability.and external validation across diverse populations. Fairness metrics, bias mitigation techniques, and inclusive development practices are being incorporated into newer AI frameworks, but ensuring true equity remains an ongoing challenge.Integration into clinical workflow also poses a significant hurdle. Even well-performing AI tools can fail if they disrupt established routines or require clinicians to learn new systems. Resistance to change, lack of time for training, or insufficient IT infrastructure can impede successful adoption. AI tools must be user-friendly, fast, and interoperable with existing systems such as PACS, RIS, and EHRs. Importantly, they should provide actionable insights rather than just additional information, helping clinicians make better decisions without increasing cognitive load. Collaborating with end users throughout the development process, from interface design to usability testing, ensures that AI tools meet real-world needs and are more likely to be embraced.

## OPPORTUNITIES FOR AI IN MEDICAL IMAGING: IMPROVED DIAGNOSTIC ACCURACY AND PATIENT OUTCOMES

The ability of AI to identify subtle patterns in medical images, often invisible to the human eye, offers profound benefits. Early detection of conditions such as cancer (including lung, breast, and prostate cancer) and neurological disorders (such as Alzheimer's and stroke) can drastically improve treatment outcomes. For instance, AI algorithms used in oncology can assist in detecting microcalcifications and irregularities in tumor structure at an early stage, leading to earlier intervention. In the case of neuroimaging, AI tools can identify even slight changes in brain structures that might signal early-onset neurological diseases, facilitating earlier and more accurate diagnoses. (Vijayakumar et al., 2024)The earlier diseases are detected, the more effective treatments can be, reducing morbidity and improving overall survival rates.Enhancing diagnostic consistency is another significant opportunity that AI provides. Human error, especially fatigue and variability among clinicians, can contribute to inconsistent diagnoses. AI systems offer a level of consistency by applying the same criteria to every image, removing the subjective variation that often occurs among different radiologists or practitioners. Moreover, AI can act as a “second reader” for medical images, providing an additional layer of review. This dual-check approach has been shown to improve diagnostic accuracy, particularly in high-volume settings, where radiologists may be overwhelmed with the number of images they need to interpret. The use of AI as a second reader reduces the likelihood of missed diagnoses, enhancing overall quality control within healthcare institutions. of a disease, allowing for more tailored treatment plans.

For instance, in oncology, AI-driven imaging techniques can help determine whether a tumor is benign or malignant, the exact stage of cancer, and its likely response to specific treatments, facilitating more precise interventions. AI’s ability to analyze large volumes of data—combining imaging, genomics, and patient history—opens the door to personalized treatment strategies that are more effective and less invasive, improving patient outcomes and minimizing the risks of overtreatmentinterest in images, highlight abnormalities, and even generate preliminary reports, accelerating the workflow and reducing bottlenecks in diagnostic processes. For example, AI-powered systems used in chest X-ray analysis or CT scans can flag abnormal areas for immediate attention, allowing radiologists to prioritize critical cases. Faster processing times enable quicker diagnoses, facilitating early treatment interventions and improving patient prognosis scans with functional data from fMRI or PET scans, providing more insights into both the anatomical and functional aspects of neurological disorders. This multidimensional approach can greatly enhance the accuracy and depth of diagnostic assessments, ultimately leading to more informed clinical decisions.and better patient management. These predictive capabilities can be used not only to improve outcomes for individual patients but also to optimize population health management strategies.improving the efficiency of medical imaging workflows, reducing the need for unnecessary tests or procedures, and minimizing diagnostic errors, AI can reduce healthcare spending while maintaining or improving care quality.ms. be user-friendly and requiring minimal training, can be utilized by clinicians with varying levels of experience. In resource-constrained settings, AI can enable early disease detection, improving healthcare outcomes in underserved populations and reducing disparities in access to high-quality medical care. learning, can be applied to update models with real-world clinical data while maintaining patient privacy, making the AI more robust and reliable with each use. As more data is collected, AI systems can fine-tune their predictions, becoming increasingly accurate and effective in real-world setting

## FUTURE DIRECTIONS FOR AI IN MEDICAL IMAGING: EMERGING TRENDS AND TECHNOLOGIES

Another key area for the future of AI in medical imaging is the application of real-time image analysis and decision support. Traditionally, medical imaging has been a retrospective process, where clinicians analyze images after they are acquired. However, AI has the potential to enable real-time, on-the-fly analysis of medical images as they are captured. This could dramatically speed up the diagnostic process, allowing clinicians to make instant decisions during procedures such as surgeries, biopsies, or interventional radiology. For example, AI tools integrated into imaging equipment, such as CT scanners or MRIs, could provide immediate feedback to clinicians on potential abnormalities, guiding them toward optimal clinical decisions while the patient is still on the table. This real-time analysis could also assist in image-guided interventions, where AI can help refine the navigation of medical instruments, increasing accuracy and reducing the risk of complications. AI could use imaging data to predict the likelihood of metastasis or recurrence of tumors, helping clinicians tailor individualized treatment plans. Similarly, in cardiology, AI could analyze imaging data to predict heart failure risk, guiding early interventions and preventive care. The a decision support tool rather than a replacement for their expertise. This collaborative approach, where AI aids clinicians in understanding complex data and making informed decisions, will be essential for ensuring safe and effective implementation of AI in medical imaging.Federated learning and privacy-preserving AI are also poised to play a significant role in the future of medical enabling collaboration across institutions while safeguarding patient confidentiality and privacy.(World Health Organization, 2021) As data privacy concerns remain central to healthcare, the ability to build effective, scalable AI systems while preserving patient rights will be crucial for the widespread adoption of AI.Additionally, This integration could also support clinical decision support systems (CDSS), where AI algorithms assist in generating differential diagnoses, suggesting treatment options, or identifying potential drug interactions, enhancing decision-making at every stage of patient care.This automation could reduce scan times, lower the burden on technicians, and ultimately improve the overall efficiency of medical imaging departments. Furthermore, it could allow radiologists to focus more on interpretation and decision-making rather than the technical aspects of image acquisition.In addition to enhancing the accuracy of medical imaging, the personalized care enabled by AI offers tremendous potential. treatment plans based on a patient's unique condition, genetics, and imaging profile.

## CONCLUSION

The rise of AI in medical imaging represents a shift from traditional methods to innovative, data-driven approaches that promise not only enhanced diagnostic accuracy but also greater efficiencies, cost reductions, and, most importantly, improved patient outcomes. takeaways from this exploration is AI's ability to significantly enhance diagnostic accuracy. Medical imaging has always been a cornerstone of disease detection and management, yet human error, variability in interpretation, and high workloads have posed challenges for radiologists. AI models, especially eye, leading to more accurate and earlier detection of diseases such as cancer, cardiovascular conditions, and neurological disorders. Furthermore, AI's ability to learn from vast datasets allows it to improve over time, continuously refining its ability to assist radiologists in making precise diagnoses and treatment decisions. Another key takeaway is the profound impact AI has on workflow efficiency and automation in medical imaging. AI is not just augmenting the decision-making capabilities of clinicians but is also streamlining many of the time-consuming and repetitive tasks associated with image acquisition, processing, and interpretation. Tasks such as image pre-processing, segmentation, and post-processing can be automated with can lead to better resource allocation, reduced turnaround times for diagnoses, and lower healthcare costs in the long term. represent a significant leap forward in how clinicians can anticipate and address patient needstypes of data, along with the power of AI to interpret complex patterns across different modalities, represents a significant step forward in the development of personalized medicine. Furthermore, the collaboration between AI and human radiologists is critical to its success and implementation in more informed, evidence-based decisions while enhancing their diagnostic capabilities.AI-driven medical imaging systems can be deployed in remote locations, where they can be accessed via cloud platforms or portable imaging devices, democratizing access to high-quality diagnostic tools. As AI technologies become more affordable and accessible, they have the potential to reduce disparities in healthcare access, ensuring that patients in even the most resource-limited areas receive the best possible care. closely monitored to ensure that AI applications do not inadvertently exacerbate healthcare inequities or compromise patient confidentiality.Another challenge is the adoption and training required for AI systems to be fully integrated into the radiology workflow. Radiologists must be trained not only to interpret AI-generated findings but also to understand the strengths and limitations of the AI models they work with. This involves a shift in how radiologists view their role, from simply interpreting images to becoming key players in managing AI-driven diagnostic workflows. Hospitals and healthcare institutions must invest in training programs and infrastructure that support the

## REFERENCES


Agboklu, M. (2024). The impact of Artificial Intelligence on innovative nanotechnologies for Advanced Medical diagnosis. *Journal of Nanotechnology Research*, *6*, 1–5.

Agboklu, M., Adrah, F. A., & Agbenyo, P. M. (2024). Hope Nyavor. From bits to atoms: Machine learning and nanotechnology for Cancer Therapy. *Journal of Nanotechnology Research*, *6*, 16–26.

Ahmed, Z., Mohamed, K., Zeeshan, S., & Dong, X. (2020). Artificial Intelligence with Multi-functional Machine Learning Platform Development for Better Healthcare and Precision Medicine. *Database : The Journal of Biological Databases and Curation*, *2020*, baaa010. PMID: 32185396

Anderson, J., & Raine, L. (2018). Artificial intelligence and the future of humans. Pew Research Center. https://www.pewresearch.org/internet/2018/12/10/artificial-intelligence-and-the-future-of-humans/

Chowdhury, F., & Link, A. N. (2022a). Public Support for Research in Artificial Intelligence: A descriptive study of U.S. Department of Defense SBIR projects. [van.]. *The Journal of Technology Transfer*, *47*, 762–774.

Chowdhury, F., & Link, A. N. (2022b). The spatial distribution of public support for AI research. [van.]. *Science & Public Policy*, *49*, 573–579.

Flower, M. A. (2012). *Webb's physics of Medical Imaging*. CRC.

Gore, J. C. (2020). Artificial Intelligence in Medical Imaging. *Magnetic Resonance Imaging*, *68*, A1–A4. PMID: 31857130

Harris, L. A. (2023). Artificial Intelligence: Overview, Recent Advances, and Considerations for the 118th Congress, https://crsreports.congress.gov

Hazarika, I. (2020). Artificial Intelligence: Opportunities and implications for the Health workforce. *International Health*, *12*, 241–245. PMID: 32300794

Kannelønning, M. S. (2024). Navigating uncertainties of introducing Artificial Intelligence (AI) in Healthcare: The role of a Norwegian network of professionals. *Technology in Society*, *76*, 102432.

Kendall, J. L., Hoffenberg, S. R., & Smith, R. S. (2007). History of emergency and critical care Ultrasound: The evolution of a New Imaging paradigm. *Critical Care Medicine*, *35*, S126–S130. PMID: 17446770

Laal, M. (2013). Innovation process in Medical Imaging. *Procedia: Social and Behavioral Sciences*, *81*, 60–64.

Lartey, B., Adrah, K., Adrah, F., & Isichei, J. (2023). Application of Machine Learning for Predicting the occurrence of Nephropathy in Diabetic patients. *International Journal of Computer Applications*, *975*, 8887.

Mayo, R. C., Sen, L. Q. C., & Leung, J. W. (2020). Financing Artificial Intelligence in Medical Imaging: Show me the money. *Journal of the American College of Radiology*, *17*, 175–177. PMID: 31918877

McGinnis, J. M., Stuckhardt, L., Saunders, R., & Smith, M. (2013). *Best care at lower cost: The path to Continuously Learning Health Care in America*. National Academy.

Najjar, R. (2023). Redefining Radiology: A review of Artificial Intelligence Integration in Medical Imaging. *Diagnostics (Basel)*, *13*, 2760. PMID: 37685300

OECD. (2023). OECD Employment Outlook 2023. https://www.oecd-ilibrary.org/content/publication/08785bba-en

Pagallo, U., O'Sullivan, S., Nevejans, N., Holzinger, A., Friebe, M., Jeanquartie, F., Jean-Quartier, C., & Miernik, A. (2023). The underuse of AI in the Health Sector: Opportunity costs, success stories, risks and recommendations. *Health and Technology*. Advance online publication. DOI: 10.1007/s12553-023-00806-7 PMID: 38229886

Pakdemirli, E. (2019). New Subspecialty or Close Ally emerging on the Radiology Horizon: Artificial Intelligence. *Acta Radiologica Open*, *8*, 2058460119837498. PMID: 30923633

Panayides, A. S., Amini, A., Filipovic, N. D., Sharma, A., Tsaftaris, S. A., Young, A., Foran, D., Do, N., Golemati, S., & Kurc, T. (2020). AI in Medical Imaging Informatics: Current challenges and future directions. *IEEE Journal of Biomedical and Health Informatics*, *24*, 1837–1857. PMID: 32609615

Rajpurkar, P., & Lungren, M. P. (2023). The current and future state of AI interpretation of medical images. *The New England Journal of Medicine*, *388*, 1981–1990. PMID: 37224199

Ramakrishnan, T., Mohan Gift, M. D., Chitradevi, S., Jegan, R., & Subha Hency Jose, P. Nagaraja, Rajneesh Sharma H.N., Selvakumar P., Sintayehu Mekuria Hailegiorgis, (2022). "Study of Numerous Resins Used in Polymer Matrix Composite Materials", Advances in Materials Science and Engineering, vol. 2022, Article ID 1088926, 8 pages, 2022. https://doi.org/DOI: 10.1155/2022/1088926

Shamshad, F., Khan, S., Zamir, S. W., Khan, M. H., Hayat, M., Khan, F. S., & Fu, H. (2023). Transformers in medical imaging: A survey. *Medical Image Analysis*, *88*, 102802. DOI: 10.1016/j.media.2023.102802 PMID: 37315483

Shen, Y. T., Chen, L., Yue, W. W., & Xu, H. X. (2021). Artificial intelligence in ultrasound. *European Journal of Radiology*, *139*, 109717. PMID: 33962110

Sreenivasulu, A., & Manimozhi, T. Satheesh kumar P., Selvakumar P. and Singh P. (2022). "The Model of Smart Sensing Device For Sensitive Nanoclusters Modification in Sensing Properties," 2022 2nd International Conference on Advance Computing and Innovative Technologies in Engineering (ICACITE), Greater Noida, India, 2022, pp. 1043-1047, doi: DOI: 10.1109/ICACITE53722.2022.9823846

Sugumaran, K. M. D., Pandiyarajan V., Y. B S, Selvakumar P. and M. S, (2024). "Analysis of Electromyography Signals for Control of Mechanical Prosthesis using Machine Learning Techniques," 2024 2nd International Conference on Intelligent Data Communication Technologies and Internet of Things (IDCIoT), Bengaluru, India, 2024, pp. 1059-1067, doi: DOI: 10.1109/IDCIoT59759.2024.10467707

Vijayakumar, G. (2024). Muniyandi Rajkumar, Rajiv Chandar N, Selvakumar P and Ramesh Duraisamy, (2024). Environmentally friendly TDS removal from waste water by electrochemical ion exchange batch-type recirculation (EIR) technique. *Environmental Science. Water Research & Technology*, *10*, 826–835. DOI: 10.1039/D3EW00793F

World Health Organization. (2021). Ethics and Governance of Artificial Intelligence for Health: WHO Guidance, Geneva.

Chapter 9

# AI-Driven Clinical Decision Support Systems Enhancing Decision-Making in Modern Healthcare

**Vikas Sharma**
https://orcid.org/0000-0001-8173-4548
*SRM Institute of Science and Technology, Delhi, India*

**Tarun Kumar Vashishth**
https://orcid.org/0000-0001-9916-9575
*IIMT Univeristy, Meerut, India*

**Renu Kumar**
*IIMT Engineering College, Meerut, India*

**Sanjukta Vidyant**
*Shobhit University, Meerut, India*

**Asheesh Pandey**
*ABES Engineering College, Ghaziabad, India*

**Barkha Samania**
https://orcid.org/0009-0006-7824-1658
*SRM Institute of Science and Technology, Delhi, India*

## ABSTRACT

*The incorporation of AI into clinical CDSS enables real-time insights which can be acted upon, thus improving the quality of care provided to the patients. The architecture as well as the features and development methods of CDSS focusing on machine learning and natural language processing as well as other predictive analytics capabilities are analysed. It discusses relevant cases that allow performing medical diagnosis and prescription of medicines so as to mitigate automation-enabled medical negligence and malpractice. Also, it addresses concerns with integration of*

DOI: 10.4018/979-8-3373-3311-3.ch009

*AI into clinical workflows such as data silos, clinician gatekeeping, social contexts, and legal contexts. With the use of case studies, this chapter illustrates the effect of AI tools on CDSS by showing the improvement in the heightened healthcare opportunities that are readily available after the use of AI, as well as the provision of individualized treatment meant for specific unique patients due to the flexible nature offered by AI.*

## 1. INTRODUCTION

The introduction of Clinical Decision Support Systems (CDSS) has revolutionized healthcare in the 21st century due to sophisticated functions directly engineered to aid a healthcare worker in making clinical decisions. These systems employ intricate algorithms to retrieve pertinent medical information and provide suggestions that enhance the accuracy, efficiency, and overall quality of care administered to patients (Vashishth et al., 2024). Bringing together Artificial Intelligence (AI) technologies with CDSS has further advanced these systems due to the ability to analyze large datasets in real time, reveal underlying patterns, and provide specific recommendations. AI integrated CDSS can offer aid in various aspects of clinical activities including but not limited to diagnosing, treatment designing, and risk evaluation which lightens the responsibility of clinicians while improving patient outcomes. Given the intricate nature and overwhelming volume of information within health systems, the demand for such adaptive and intelligent tools is exceedingly high. This chapter examines how AI technologies such as machine learning, natural language processes, and predictive analytics are used to expand the limits of CDSS (Mitra and Rehman, 2025). It lays the foundation on understanding how AI-based decision support systems are transforming clinical workflows, enabling precision medicine, and addressing long-standing issues concerning the provision of quality healthcare services (Ahsan and Damaševičius, 2024).

### 1.1 Overview of Clinical Decision Support Systems (CDSS)

A Clinical Decision Support System (CDSS) is a subcategory of health informatics systems designed to assist a clinician or any other healthcare worker or the patients themselves in performing relevant medical actions. These systems operate by comparing the clinical specifics of a patient with the body of medical knowledge, evidence-based guidelines, and rules of experts in order to provide intelligent suggestions, alerts, or even reminders that can enhance the effectiveness of the patient's treatment through timely and tactful intervention at the clinical decision-making point. Figure 2 depicts the clinical support and alert system with clinical and patient interface. The CDSS has as its main goals the improvement of health care services to increase their quality, the reduction of clinical practice errors, the enhancement of standardization in the practice of medicine and, above all, the protection of patients. Generally speaking, CDSS encompasses many helpful devices, such as diagnostic assistance, warning systems for drug interactions, preventative care reminders, disease risk assessments, and compliance checks with clinical guidelines (L Pohane et al., 2025).

*Figure 1. Clinical Decision Support Systems*

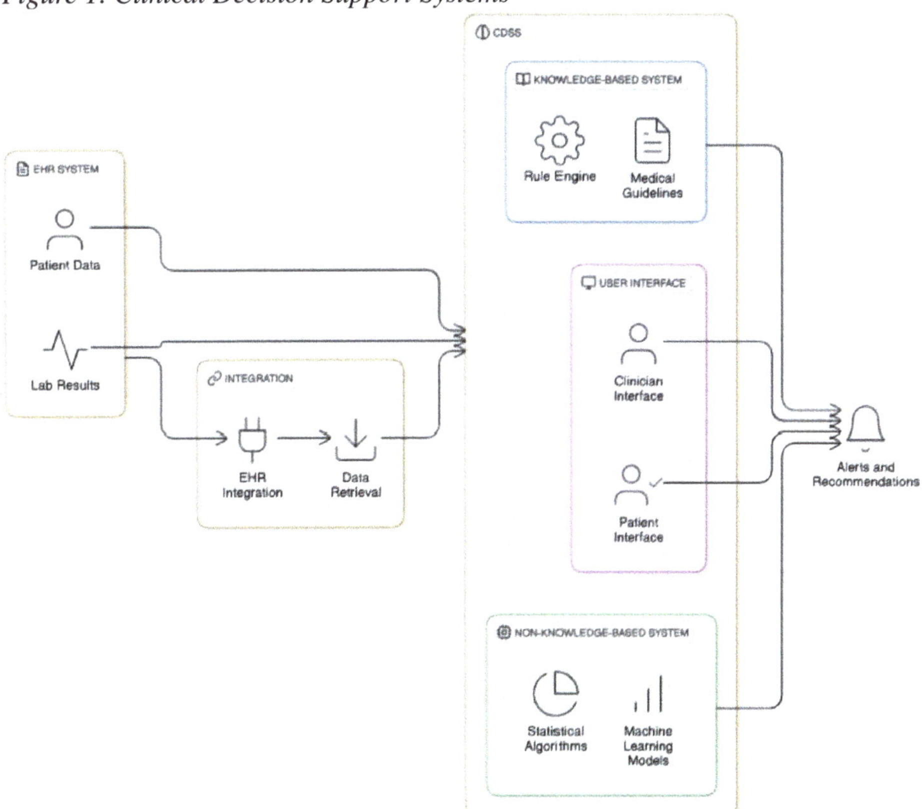


For instance, upon receiving a patient's symptoms and lab test results, a physician could access an EHR system, where a CDSS might offer a ranked list of likely diagnoses whilst also suggesting relevant tests or updated treatment protocols to the clinician (Edison, 2023). The effectiveness of a CDSS depends significantly on how well it is integrated into clinical workflows. When properly implemented, CDSS can provide real-time, context-aware support that does not disrupt but rather enhances the natural flow of healthcare delivery. Integration with EHRs allows for seamless data retrieval and decision support without requiring the clinician to switch platforms or re-enter information, which increases usability and adoption (Ouanes and Farhah, 2024).

## 1.2 Role of Artificial Intelligence in Healthcare

AI is changing how healthcare is practised today for the better. AI improves diagnosis, patient care, and operational activities within the healthcare system (Salehi, 2024). AI, or artificial intelligence, refers to the ability of a machine to imitate human actions such as learning, reasoning, and self-correction, all of which fall under human intelligence. In medicine, AI systems use large datasets of clinical data, medical files, imaging records, and patient histories to analyze, predict, and aid in decision making in real-time and with great precision. The roles of AI in healthcare are as follows:

1. **Early Detection and Disease Diagnosis:** AI has made it possible to advance early and accurate diagnosis by performing complex analyses on imaging scans, pathology reports, and even genetic profiles. Machine learning approaches can identify conditions such as cancer, heart ailments, and neurological disorders at stages where humans face difficulties detecting them. This enhances the survival rates of patients tremendously (Comito et al., 2022).
2. **Individualized Treatment Plans:** AI lends a hand in precision medicine through developing individual treatment plans as per a patient's genetic data, lifestyle, and medical history. It also predicts how patients are likely to respond to certain treatment allowing clinicians to minimize the risk of prescribing harmful therapies and use the most effective ones instead (Khalifa et al., 2024).
3. **Natural Language Processing (NLP):** AI-enabled NLP tools automatically extract information from clinical records like doctors' notes, prescriptions, and discharge summaries containing unstructured data. These tools assist in faster retrieval of vital information, support automation of documentation, enable decision-making by large volume clinical text summarization, and improve clinical practices.
4. **Operational and Administrative Efficiency:** AI systems simplify monotonous administrative work like managing appointments, billing patients, processing claims, and managing stock inventories. This helps in the operational efficiency of these health facilities, saves time, and lowers human error through automation in repetitive tasks (Pathan et al., 2025).
5. **Public Health Surveillance and Epidemic Management:** AI models monitor and assess the dynamics of infectious diseases using real-time population data to predict their spread. In times of health emergencies like the COVID-19 pan-

demic, AI was used for forecasting outbreaks, modeling the progression of the disease, and guiding vaccine and resource distribution (Sharma et al., 2023).

That said, Artificial Intelligence is more than just a technological advancement; it is changing the dynamics of healthcare. It's predictive and personal care algorithms, alongside analytics, revolutionize the practice and delivery of medicine toward far more sophisticated, intelligent, and patient-centric healthcare systems.

## 2. STRUCTURAL DESIGN AND CORE COMPONENTS OF CDSS

The effectiveness of a Clinical Decision Support System (CDSS) relies upon the design and integration of its basic components which guarantee accuracy, timeliness, and relevance within context of clinical decision making. Rather than a monolithic unit, CDSS is an elaborate system that integrates an Electronic Health Record (EHR), a medical database, and an interface to assist users during their clinical workflows.

1. **Knowledge Base:** A Clinical Decision Support System (CDSS) will not function or provide useful recommendations without a database, which serves as the key underpinning of supportive recommendations for clinical decision making. The knowledge base includes medical guidelines, clinical protocols, information on drug interactions, and all other practices necessary in performing Evidence-Based Medicine. Because of continuous updates, this knowledge base is in the process of change due to new research, treatment innovations, and changes in clinical practice. In simpler systems, the knowledge base utilizes static databases created by healthcare workers through manual updates. In more sophisticated AI systems, the knowledge base has the ability to dynamically update using patient record information, relevant literature, and clinician comments.
2. **The Inference Engine or Reasoning Engine:** One of the most important components of the system is the reasoner or inference engine, which analyses the stored data in the knowledge base and issues recommendations for action to be taken by the clinician. The inference engine decides or recommendation usually based on some patient data. For diagnostic systems with CDSS rules, the inference engine uses "if-then" rules (deterministic logic). An example of this would be a system which suggests a patient's blood pressure intervention when it is higher than a certain threshold. However, with AI-enabled CDSS, the inference engine is far more sophisticated; it applies machine learning (ML) and deep learning (DL) algorithms that deal with vast amounts of complicated data sets at once, identify trends within, and come up with probabilistic outcomes. These algorithms receive and respond to extensive data sets, progressively re-

fining their recommendations through continuous interaction with new clinical cases, thus tailoring them more accurately to the patient's unique requirements (Vashishth et al., 2024).

3. **Patient Data Module:** This module's purpose centers around acquiring, organizing, and assimilating patient information data from different sources which include Electronic Health Records (EHRs), other diagnostic tests, medical imaging, and medical histories. Other than that, it is also worthwhile to mention this module enables making available current and correct real-time data to the CDSS about the patient's health status. The data may indeed be structured like numerical results from laboratory medicine or vital signs or unstructured like note texts from doctors. The capture of this entire set is therefore important because the system is able to provide more comprehensive recommendations. Integration of data, especially patient data, is most needed if the system is going to utilize the information to provide system recommendations which are based on devices.
4. **User Interface (UI):** The user interface (UI) is the point of interaction between the clinician and the CDSS, providing an intuitive and accessible way for healthcare professionals to receive recommendations, alerts, and guidance. A well-designed UI presents complex data and decision support information in an understandable, easy-to-navigate format, without overwhelming the user. It often incorporates graphical representations of patient information, clinical opinion suggestions, treatment regimen recommendations, and warning notifications of risks such as medical interacting substances or abnormalities in different tests. For a CDSS to be effective, the complete user interface (UI) must be part of the clinician's workflow so that proper assistance is provided without interfering with the process of planning. The design should guarantee a helpful interface with features such as specific and relevant instructions, unobstructed workflows, and adjustable profile options that cater to various specialties and other areas of medicine (Nivedhaa, 2024).
5. **Feedback and Learning Module:** This AI powered feedback and learning module is sophisticated and intelligently learns from its user's input, new data, clinical outcomes, and user interaction. Clinicians' feedback considering the outcomes of previous recommendations helps the system evaluate its algorithm and adjust like in the aforementioned example where a system recommendation leads to positive clinical outcomes. This feedback evaluation loop coupled with the clinician's insights permits the CDSS to keep up with modern shifts or updates in surgical procedures, changing patient conditions, and newly emerging clinical practices pertinent to medicine while maintaining accuracy and relevance in evolving medical environments (Vashishth et al., 2024).

The cited CDSS set to achieve an applicable goal needs a maintenance free user's keen interactive interface framework for security, privacy, and to stop unwanted data leaks while having easy access to a current database of knowledge, a fluent inference engine, and ensuring data collaboration is multi-faceted. Streamlining these aspects permits CDSS to not only streamline clinical tasks and enhance patient satisfaction but also enable healthcare specialists to make reliable medically sound decisions (Vashishth et al., 2025).

## 2.1 Types of CDSS: Diagnostic, Therapeutic, and Preventive Systems

The Clinical Decision Support Systems (CDSS) were developed to aid a user with adequate and reliable based recommendations so that the practitioner can make the appropriate decision. The systems in question can be classified as being either active of passive depending on their role in the surgical decision-making process. Figure 2 illustrates the three types of CDSS are diagnostic, therapeutic, and preventive systems which each serve a unique function in patient care.

*Figure 2. Three Primary Types of CDSS*

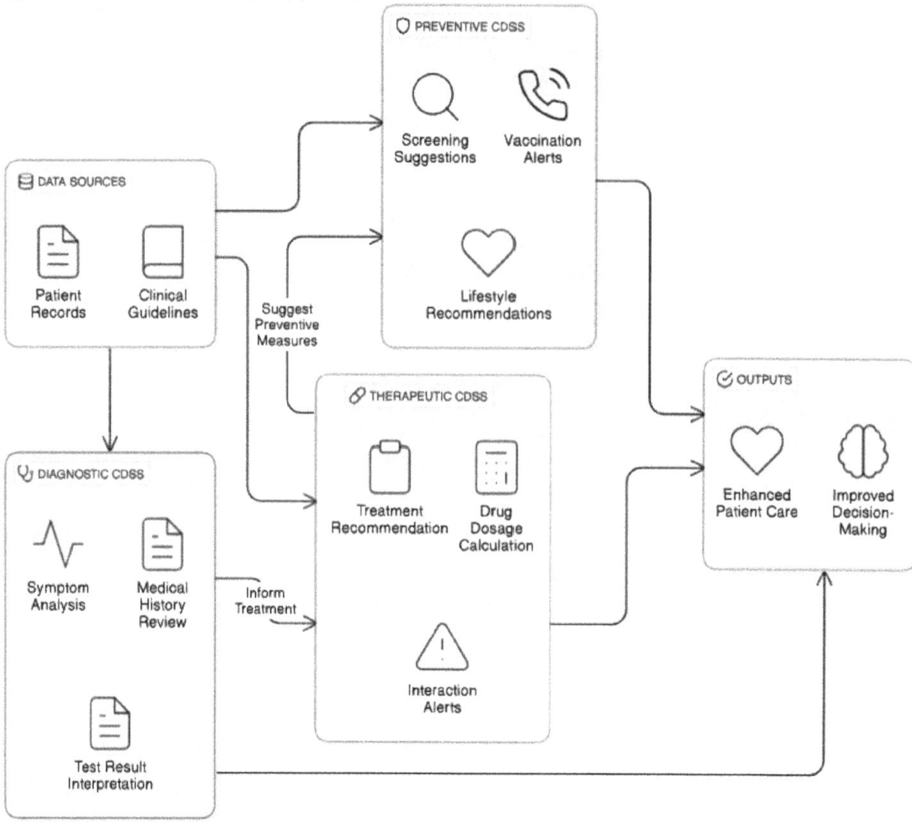


1. **Diagnostic CDSS:** The aim of diagnostic CDSS is to provide decision support to the clinicians on the most appropriate diagnosis to give a patient depending on a set of symptoms, history, medical tests and other data. CDSS assists practitioners with determination of appropriate diagnosis utilizing concepts of pattern recognition, clinical algorithms, and knowledge-based inference. By analyzing vast amounts of patient data, diagnostic CDSS can help uncover complex patterns and suggest potential diagnoses that clinicians may not have initially considered (Neravetla et al., 2024).
   - **Function**: These systems assist healthcare providers by listing different possible diagnoses and ranking them based on their clinical relevance.
   - **Data Used**: A patient's clinical history, relevant clinical signs, laboratory data, and age and sex.

- **Examples**: A diagnostic CDSS can help to diagnose diabetes, carcinoma, and even some rare diseases by evaluating a patient's data against a database containing extensive clinical data sets.

Benefits of Diagnostic CDSS:

- **Reduces Diagnostic Errors**: These systems aid in diagnosis by minimizing human error in assessing potential diagnoses that are often ignored.
- **Improves Accuracy**: These systems have access to a great proportion of datasets and medical literature; therefore, they are capable of making recommendations based on the most recent research improving diagnostic accuracy.
- **Enhances Efficiency**: Reduces the time a clinician takes to arrive at a decision by expediting the process of differential diagnosis.

2. **Therapeutic CDSS:** The main function of therapeutic CDSS is to assist healthcare specialists in determining the appropriate alias treatment techniques for a specific patient. This system combines a particular patient's information with treatment protocols, drug data, and clinical best practices to formulate suggestions that will result in better outcomes for patients. Using age, medical history, and relevant co-morbidities, a therapeutic Computerized Decision Support System (CDSS) can recommend surgical and non-invasive procedures alongside a therapeutic drug regimen.

- **Function**: Offers treatment strategies, drug therapies, and appropriate dosages for the patient.
- **Data Used**: Patient's medical history, laboratory examinations, allergic reactions, drug contraindications, and clinical protocols; checked against clinical guidelines.
- **Examples**: A therapeutic CDSS may recommend the most suitable chemotherapy regimen for patients with malignancy or formulate a pain management strategy for a patient following surgery.

Benefits of Therapeutic CDSS:

- **Personalized Treatment**: By considering individual patient factors, therapeutic CDSS can tailor treatments to the specific needs of the patient, improving outcomes.
- **Reduces Medication Errors**: These systems can alert clinicians to potential drug interactions, allergies, or contraindications, thereby reducing the risk of medication errors.

- **Optimizes Resource Utilization**: Ensures that the most effective and cost-efficient treatment options are chosen, avoiding unnecessary procedures or medications.

3. Machine Learning in CDSS

The development of Clinical Decision Support Systems (CDSS) has been enhanced by the advent of technology such as Machine Learning (ML). When given the ability to learn from experience based on massive amounts of data patient's information, systems are able to logically make better decisions over time. This allows the CDSS to better assist the clinician to care and treatment that is more accurate and improved. This section on machine learning deals with CDSS under ML wherein its functions are given, the types of ML algorithm used are given, and the areas addressed at the points of clinical decision making are specified.

## 3.1 Introduction to Machine Learning Techniques in Healthcare

The use of Machine Learning (ML) in the field of healthcare has grown tremendously, especially concerning clinical decision making. With the application of statistical models and algorithms on massive datasets, ML has the capacity for pattern recognition, predictive analysis, and decision-making facilitation. The incorporation of ML in Clinical Decision Support Systems (CDSS) provides real-time data insights which result in better patient care, lower error rates, and streamlined processes in the healthcare system. Because healthcare data is inherently complex because of its multidimensional features that include, but are not limited to, electronic health records (EHRs), lab results, medical imaging, self-reports, and data from wearables (Almadani et al., 2025), it is complicated. These tasks can be accomplished using modular ML techniques, enabling the simplification of complex data through the recognition of hidden patterns, trends, or correlations. This allows for enhanced decision support from CDSS throughout the entire healthcare process continuum, including diagnosis, treatment, and prevention (Vashishth et al., 2024). There are many ML techniques that have particular relevance in the setting of healthcare:

1. **Supervised Learning in Healthcare:** This kind of supervised learning is a popular ML technique used in the healthcare field. In this case, the model is trained on labelled data where every input has a corresponding output. For instance, demographic and clinical history of patients with their corresponding disease diagnosis and treatment plan may have lots of patient data. The model will now be able to predict the output for the new, never before seen novel data after training. Carrying out supervised learning therefore leads to the improved

classifying diseases from medical images, outcome prediction for patients, and in risk assessments. With this method, advanced CDSS can enable the health care professionals to make precise identifications through the analytical data and clear, objective methods aided by the information that are available from the historical data vertices (Vashishth et al., 2025).

2. **Unsupervised Learning in Healthcare:** With unsupervised learning, we train the algorithm without pre-assigned outcomes or results. Instead of trying to achieve a given outcome, the algorithm attempts to discover hidden patterns or structures in the data. This method is useful in situations where no set labels or outcomes exist. In healthcare, this form of learning is primarily used in clustering which aims at associating patients or medical conditions with common characteristics. It is also commonly used for abnormality detection which can identify atypical or rare cases like unusual diseases or rare conditions in patients. This is useful in uncovering new disease subtypes that are latent and may not be obvious to clinicians or found from other health care data sets.
3. **Healthcare Applications of Reinforcement Learning:** One distinguishing feature in machine learning is the use of a method called Reinforcement Learning (RL), which allows a system to learn from the environment via interactions using rewards or penalties commensurate with feedback. In healthcare, RL can assist in optimizing tasks that are performed over a duration of time by multiple decisions. For instance, in adaptive treatment scheduling, RL can help in selection and change of treatment actions depending on how the patient is responding to treatment. The model "picks" the possible actions (e.g. changes to the medication) which are the most fitting and yield an optimal self-reinforcing return value, make the most 'decisions' at each 'step' a system to maximize rewards. Perpetual feedback loops paired with changes, like in robotic surgeries and real-time clinical decision making, are very promising for reinforcement learning.
4. **Deep Learning in Medicine:** Deep learning is a subfield of machine learning which involves the use of several layers of neural networks to identify and extract intricate patterns from large quantities of data. The methodology is particularly adept at analyzing and interpreting dimensional data such as images and text in the medical field. Tasks like medical image diagnostics have benefited greatly from deep learning technology, with models now proficient at spotting and flagging tumours or lesions in X-rays and MRIs. Structures concerned with deep learning are also employed in natural language processing (NLP) to retrieve pertinent information archived in clinical notes or electronic health records. Its ability to work with vast and intricate datasets renders deep learning indispensable in enhancing the accuracy of diagnostics and the depth of clinical decision-making (Vashishth et al., 2024).

5. **Healthcare Applications of Transfer Learning:** Transfer learning is the use of previously designed models to tackle new tasks that are similar in nature. Unlike the majority of algorithms, which require extensive amounts of data to be collected and organized into a complete training set, transfer learning lets healthcare systems utilize information derived from one task (like general image classification) for an associated task (such as tumour detection). This is very useful for the field of medicine, where the amount of available labelled data is scarce. For instance, a model designed to recognize certain patterns in medical images may be adjusted to show more specific conditions, like lung cancer, in chest X-rays. The application of transfer learning achieves faster and more effective implementation of models in practice, especially in the context of specialized medical fields where data is limited.

## 3.2 Applications in Disease Prediction and Risk Assessment

As a subsystem of CDSS, machine learning (ML) algorithms perform a crucial role in risk assessment and disease prediction, increasing the precision and speed of the diagnosis and medical action taken. With ML, the numerous sets of patient data such as medical histories, laboratory results, imaging data, and even genetic data can be analysed in order to predict certain diseases and determine risks on an individual basis for specific treatment and early intervention.

1. **Disease Prediction:** With the ever-increasing amount of accumulated historical data such as the medical history, lab results, and lifestyle factors of patients, predicting the onset of a disease with machine learning techniques becomes increasingly easier. With trained ML models, correlations and patterns within the data that would otherwise go unnoticed by clinicians can unveil predicting capabilities for chronic diseases such as diabetes, heart disease, and certain types of cancer. Ascertaining the patient's risk is crucial since it helps healthcare professionals in planning resource allocation, determining the risk groups to monitor, and customizing the monitoring processes. Those patients identified to be as high risk through the use of these ML prediction models can receive targeted monitoring and timely treatment even before the symptoms are manifested. Proactive approaches like early intervention, lifestyle changes, treatment commencement, or, most importantly, proactive health measures can greatly reduce risk, hinder disease progression, and improve overall health (Shamszare and Choudhury, 2023).
2. **Predictive healthcare analytics:** AI assists in the predictive healthcare analytics domain with devising algorithms capable of novel risk stratification such as due to a clinical snapshot that enables setting optimal treatment plans

tailored to individual patient needs. Machine learning improves risk evaluation by calculating an individual's risk factors related to the rest of the population with their age, gender, medical and family history, and lifestyle habits. For example, ML models can estimate the likelihood of a patient experiencing a heart attack, stroke, or any other health issue using blood pressure, cholesterol levels, and BMI. Understanding these factors aids healthcare practitioners in directing proactive clinical attention toward the patients who would suffer the most from adverse health effects and the most effective alleviation.

3. **In Oncology:** For several oncology concerns, early detection is a critical aspect which remains a key area for outcome enhancement through machine learning integration. ML algorithms are able to analyze imaging data such as X-rays, mammograms, and CT scans and are capable of learning to detect early signs of carcinoma. The application of such advanced technology to medical imaging provides earlier recognition of tumours and other changes, making it possible to administer timely and effective health care, thus, promoting better outcomes and successful intervention methods.
4. **Prognosis Prediction:** ML algorithms are extremely helpful in estimating the course of diseases over time as well. By leveraging data from several patient visits, these models are able to make predictions concerning the progression of cancer, diabetes, or cardio vascular diseases (Abirami, 2023). For instance, it is possible to use machine learning algorithms to predict the rate of spread of cancer or the decline in health due to chronic disease. Being able to anticipate how a disease progresses enables clinicians to treat patients proactively in order to prevent complications, and to provide the best care possible based on a patient's health condition.
5. **Customized Treatment Strategies:** As with other sectors, the greatest ML (Machine Learning) achievements in healthcare came with personalizing treatment strategies concerning the precise risk factors and predictions of the patient. With modern technology, there is ease in understanding a patient's medical history, their genetic information, or even their lifestyle choices. Such a level of personalization ensures that there will be an increased treatment success rate, satisfaction, and better health outcomes for the patients within a favourable prolonged time frame. Monotonically directed interventions that target specific individuals enhance the probability of improving a patient's health state very greatly.
6. **Optimal Resource Distribution:** The use of machine learning in disease prediction and risk stratification comes with many benefits, one of them being the efficient allocation of healthcare resources. Recognizing patients who are very likely to experience certain diseases or health events enables healthcare systems to precisely direct interventions and resources. Patients who are likely

to suffer may require complete remediation, while patients who are less likely to suffer may require only preventive care. This approach is effective in preventing unnecessary examinations, overtreatment avoidance, and facilitating targeted healthcare services distribution. This improves the overall effectiveness and resulting outcomes of care in the healthcare system (Elgin and Elgin, 2024).

In this manner, machine learning enhances the prediction of diseases and risk factors by providing the right information at the right time enabling early actions, treatment customization, and positive outcomes.

## 3.3 Case Examples: AI in Early Detection of Sepsis, Cancer Prediction

Artificial Intelligence (AI) technologies have changed the landscape of using Clinical Decision Support Systems (CDSS)in the early detection of life-threatening conditions including sepsis and other cancers. Through the use of AI, systems powered by big data technology can process vast amounts of patient data in real time, detecting subtle changes that occur prior to the appearance of clinical signs and treating them. AI ensures early action which can result in better outcomes for patients.

1. **Understanding Sepsis and Its Early Detection:** Once believed to be an uncommon phenomenon, sepsis today stands as one of the major causes of mortality among ICU patients. The condition reflects the body's extreme response to infection, as in the case of severe bacterial infection across different organ systems, or multi-organ failure. Timely detection of the said condition is essential in ensuring the patients do not go under life threatening medical emergencies. Most of the traditional approaches used tend to focus on gross signs of the condition that appear towards the later stages of the disease. Unlike AI based CDSS which has the capability to analyze the data streams of a patient, including vital signs, lab results, and clinical notes—in order to detect signs of sepsis several hours before it is clinically visible. For example, Epic Sepsis Model and Targeted Real-time Early Warning System (TREWS) are implemented in hundreds of schools across the country which helps in monitoring patients continuously, and alerting clinicians when some preliminary indicators of sepsis are observed. According to research, these tools mitigate the risks of long term and lifelong disabilities achieved through better outcomes, while also reducing the duration of unnecessary hospital stays thereby effectively cutting down the overall healthcare costs (Vashishth et al., 2023).
2. **Predication and Diagnosis of Cancer:** AI models have shown unparalleled accuracy in the detection of various cancers such as breast, lung, and skin cancer.

These models incorporate with medical imaging, histopathology, and genome datasets. As an example, Google AI's breast cancer detection model has been proven to exceed the ability of radiologists to detect cancer through mammograms as it has lower false positive and false negative results. Furthermore, IBM Watson for Oncology passes patient records through natural language processing and machine learning to analyze and prescribe based on evidence cancer treatment suggestions. In dermatology, modern-day convolutional neural networks (CNNs) have been able to match dermatologists' level in skills of malignant skin lesions identification via thermoscopic imagery.

AI assists in improving accuracy on the diagnosis while reducing the time taken to make decisions enabling clinicians to start treatment significantly earlier and optimizing care tailored to the patient's predicted risk. Such implementations demonstrate the success and positive impact AI has had in shifting early detection of disease ai systems and changing the standard of care expected in clinical settings.

## 4. PREDICTIVE ANALYTICS AND PERSONALIZED MEDICINE

The combination of predictive analytics and personalized medicine within fully automated CDSS interfaces is transforming contemporary healthcare. Advanced algorithms along with previous records of a patient's health are utilized in predictive analytics to predict impending health events, this allows clinicians to take decisions that are proactive as opposed to reactive (Elhaddad and Hamam, 2024). Personalized medicine, however, seeks to consider the patient's specific attributes like their genetics, lifestyle, and environment while tailoring medical directions meant to treat them. Utilizing AI methods like machine learning, deep learning, and data mining allows creating models that can accurately forecast the risks and advancement of diseases alongside potential treatment outcomes. Such information assists healthcare practitioners in identifying patients who are most likely to develop chronic diseases, for example, diabetes or cardiovascular diseases, so they can initiate advanced steps. For example, AI can estimate the chance of outpatient appointments being missed or issues occurring after surgical procedures, thus optimally guiding the supervision and allocation of resources related to patients care (Yingngam et al., 2024).

### 4.1 From Population-Based to Individualized Treatment

In the past, primary medicine and secondary care services procedures have primarily relied on population statistics, or treated average patients within a given population, offering what is termed "one size fits all" healthcare. Although there have been tremendous advancements in public health systems, this approach tends to ignore the unique biological differences, lifestyle as well as the environment of people. Consequently, approaches that might work well for some patients might be wholly unhelpful or, worse, detrimental for others. This is likely to happen in a purely population-based method and in cases when an individual's clinical profile is far from the average. In contemporaneous times, there is a paradigm shift in medicine from a reactive response to health issues to a pre-emptive model by employing AI technologies, data science, and genomic sequencing. Artificial Intelligence (AI) has transformed the way we personalize medicine. AI tools can analyze huge heterogeneous collections of data such as electronic health records (EHRs), genetics, lab work, and even data captured directly from patients. These tools strive to make sense of the overwhelming array of information, ensuring no individual specifics are overlooked (Attiwi et al., 2024).

AI assists in matching therapies to patients by using advanced techniques analyzing the genetic mutations in their tumours which is more effective than simply looking at the type of cancer. AI also functions in cardiology by forecasting the response of a patient to given medications which helps to improve results and minimize adverse effects. It is clear that moving away from the population-based approach and a uniform method of treatment to a more personalized and sophisticated approach which incorporates the individual's information and behaviours turns out to be more effective while minimizing adverse effects at the same time. This shift in thinking enables specialists to apply precision medicine – advanced medicine that seeks to harm as little as possible, while, maximize effectiveness, improve clinical outcomes, and ensure patient satisfaction without compromises (Asiri et al., 2024).

## 4.2 Leveraging Predictive Models for Clinical Insights

Clinical practice is integrating these predictive models into their workflow, and as a result, they are recasting the value proposition of a patient's data by creating value out of it. The application of AI and ML techniques to vast and complex datasets that include EHRs, genetics, imaging studies, lab data, and even real-time biometrics captured through wearable devices results in the creation of predictive models. Predictive models facilitate risk prognosis, accurate forecasting of disease progression, and development of individualized specific treatment recommendations by means of identifying trends, patterns, and relationships within the data (Kukreti et al., 2025). The most important aspect of these models is their ability to pre-emptively predict critical illness conditions. For instance, sepsis, heart failure as well as distress syndrome can be detected by minute physiological changes several hours before these changes can be noted clinically. This enables interventions to be performed in a timely manner which improves patient outcomes and lowers the mortality rates significantly. In a similar fashion, these models are widely used for predicting hospital readmission and thus assisting the healthcare providers in formulating timely follow-up care, discharge plans, and enhancing resource utilization and patient satisfaction. Alongside aiding in risk stratification, these treatment pathways are guided through predictive models which enable optimization. With the aid of powered systems, the amalgamation of age, medical history, genetic data, and lifestyle make the identification of optimal treatment options tailored to each individual patient. This paradigm shift enhances medicine toward precision medicine, wherein not only effective but far safer, targeted treatments are administered. Algorithms can foresee changes in blood sugar levels and adapt insulin recommendations accordingly for diabetes care, while chemotherapy suggestions can be tailored to the tumour's genomic profile in oncology. In addition, predictive models have a positive impact on the efficiency in the management of healthcare systems. They enable administrators to more accurately predict the number of patients who will come in, so that resources can be optimally allocated and staffing levels managed according to the expected demand. They also assist in health population management by identifying some members of the population as high risk and enabling prevention outreach programs to be focused on them (Amiri, 2024).

Change and improvement within a clinical setup is powered by data intelligence gathered through predictive algorithms. Such models provide a more profound understanding of the patients, improve the accuracy of diagnosis on both the therapeutic and operational dimensions, and ensures streamlined processes thereby establishing a more effective and antagonistic approach to tailored and personalized healthcare on a case basis building an optimal healthcare ecosystem.

## 4.3 AI in Genomics and Tailored Drug Recommendations

AI is transforming the field of genomics and personalized medicine, reshaping the treatment paradigm for many diseases. Genomics is the scientific discipline that focuses on the studying of an individual's genes and their functions; when combined with AI technologies, genomics is able to provide highly individualized and precise cures. The integration of AI algorithms makes it possible to compute vast genomic datasets within a very short time and do so accurately. These algorithms are very good at finding mutations and genetic markers along with inherited traits that have a bearing on the likelihood of a person getting certain diseases. AI is capable of untangling the intricate genetic patterns using deep learning and machine learning models which no human genius could ever hope to figure out. Understanding these patterns helps in the prediction of risks of genetic disorders, early-stage identification of diseases, and tailoring the medications to be administers to the patient depending on the genetic makeup of the patient. Such practices are incredibly valuable in the field of oncology, where AI identifies important genomic changes in tumours and proposes far more effective and less harmful alternatives to traditional medicine. AI also assists in pharmacogenomics—concerning the interaction between a person's genetics and their medications—by interpreting genetic and clinical datasets. AI, considering polymorphisms in genes that code for drug-metabolizing enzymes, can aid physicians in the precise administration of certain drugs at specific doses tailored to a patient's individual genetic makeup, thereby reducing adverse effects and increasing effectiveness. For instance, AI systems can offer alternative treatment strategies for patients whose genetic profiles predispose them to adverse effects from standard treatment protocols. Moreover, AI technologies in genomics are revolutionizing biopharmaceutical research and development. AI aids in the identification of potential pharmaceutical targets, modeling the interaction of drugs with genes, and predicting the reaction to new treatment strategies in different population groups which lowers the costs and time to produce new drugs. New interventions for chronic and multi-faceted genetically complex diseases like cancer, diabetes, and other rare genetic disorders are made possible due to these advanced technologies.

*Figure 3. Drug Recommendation through AI*

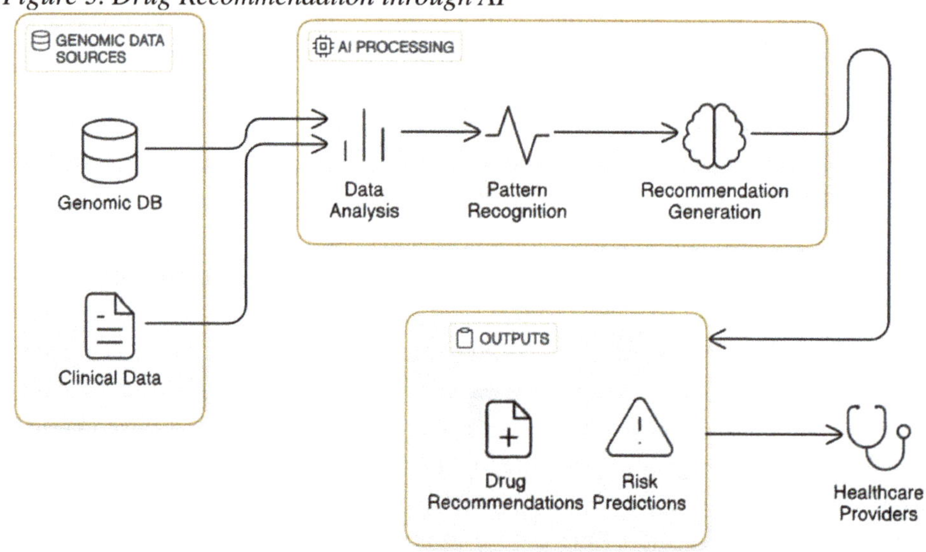


Thus, the incorporation of Artificial Intelligence into genomic sciences is a step forward towards personalized medicine. Figure 3 depicts the integration of drug recommendation with artificial intelligence. AI improves therapeutic recommendations by making them safer and more effective in accordance with an individual's genetic makeup. This moves away from treatment approaches based on population averages towards a treatment philosophy where every patient is catered to uniquely designed care pathways.

## 5. CASE STUDIES OF AI-DRIVEN CDSS IN PRACTICE

The listed case studies collectively demonstrate the transformative potential of AI-driven CDSS in enhancing diagnostic accuracy, enabling early interventions, and supporting personalized treatment decisions across various domains of medicine.

**5.1 IBM Watson for Oncology:** The has broadened the integration of Artificial Intelligence and Oncology clinical workflows with decision support systems in cancer treatment planning. In collaboration with Memorial Sloan Kettering Cancer Center, Watson develops sophisticated natural language processing (NLP) and machine learning algorithms that analyze bulk volumes of medical literature, clinical trial records, and patient health data. Watson processes medical literature alongside patient-specific data and clinical documents of trust accounts, providing tailored treatment recommendations that are ranked and justified. Watson has the ability to profile patients and their genetic mutations, pathology reports, and their medical history alongside the available oncology research for the best treatment options. This CDSS for oncology improves the accessibility, reliability, and standardization of cancer care delivery, especially for complicated cases with numerous possible interventions. It was often criticized for limited region-specific tailoring, overly passive prompts, and preset templates to assist users, resulting in patients lacking contextual relevance and setting trust clinical contextual reliance. With clinician-customized updates and ongoing progression documentation, its contextual accuracy has sustained improvement to ensure dependability in real clinical environments.

**5.2 Google DeepMind's Streams in Acute Kidney Injury:** The Streams application by Google DeepMind, developed alongside the UK's National Health Service (NHS), serves as a testament to the efficacy of AI in the management and triaging of acute kidney injury (AKI). Nurse practitioners and junior doctors engage with the platform on a daily basis and seamlessly navigate through various interfaces including patient notes and outline grader. The system performs predictive analytics of the patient's data recorded within the electronic health file and predicts the development of AKI signs long before the patient starts exhibiting clinical signs. Streams applies machine learning methodologies for detecting blood test and vital sign changes suggestive of possible kidney injury. Interventions can be done promptly since the system sends alerts to clinicians through a secured mobile gateway. This level of care eliminates chronic delays in AKI treatment because organ injury, hospital stays, and the patient's health outcomes are improved when AKI is treated early. The results of Streams showed the extent to which AI could be integrated into CDSS and used to facilitate work and responsiveness to patient needs in critically responsive areas, but it also raised key privacy and data transparency concerns within the context of health AI (Patil and Shankar, 2023).

**5.3 Predicting Cardiovascular Risks with AI at Mayo Clinic:** Through the use of AI, the Mayo Clinic has enhanced cardiovascular risk prediction by integrating it with ECG (electrocardiogram) data. By employing deep learning on extensive datasets containing records of ECGs and clinical outcomes, the system is capable of detecting markers of risk for atrial fibrillation, heart failure, and even sudden cardiac death. Unlike traditional risk calculators that depend on known clinical factors such as cholesterol levels and blood pressure, this model identifies concealed markers within the ECG patterns that even trained specialists are unable to perceive. This permits the forecasting of cardiovascular complications long before symptoms are observable, facilitating earlier interventional and preventive measures. The CDSS approach developed by Mayo Clinic demonstrates the potential for AI to be incorporated into routine diagnostics for providing real-time, advanced—individualized—risk evaluations. Such success has sparked the use of other AI applications in diagnostic and preventive cardiology, signifying a shift toward proactive personalized healthcare.

## 6. CHALLENGES AND CONCERNS IN INTEGRATING AI IN CLINICAL WORKFLOWS

Despite the advancements in healthcare that AI has brought about through CDSS systems, clinical workflows have not integrated AI systems into their practice due to numerous issues that need to be addressed.

1. **Data Compatibility Issues:** One of the particular concerns is the compatibility of data sets in relation to AI's integration into clinical workflows. Patient health information is frequently captured and stored in unique, proprietary EHR systems or other departmental silos, restricting access. AI tools that predict offers insightful recommendations based on the vast knowledge accessible, including patient medical histories, lab examinations, and current imaging studies. However, if the data is housed in incompatible, siloed systems, there are serious challenges to AI's ability to process and integrate this data restricting its usefulness. Ensuring that healthcare institutions adopt uniform data standards and facilitate cross-platform data sharing will transform the capability of AI-dependent CDSS (Chen et al., 2023).
2. **Clinician Acceptance and Trust:** Clinician trust remains a barrier towards the integration of AI into clinical workflows. Although AI renders useful information, most of the healthcare providers still tend to avoid using these systems,

particularly when the logic behind an AI's decision is not evident (Annamalai et al., 2024). AI systems that operate as "black boxes" wherein the logic behind the recommendations is obscured foster scepticism and anxiety. Clinicians may be hesitant to incorporate AI systems because they do not feel comfortable utilizing a system with unclear reasoning that starkly diverges from their clinical and ethical reasoning. This challenge can be mitigated by creating AI systems that clinical professionals are able to comprehend and interpret, therefore enabling them to trust the model's decisions fully, making sure that AI is an aid and not a supplantation of human intelligence (Ratta et al., 2025).

3. **Training and Change:** The incorporation of technology as well as AI systems into everyday clinical practice requires training, which is often a difficult task for healthcare professionals. Most clinicians lack some degree of knowledge regarding AI, and incorporating these systems poses a significant threat to their workflows. A proper training course needs to be developed to facilitate AI tool user competence among clinicians. This step needs to be structured in a way that reduces the burden posed in the attempt to learn new technologies. AI systems also need to be designed in a way that enables easy use and integration with clinical environments, which greatly prevents workflow disruption and enables the continuous focus on patient care.
4. **Privacy and Security of Data:** The accuracy of AI recommendations is often predicated on the availability of sensitive patient data. This creates challenges regarding data privacy and security because healthcare data is very confidential. The legal and ethical implications resulting from breaches in patient data, if any, misappropriation, or exploitation are extremely damaging. Furthermore, since the applications of AI in medicine tend to be cloud-based or facilitate inter-organizational data sharing, compliance with strict guidelines such as HIPAA is vital. Organizations also need to devise effective cybersecurity policies and frameworks to safeguard the AI from vulnerabilities and cyberattacks, thereby securing the protected health information, termed as PHI, from unauthorized access (Vashishth et al., 2024).
5. **Regulatory and Ethical Aspects:** There are numerous regulatory and ethical ramifications associated with the incorporating AI into healthcare processes. The controversy of how to govern AI applications is still open as the existing regulations for medical equipment do not seem to cover the complexities of AI systems adequately. Other liability issues emerge: in the case that an AI system makes an inappropriate recommendation which results in patient injury, assigning responsibility is very challenging. Even more disturbing are the ethical issues with AI replacing human ability to reason and show compassion, considering human discernment necessary for caregiving at the end-of-life or managing

complex rare conditions. Forming such frameworks will be pivotal to support the sustainable development of AI technology in healthcare (Bertl et al., 2023).

While AI is capable of significantly improving clinical decision making and patient care, its integration into healthcare systems is entangled with several issues. The most important open questions of AI-enabled CDSS focus on data interoperability with trust, training, privacy, regulation, bias, and cost (Mohammed et al., 2024).

## 7. STRATEGIES FOR EFFECTIVE IMPLEMENTATION OF INTELLIGENT CDSS

The effective implementation of intelligent Clinical Decision Support Systems (CDSS) requires detailed planning and different strategies for different healthcare contexts. The measures listed below will enhance the usefulness of AI-powered CDSS for clinicians while avoiding many challenges associated with incorporation into clinical practice.

1. **Streamlining Data Compatibility:** One of the other steps in the implementation process is the standardization and compatibility of the data with the AI system. According to estimates, healthcare organizations need to spend resources to create standardized data schemas, implement relevant health information exchange standards such as HL7 and FHIR, and facilitate system integration, including with EHRs and laboratory information systems. This investment, however, will empower AI-based CDSS systems with accurate, complete, and current patient data, which in turn enhances clinical insights for better decision-making (Jayaprakasam, 2025).
2. **Integrate Decision Support Systems for Clinician Participation:** The active participation and engagement of healthcare providers with the intelligent CDSS needs to occur prior to the deployment of the system. In as much as healthcare professionals are in the design and customization phases of these systems, they will be able to align clinical practices and workflows, accordingly. Furthermore, such extensive systems as the one proposed will require sophisticated training for clinicians to appreciate the functions and scope boundaries of the AI embedded in the system. Granting clinician's immediate access to operational support will enable them to incorporate the tools and confidently streamline their decision-making processes while ensuring they retain authoritative control over their final medical judgements.
3. **Formulate Adequate Protocols on Data Privacy and Security:** When it comes to AI integration in the medical field, patient's data privacy and security

is crucial. Healthcare organizations need to implement strong cyber security policies such as encryption, secure data storage, and limited access to sensitive information files. So as to guarantee confidentiality of the data, compliance with set guidelines like HIPAA in the U.S. is highly essential. Regular audits and updating the security framework can curb breaches and ensure that AI systems function within the confines of data laws (Vashishth et al., 2025).

4. **Iterative Development and Continuous Improvement:** AI-enhanced CDSS solutions should grow over time with the use of iterative processes. After first implementing the system, feedback sessions should be conducted continuously with the clinicians to improve and modify the system. The system's machine learning algorithms should be updated with data from additional patients, clinical evaluations, and contemporary research to ensure optimal AI performance. Implementing systems based on actual user feedback will maintain congruence with clinical practices, thereby improving predictive precision.
5. **Ensure Legal and Ethical Compliance:** Protecting the legal and ethical boundaries of an AI-assisted CDSS has to be considered. Healthcare institutions need to collaborate with lawyers to define the boundaries of responsibility on the part of the AI in its recommendations, and the role that human practitioners have in the final decision. There are ethical issues around AI like biases that exist in its ML algorithms, and over-dependence on machines that need careful scrutiny. Policymakers might need to create and adopt new regulations concerning the application of AI in healthcare to ensure that these technologies and their unintended consequences do not harm patients (Dlugatch et al., 2024).

The implementation of intelligent CDSS should be systematic in nature for it to be useful in the healthcare sector to ensure involvement of data consolidation, clinician participation, system transparency, data privacy, system enhancements, regulatory compliance, performance auditing, and stakeholder alliances. With these strategies, AI integration in clinical decision-making will lead to better care outcomes and improved care delivery.

## 8. FUTURE DIRECTIONS OF CLINICAL DECISION SUPPORT SYSTEMS

The future advancements in technology, modernization in healthcare, as well as the functionality of AI, Machine Learning, and Data analytics will greatly have an impact in Clinical Decision Support Systems (CDSS) as we know it. Below are some of the factors which are most likely to change the landscape of CDSS:

1. **Incorporation of Multi-Model Data Sources:** As the healthcare ecosystem advances, there will be an increased emphasis on the incorporation of multi-model data sources CDSS. Inclusion of these data sources will open doors to much real time information which comes from wearable devices like sensors, and social heuristics. Not only is it helpful in getting advanced real time and comprehensive insights but also enhances lab results, medical history, images, and any other patient related data. All these aspects will enhance CDSS and make it much more robust, improve patient outcomes, and ease clinical decisions (Vashishth et al., 2024).
2. **Improved Predictive Functions with Artificial Intelligence and Big Data:** In the years to come, the CDSS system will greatly improve its predictive capabilities as a result of the incorporation of big data and AI logic. By harnessing extensive datasets from various domains, CDSS will enhance its accuracy in anticipating patient outcomes, the progression of diseases, and responses to treatments. Machine learning algorithms will perpetually update and refine their accuracy by studying patterns in patient data. Healthcare providers will be able to use these predictions to help avert complications, which will tremendously improve care.
3. **Personalized and Targeted Healthcare:** With the increased usage of AI in CDSS, there is a chance that the shift towards personalized medicine will happen much faster. AI CDSS will analyze genomic data along with the lifestyle and environment of the patient to create tailored treatment plans with outmost precision for each patient. Such treatment optimization will improve efficacy but also reduce unnecessary procedures, enhancing the cost-efficiency of healthcare. The change will enable clinicians to apply targeted interventions which will radically change the approach to diagnosis and treatment from a generic model.
4. **AI-Operated Automation of Clinical Workflows:** These future user CDSS systems will more likely incorporate the automation of clinical workflows at various levels. The administrative work for healthcare providers will be less burdensome. AI can perform better sophisticated tasks like documentation, medical coding, and even scheduling thereby giving more room to clinicians to attend patients. Removing routine tasks from humans can reduce errors and contribute to system efficacy. AI integrated CDSS will optimize workflows and improve the delivery of healthcare services, productivity, patient satisfaction and well-being.
5. **Improving Clinical Communication and Developing NLP CDSS:** As we discussed before, the functionalities NLP will have on CDSS will be massive, especially to advance communication. Other strategies will look at how NLP can enable extraction of relevant information from semi-structured clinical text, hence enhancing the functionality of already structured information like notes,

discharge summaries, and research papers. Such improvements in information access will aid speedy and precise clinical decision-making by guaranteeing a wider range of actionable information. Automating the verbatim capture of information reduces paperwork and mitigates clinician fatigue to improve performance in clinical environments.

## 9. CONCLUSION

The application of artificial intelligence in Clinical Decision Support Systems (CDSS) signifies the next era for healthcare, providing advanced technologies that enhance the precision of diagnostics, tailor treatments, and optimally improve patient results. With the incorporation of machine learning, predictive analytics, and natural language processing, CDSS can automate clinical-sphere workflows, real-time updates, and offer better informed decision-making during patient care. The use of AI tools in clinical setup poses difficulties in data fusion, integration, clinician buy-in, and ethical issues. There is little doubt that as AI systems become more sophisticated, their use in healthcare will expand and provide novel solutions for managing precision medicine, detecting diseases at an early stage, and providing tailored treatment strategies. Striking a balance between deploying them responsibly, ethically, and incorporating them effectively, will be the primary challenge faced in unleashing the potential of AI-enhanced CDSS aimed at transforming healthcare.

## REFERENCES

Abirami, M. S. (2023, October). AI clinical decision support system (AI-CDSS) for cardiovascular diseases. In *2023 International Conference on Computer Science and Emerging Technologies (CSET)* (pp. 1-7). IEEE.

Ahsan, M., & Damaševičius, R. (2024, October). AI-Based Decision Support Systems to Improve Diagnostic Accuracy via Medical Imaging. In International Conference on Advanced Research in Technologies, Information, Innovation and Sustainability (pp. 197-208). Cham: Springer Nature Switzerland.

Almadani, B., Kaisar, H., Thoker, I. R., & Aliyu, F. (2025). A Systematic Survey of Distributed Decision Support Systems in Healthcare. *Systems*, *13*(3), 157.

Amiri, Z. (2024). Leveraging AI-Enabled Information Systems for Healthcare Management. *Journal of Computer Information Systems*, 1–28.

Annamalai, M., Mittal, T., Sunkara, K. C., Pandey, H., Jadhav, G., & Nemane, V. (2024, December). Revolutionizing Medical Diagnostics with Transparent AI-Driven Decision Support Systems. In 2024 4th International Conference on Mobile Networks and Wireless Communications (ICMNWC) (pp. 1-7). IEEE.

Asiri, M. A., Almutairi, A. D., Ozam, T. S., Al Ahmari, R. Y., Alhazmi, S. M., Al-moudhi, A. A., & Alqahtani, N. M. (2024). AI-Driven Decision Support Systems: Transforming Hospital Management Strategies. [JICRCR]. *Journal of International Crisis & Risk Communication Research*, *7*(3).

Attiwi, M. H., Almass, J. O., Roukiah, A. S. F., Shakir, K. H., Asaad, L. I., Alab-deli, H., & Hassan, E. (2024, November). Unremarkable AI: Intelligent Decision Support in Critical Clinical Decision-Making. In 2024 International Conference on IoT, Communication and Automation Technology (ICICAT) (pp. 610-616). IEEE.

Bertl, M., Ross, P., & Draheim, D. (2023). Systematic AI support for decision-making in the healthcare sector: Obstacles and success factors. *Health Policy and Technology*, *12*(3), 100748.

Chen, Z., Liang, N., Zhang, H., Li, H., Yang, Y., Zong, X., & Shi, N. (2023). Harnessing the power of clinical decision support systems: Challenges and opportunities. *Open Heart*, *10*(2), e002432. PMID: 38016787

Comito, C., Falcone, D., & Forestiero, A. (2022). AI-driven clinical decision support: Enhancing disease diagnosis exploiting patients similarity. *IEEE Access : Practical Innovations, Open Solutions*, *10*, 6878–6888.

Dlugatch, R., Georgieva, A., & Kerasidou, A. (2024). AI-driven decision support systems and epistemic reliance: A qualitative study on obstetricians' and midwives' perspectives on integrating AI-driven CTG into clinical decision making. *BMC Medical Ethics*, *25*(1), 6. PMID: 38184595

Edison, G. (2023). Transforming Medical Decision-Making: A Comprehensive Review of AI's Impact on Diagnostics and Treatment. *BULLET: Jurnal Multidisiplin Ilmu*, *2*(4), 1121–1133.

Elgin, C. Y., & Elgin, C. (2024). Ethical implications of AI-driven clinical decision support systems on healthcare resource allocation: A qualitative study of healthcare professionals' perspectives. *BMC Medical Ethics*, *25*(1), 148. PMID: 39707327

Elhaddad, M., & Hamam, S. (2024). AI-driven clinical decision support systems: An ongoing pursuit of potential. *Cureus*, *16*(4). PMID: 38711724

Jayaprakasam, B. S. (2025). AI and Big Data-Driven m-Health: Integrating Cloud Computing, Remote Patient Monitoring, Clinical Decision Support Systems, and Self-Supervised Learning with FHIR for Scalable Healthcare Systems. *Indo-American Journal of Life Sciences and Biotechnology*, *22*(1), 11–25.

Khalifa, M., Albadawy, M., & Iqbal, U. (2024). Advancing clinical decision support: The role of artificial intelligence across six domains. *Computer Methods and Programs in Biomedicine Update*, *5*, 100142.

Kukreti, S., Shrivastava, A., Chandrashekar, R., Rani, K. P., Badhoutiya, A., & Lakhanpal, S. (2025, February). AI-Driven Clinical Decision Support Systems: Revolutionizing Healthcare with Predictive Models. In *2025 International Conference on Computational, Communication and Information Technology (ICCCIT)* (pp. 560-565). IEEE.

Mitra, U., & Rehman, S. U. (2025). Leveraging AI and Machine Learning for Next-Generation Clinical Decision Support Systems (CDSS). In AI-Driven Innovation in Healthcare Data Analytics (pp. 83-112). IGI Global Scientific Publishing.

Mohammed, A. S., Neravetla, A. R., Nomula, V. K., Gupta, K., & Dhanasekaran, S. (2024, June). Understanding the Impact of AI-driven Clinical Decision Support Systems. In 2024 15th International Conference on Computing Communication and Networking Technologies (ICCCNT) (pp. 1-6). IEEE.

Neravetla, A. R., Nomula, V. K., Mohammed, A. S., & Dhanasekaran, S. (2024, June). Implementing AI-driven Diagnostic Decision Support Systems for Smart Healthcare. In 2024 15th International Conference on Computing Communication and Networking Technologies (ICCCNT) (pp. 1-6). IEEE.

Nivedhaa, N. (2024). A comprehensive study of artificial intelligence's contribution to streamlining healthcare workflows and enhancing decision-making practices. [IJITEE]. *International Journal of Information Technology and Electrical Engineering*, *13*(5), 1–7.

Ouanes, K., & Farhah, N. (2024). Effectiveness of Artificial Intelligence (AI) in clinical decision support systems and care delivery. *Journal of Medical Systems*, *48*(1), 74. PMID: 39133332

Pathan, R. R., Osei-Asiamah, J., Jadhav, P. N., Saravanan, S., Singh, A. K., & Sahoo, S. K. (2025). Developing Decision Support Systems for Healthcare Administration using AI. *Journal of Neonatal Surgery*, *14*(10s).

Patil, S., & Shankar, H. (2023). Transforming healthcare: Harnessing the power of AI in the modern era. *International Journal of Multidisciplinary Sciences and Arts*, *2*(2), 60–70.

Pohane, L, A., J Dighade, S., S Rithe, E., R Mangwani, R., S Raut, A., & S Bhamburkar, S. (2025). AI-Driven Advancements in Pharmacy: Enhancing Drug Discovery, Optimization and Clinical Decision-Making. *International Journal of Innovative Science and Research Technology*, *10*(3), 615–626.

Ratta, R., Sodhi, J., & Saxana, U. (2025). The Relevance of Trust in the Implementation of AI-Driven Clinical Decision Support Systems by Healthcare Professionals: An Extended UTAUT Model. *Electronic Journal of Knowledge Management*, *23*(1), 47–66.

Salehi, F. (2024). The transformative role of artificial intelligence in the healthcare industry: A comprehensive analysis. *Asian Journal of Research in Medicine and Medical Science*, *6*(1), 62–70.

Shamszare, H., & Choudhury, A. (2023, August). Clinicians' perceptions of artificial intelligence: focus on workload, risk, trust, clinical decision making, and clinical integration. In Healthcare (Vol. 11, No. 16, p. 2308). MDPI.

Sharma, V., Vashishth, T. K., Kumar, B., Sharma, K. K., Vidyant, S., & Chaudhary, S. (2023, December). Health Interpretation of Covid-19 Patients using Artificial Intelligence. In *2023 International Conference on Artificial Intelligence for Innovations in Healthcare Industries (ICAIIHI)* (Vol. 1, pp. 1-5). IEEE Computer Society.

Vashishth, T. K., Chaudhary, S., & Sharma, V. (2023). Optimum Utilization of Bed Resources in Hospitals: A Stochastic Approach. In: Manju, Kumar, S., Islam, S.M.N. (eds) Artificial Intelligence-based Healthcare Systems. The Springer Series in Applied Machine Learning. Springer, Cham.

. Vashishth, T. K., Sharma, V., Kumar, B., Panwar, R., Sharma, K. K., & Chaudhary, S. (2024). AI-Integrated IoT in Healthcare Ecosystem: Opportunities, Challenges, and Future Directions. AI and IoT Technology and Applications for Smart Healthcare Systems, 37-54.

Vashishth, T. K., Sharma, V., Kumar, S., Verma, N., Vidyant, S., & Kaushik, S. (2025). The Integration of AI in Telemedicine Transforming Healthcare Delivery and Patient Outcomes. In *AI-Driven Personalized Healthcare Solutions* (pp. 71–98). IGI Global Scientific Publishing.

Vashishth, T. K., Sharma, V., Sharma, K. K., Chaudhary, S., Kumar, B., & Panwar, R. (2024, March). Artificial neural networks & discrete Wavelet transform enabled healthcare model for stress and emotion assessment using speech signal recognition. In AIP Conference Proceedings (Vol. 3072, No. 1). AIP Publishing.

Vashishth, T. K., Sharma, V., Sharma, K. K., & Kumar, B. (2024). Elevating healthcare services: The integration of cloud with fog computing. In *Web 3.0* (pp. 54–75). CRC Press.

Vashishth, T. K., Sharma, V., Sharma, K. K., Kumar, B., Chaudhary, S., & Panwar, R. (2024). Intrusion Detection and Prevention Techniques in FL Cloud-Based Healthcare 5.0: A Comprehensive Review. Pioneering Smart Healthcare 5.0 with IoT, Federated Learning, and Cloud Security, 152-174.

Vashishth, T. K., Sharma, V., Sharma, K. K., Kumar, B., Chaudhary, S., & Panwar, R. (2024). Security Challenges in Storing and Exchanging Medical Information. In *Medical Robotics and AI-Assisted Diagnostics for a High-Tech Healthcare Industry* (pp. 378–402). IGI Global.

Vashishth, T. K., Sharma, V., Sharma, K. K., Kumar, B., Chaudhary, S., & Panwar, R. (2024). Enhancing biomedical signal processing with machine learning: A comprehensive review. Digital Transformation in Healthcare 5.0: Volume 1: IoT, AI and Digital Twin, 277.

Vashishth, T. K., Sharma, V., Sharma, K. K., Kumar, B., Chaudhary, S., & Panwar, R. (2025). Data-driven healthcare: Leveraging AoT and metaverse for better diagnosis. In *Leveraging Metaverse and Analytics of Things (AoT) in Medical Systems* (pp. 41–60). Academic Press.

Vashishth, T. K., Sharma, V., Sharma, K. K., Sethi, P., Chaudhary, T., & Bhardwaj, A. (2024). Future Implications of Blockchain for Biomedical and Healthcare. In *Blockchain for Biomedical Research and Healthcare: Concept, Trends, and Future Implications* (pp. 367–404). Springer Nature Singapore.

Vashishth, T. K., Sharma, V., Sharma, M. K., & Sharma, R. (2025). Healthcare and Smart Cities Applications of Secure 6G Infrastructure. In Building Tomorrow's Smart Cities With 6G Infrastructure Technology (pp. 399-432). IGI Global Scientific Publishing.

Yingngam, B., Navabhatra, A., & Sillapapibool, P. (2024). AI-Driven Decision-Making Applications in Pharmaceutical Sciences. In Using Traditional Design Methods to Enhance AI-Driven Decision Making (pp. 1-63). IGI Global Scientific Publishing.

Chapter 10

# AI-Enhanced Clinical Decision-Making Through a Collaborative Approach

**Ravikumar R. N.**
https://orcid.org/0009-0009-3705-1681
*Marwadi University, Rajkot, India*

**Satheesh Kumar A.**
*Nandha Engineering College, Erode, India*

**S. Aarthi**
https://orcid.org/0009-0006-9064-2091
*Marwadi University, Rajkot, India*

**Muhabbat Jumaniyozova**
*Urgench State University, Urgench, Uzbekistan*

**Bekhzod Ruzimbaev Saparbaevich**
*Mamun University, Khiva, Uzbekistan*

**Shakhnoza Toshova**
*Termez University of Economics and Service, Termez, Uzbekistan*

## ABSTRACT

*AI integration in healthcare transforms medical decision-making and treatment processes, enhancing patient care and advancing research. Deep Q-Networks (DQNs) with reinforcement learning help healthcare professionals analyze data for personalized treatment plans. AI automation boosts diagnostic accuracy and operational efficiency through collaboration between humans and machines. This chapter focuses on AI-powered clinical decision support systems that assist in diagnosing complex diseases and developing treatment strategies. Real-time analysis of medical imaging and health records enables early detection of cancers, cardiovascular disorders, and neurological disorders. Reinforcement learning also streamlines hospital resource use and cuts costs. Despite progress, ethical oversight is essential to address privacy,*

DOI: 10.4018/979-8-3373-3311-3.ch010

*algorithmic bias, and ensure transparency. This study explores human-AI synergy in clinical settings, pointing out the importance of trustworthy, ethically guided AI that complements human intuition for improved patient outcomes.*

## 1. INTRODUCTION TO AI-ENHANCED CLINICAL DECISION-MAKING

Healthcare organizations in the present day use Artificial Intelligence to improve their clinical decision-making procedures. AI technologies facilitated advanced healthcare solutions for professionals through providing both sophisticated medical data requirements and individual patient care specifications. Deep Q-Networks (DQNs) produce the most effective outcomes from reinforcement learning-based models because they demonstrate superiority at optimizing environment interactions for decision-making. Traditional clinical decision-making relies heavily on physicians' expertise, historical knowledge, and intuition (Amann et al., 2020). The success rates of traditional human-based healthcare choices decrease when patients require specific medical treatments for effective responses to state-of-the-art diagnostic procedures. Medical professionals use AI data processing tools with pattern detection procedures to generate knowledgeable decisions from validated data findings in medical information-heavy situations. AI-generated data views provide healthcare professionals with better working capabilities but do not weaken their clinical expertise. Joint work processes between healthcare providers allow them to develop precise decisions.

The healthcare Clinical Decision Support Systems (CDSS) implement AI technologies to detect complete diseases then produce therapeutic estimates and customized treatments for patients. The implementation of DQNs with intelligent models activates both practice guideline modifications and patient-directed data entry systems which enable healthcare staff continuous educational development. Healthcare organizations need adjustability to maintain necessary functionality when dealing with two key areas which constantly change: critical care units and oncology departments and the management of chronic diseases (Asan et al., 2020). This research demonstrates the enhanced medical service decision systems that occur through the use of DQNs coupled with reinforcement learning algorithms. Healthcare organizations should enable AI systems to function with medical supervision so they uphold patient trust while offering individualized care. Healthcare underwent digital change which led to artificial intelligence implementation for advanced decision systems to develop smart and long-lasting medical care.

## 1.1 Role of AI in Transforming Modern Healthcare

AI enables the modern healthcare system to transform because it enhances disease assessment and yields exact medical evaluations that achieve treatment success. The combination of EHRs and wearable devices with other diagnostic tools and genomic sequencing produces large amounts of patient healthcare data in modern medicine. The standard analytical systems cannot manage current healthcare situations appropriately. Healthcare systems convert big data into useful information through the implementation of AI data conversion functionality (Charow et al., 2021).

The integration between latent pattern detection and anomaly detection and predictive forecasting systems gives AI algorithms superior diagnostic capabilities than those of human professionals. Medical organizations succeed in deploying these technological features to discover diseases early and create accurate treatment strategies and emerge with new pharmaceutical discoveries by making model-based predictions. The system analyses early-stage cancers through medical imaging AI before performing hospital readmission prediction using historical treatment data which enables healthcare staff to plan preventive measures (Giordano et al., 2021).

The innovative administration of medical services coupled with strategic resource capabilities produces better results with a reduced probability of clinical misdiagnoses. Through AI tools medical facilities can produce emergency decision-support recommendations to speed up both decision processes and enhance precision. The deployment of Artificial Intelligence technologies modifies technical medical infrastructure and social healthcare systems simultaneously. Fundamental shifts occur throughout the healthcare delivery models because this technology improves healthcare provider skills while building a preventive healthcare system that surpasses basic reactive treatment by using data-based methods. The capabilities of AI medical tools should advance for developing enhanced healthcare services with targeted treatment systems operated by neutral systems. A strategic implementation plan becomes essential for professional model deployment because it enables automated systems to use medical expert knowledge for creating superior patient treatment outcomes. The Fig.1 illustrates key applications of Artificial Intelligence in healthcare, including diagnostics, treatment, and data analysis. AI enhances areas like medical imaging, drug discovery, and clinical decision support for improved patient outcomes.

*Figure 1. Role of AI in Transforming Modern Healthcare*

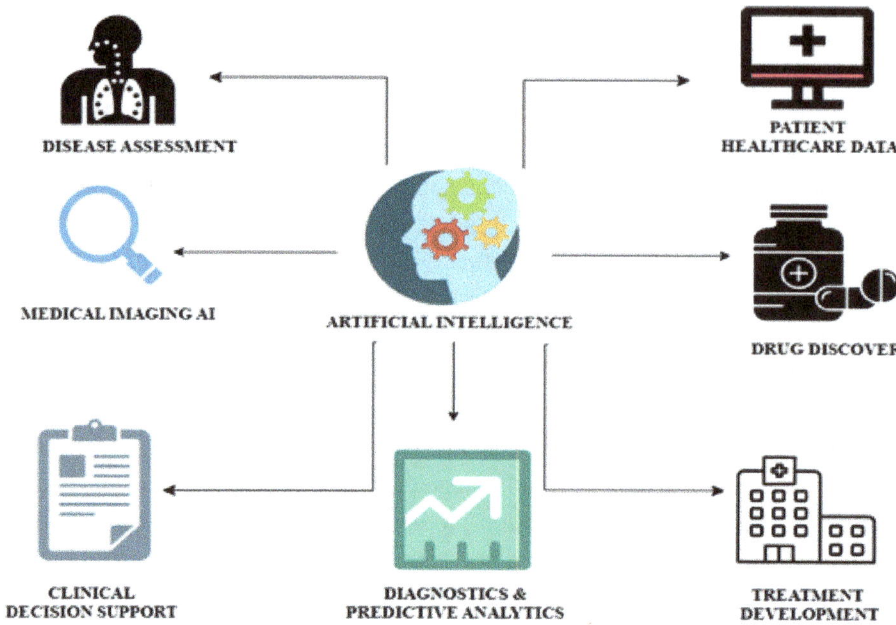


## 1.2 Importance of Collaboration Between AI Systems and Medical Professionals

For clinical application of AI systems to become effective it requires two necessary components that unite medical personnel with AI systems. Medical professionals achieve optimum AI outcomes by connecting their technical expertise to calculation functions that AI systems need help with. The medical decisions reach their optimal state when healthcare professionals collaborate with AI systems because each output type stems from necessary data while preserving patient dignity and upholding ethical medical care (Jabbour et al., 2023). Complex data processing speed of AI systems enables them to produce diagnostic information combined with prescriptive and forecasting recommendations. The algorithms that process input from training algorithms using existing data databases produce outputs which lack accurate representation of particular patient characteristics and medical situation developments. The assessment of AI outputs by medical staff requires oversight for specific patient information which controls the medical decision-making process.

Collaborative decision-making between healthcare providers enables them to trust AI systems for implementation purposes. Healthcare providers support operational systems which work in clinical practice during testing phases of tool development and deployment. The involvement of workers throughout AI technology implementation supports the execution of system integration while generating precise medical outcomes (Jhade et al., 2024). AI systems practice ethical operation when human personnel collaborate with these systems in their operational phase. The medical practice objectivity of doctors remains possible through their ability to distinguish diagnostic inputs received from the AI system. AI system integration demands human-machine teaming for creating effective collaborations between machines and humans which drives positive health care services and operational success within medical organizations. The Fig.2 presents a layered flow of factors contributing to responsible and effective AI integration. It emphasizes collaboration, speed, accuracy, trust, and ethical operation as essential components for successful human-AI teaming.

*Figure 2. AI and Medical Professionals Collaboration*

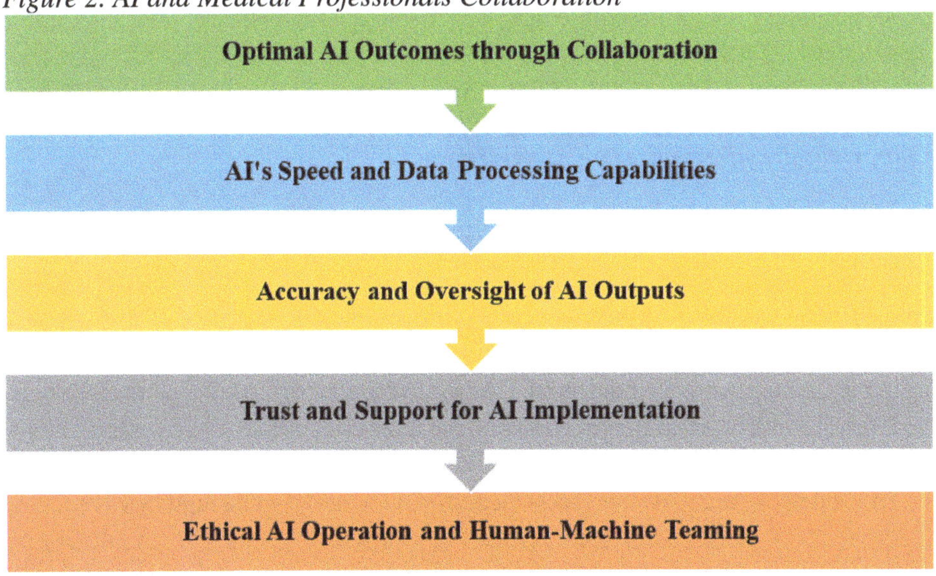


## 1.3 Introduction to Deep Q-Networks (DQNs) in Clinical Contexts

The best medical decision support system from reinforcement learning exists in its advanced approach known as Deep Q-Network. The AI system uses Q-learning agents extracted by deep neural networks from DQNs to obtain its most rewarding actions (Jain & Jaidka, 2024). The training cycle must be used by AI systems to create intelligent decision-making abilities through knowledge collection inside different healthcare centers working in challenging settings. Traditional machine learning methodologies differ from DQNs since they gain reward information through environment feedback obtained during their interactive learning process (Orji et al., 2023). These feedback systems can modify their approaches through unexpected operational conditions which leads to enhanced healthcare service quality.

The clinical functions that DQNs produce result from their ability to develop improved patient care protocols alongside facility operational strategies while forecasting important results and creating treatment strategies for chronic medical conditions. A maximum effective diabetic treatment plan results from the DQN model by fusing blood glucose data with medication details and patterns of human actions. The primary asset of DQNs results from their ability to generate decision-based solutions that mirror clinical protocols for sequential medical choices. DQNs integrated into Clinical Decision Support Systems prove vital for enhancing patient-specific medical system modifications combined with care delivery while making CDSS necessary for AI-based medical treatment development.

## 2. FOUNDATIONS OF DEEP Q-NETWORKS AND REINFORCEMENT LEARNING

Agents can obtain environmental reward feedback through experiments to learn using Deep Q-Networks which constitute specialized reinforcement learning algorithms. Q-DN works with the exact learning method that medical decision processes use. Discovering the most rewarding policy represents the fundamental operational principle of RL during evaluation of extended sequences of performance (Sorte et al., 2024). Health practitioners need to find the most effective sequence of treatments which makes this method perfectly suitable for clinical requirements.

Traditional Q-learning performs action-state pair Q-value updates by using Q-tables as its mechanism. Medical facilities present various states and actions which preclude the use of Q-tables as a practical decision-making tool. DQNs solve the scalability problem by implementing deep neural networks to function as Q-function approximators which process dynamic continuous state space arrangement. The training procedure of DQN operates by using a memory buffer which stores historical experiences to conduct experience replay functions. The target network mechanism allows stable learning performance by decreasing the unpredictable behaviours that appear during value estimation processes. DQNs become suitable for practical applications when enhancement additions are applied for improved operational functionality (Temsah et al., 2024).

Through clinical patient data processing along with treatment protocols and feedback outcomes DQNs acquire the ability to discover suitable treatment plans.

The system improves its recommended treatments during longer periods of operation by receiving feedback about patient responses changes. The advanced Clinical Decision Support Systems (CDSS) execute central support operations using this framework for delivering customized medical interventions as it functions through adaptive patient data management.

*Figure 3. DQN and Reinforcement Learning Foundations*

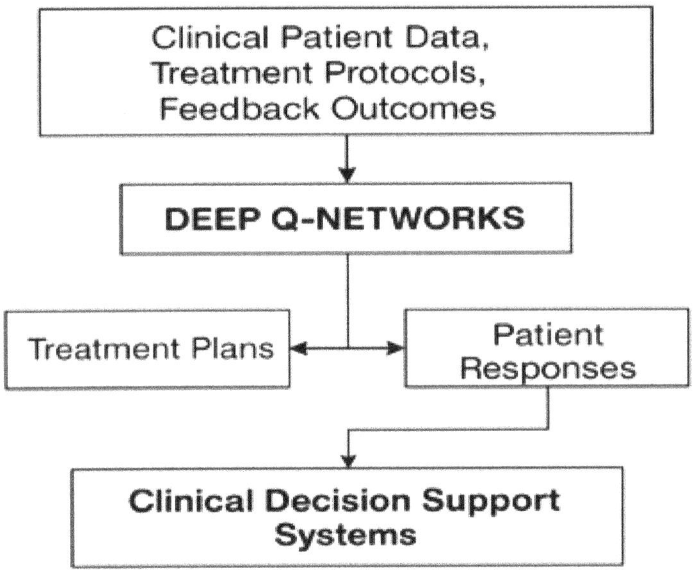


## 2.1 Overview of DQNs and How They Learn from Healthcare Data

The process of Deep Q-Network (DQN) allows systems to interact with environmental data to generate multiple sequential choices. The healthcare environment contains a combination of medical databases with patient records and feedback from intervention activities and examination outcomes (Wood et al., 2021). Deep neural networks function as approximation models for Q-function action values in the approval process when the system encounters specific states. The system structure allows it to choose actions that result in maximum clinical outcomes in the long term. DQNs acquire knowledge by tracking an exploration process which uses feedback generated from healthcare datasets in the environment. Medical processing of data shows how different treatment approaches enable the model to reach its optimal clinical results. Face the challenge of diabetic patient treatment using DQNs because these models evaluate drug modifications and lifestyle modifications methods against each other to achieve optimal blood sugar control with minimal adverse effects.

DQNs train through a process that saves Experience tuples containing present state information after linking it with preferred action selection and reward outputs and next state data into replay memory. The randomness of sampling from replay memory ensures stable training outcomes since it prevents experience data synchronization. The learning process of DQNs results in increasing effectiveness over time by performing continuous updates which enable them to learn different patient situations and complicated clinical situations (Ghavidel et al., 2024). Effective time-sensitive medical choice management becomes available for healthcare providers who employ DQNs as a solution. DQNs bring significant worth to disease treatment development and individual medicine practices by enabling the analysis of current patient information for improved treatment strategies.

## 2.2 Benefits over Traditional Machine Learning Models

The healthcare analytics systems based on original machine learning models generate single predictions from static data points at once. The models show minimal ability to adjust clinical systems while maintaining consistent optimal performance outcomes. A DQN system builds upon traditional machine learning features through reinforcement learning by implementing a sophisticated framework structure. The capability of DQNs to create procedure decision models represents their principal strength. DQNs perform complete evaluation of future action outcomes while traditional ML depends on current data to make predictive analyses. DQNs provide maximum value to medical applications by making decisions that guide medical practices which range from disease management to therapeutic development as well as drug dosage adjustments.

DQNs provide successful performance when managing information systems which consist of numerous attributes together with unpredictable features (Shao, 2024). Modern analytical methods struggle to manage large complex medical information consisting of laboratory tests and genetic data alongside radiological picture laboratory outputs. Multi-input neural networks in DQNs conduct extensive evaluations that help detect multiple patterns as well as multiple association types to generate precise responses for specific clinical applications. Moreover, DQNs are inherently adaptive. The medical model operated by DQNs produces enhanced outcomes from processing newly acquired patient data or doctor situations while maintaining operation without executing full training redesign. DQNs maintains learning persistence that helps the system develop new clinical solution capabilities during its operational phase. Through the application of experience replay with target networks the system obtains two-fold defensive training capabilities that reduce learning instability and avoid standard machine learning misfit issues (Shuford, 2024). The advanced functionality of DQNs makes them suitable novel solutions for enabling adaptive intelligent healthcare operations (Jain & Jaidka, 2023).

## 2.3 Applications in Dynamic and Complex Medical Environments

The healthcare system features multiple complex components because providing individual patient care requires ongoing adjustments of mutable variables throughout healthcare management and essential medical intervention assessment. The ability of dynamic healthcare environments to use DQNs proves suitable since these networks learn in real time while adapting to optimize system performance. The use of Deep Q-Network technology provides Clinical Decision Support Systems with adaptive recommendation solutions that serve hospital staff in their particular healthcare environments. Patient data acquisition occurs in the critical care unit to help DQNs develop optimal ventilation approaches together with medication protocols and fluid therapy protocols (Zhang, 2023). Healthcare professionals solve their urgent timing needs with reinforcement learning to produce better healthcare services and lower the number of preventable negative outcomes.

The combination of chemotherapy treatments with the design of radiation therapy plans for cancer patients now receive help from DQNs in modern medical practice. The network uses genetic indicators along with tumor measurement factors to study historical therapeutic outcomes for producing treatment protocols with lesser adverse side effects (Jain & Jain, 2023). DQNs allow healthcare staff to use their advanced modelling abilities for predicting long-term patient outcomes while allowing them to adjust diabetes and hypertension patient treatments using obtained patient forward data. Basic hospital management software development with DQN assistance enables better scheduling operations and improves urgent care procedures and patient room planning procedures (Abell et al., 2023). The performance enhancement through DQNs improves operational quality to create benefits which positively affect both medical outcomes and clinical functions. The system conducts disease predictions by integrating DQNs together with readmission pattern analysis and predicted treatment assessments. Healthcare institutions leverage DQNs to build flexible technological infrastructure through which medical staff can evaluate data with rising treatment delivery approaches. The table 1 presents various application areas where Deep Q-Networks (DQNs) enhance healthcare operations. It highlights their role in Clinical Decision Support Systems, critical care, and personalized treatment planning. DQNs assist in managing hospital operations, predicting diseases, and optimizing clinical workflows. Each entry explains how AI-driven solutions contribute to improved patient care and operational efficiency.

*Table 1. Applications of DQNs in Healthcare*

| Application Area | Description |
|---|---|
| Clinical Decision Support Systems (CDSS) | Provides adaptive, real-time recommendations customized for hospital staff and environments. |
| Critical Care Optimization | Optimizes ventilator settings, medication protocols, and fluid therapy using real-time ICU data. |
| Emergency and Time-Critical Decisions | Uses reinforcement learning to assist in rapid decisions, improving care quality and outcomes. |
| Cancer Treatment Planning | Designs radiation protocols by analyzing genetic and tumor data for fewer side effects. |
| Cancer Treatment Planning | Predicts and adjusts treatments for diabetes and hypertension using forward patient data. |
| Hospital Operations Management | Enhances scheduling, urgent care planning, and room allocation for better resource use. |
| Operational Performance Enhancement | Improves clinical workflows and medical outcomes through performance optimization. |
| Disease Prediction & Readmission Analysis | Forecasts disease progression and readmission risks using historical and treatment data. |
| Technological Infrastructure Building | Supports creation of flexible, scalable platforms for dynamic treatment delivery strategies. |

## 3. AI-DRIVEN CLINICAL DECISION SUPPORT SYSTEMS (CDSS)

The development of medical decisions for physicians depends on operational frameworks that emerge from deploying CDSS systems that utilize deep Q-Networks within healthcare facilities. Clinical Decision Support Systems (CDSS) stand as foundational healthcare devices which direct medical staff toward better clinical choices. Deep Copy-Network builds better healthcare solutions with customizability than rule-based systems through its flexible CDSS platforms (Van Cauwenberge et al., 2022).

A medical practitioner uses AI to develop diagnosis recommendations using EHR information which brings together results from clinical tests and lab results and genetic information. The diagnostic elements of DQNs enable predictive capabilities since they process diagnostic testing results for predictions. CDSS with artificial intelligence strengthens its operational capacity during learning to provide effective healthcare for difficult clinical situations. DQN-based CDSS tools establish optimal therapy approaches for complex illnesses by incorporating both medical review history procedures with patient-considered details. Fast medical processes occurring on the informational system produce exact medical evaluations combined with lower procedural errors.

Clinical Decision Support Systems enabled by AI allow healthcare personnel to deliver immediate medical services when they integrate disease forecasting capabilities with treatment outcome forecasting mechanisms. The system programs enable medical practitioners to create automatic procedures for conducting patient meetings without needing any administrative processes. Medical organizations establish effective proactive healthcare services for their healthcare systems by integrating CDSS systems with AI functionality (Elhaddad & Hamam, 2024). Healthcare staff working as a group develops professional medical alliances within these systems to produce exceptional medical decisions which boost treatment performance across different domains.

## 3.1 Functionality and Architecture of AI-Powered CDSS

Healthcare data sources move through data-driven artificial intelligence systems that use evidence-based data transmission channels to reach artificial intelligence models through their organizational structures. Every Computerized Decision Support System consists of data collection facilities with knowledge management tools and analytical engines that aid in making inferences and user interface functionality. The functionality of DQNs allows systems to establish optimal choices using their built-in clinical operational methods. Under normal operations the AI-powered CDSS System retrieves healthcare information from EHRs then integrates these records and linked lab results and device data as well as wearable device data. Standardization rules enable the conversion of front section data units into a format suitable for evaluation (Eltawil et al., 2023). The patient record assessment stage of the DQN model enables its top performance level for decision generation. Virtual testing's advanced methodology examines long-term advantages that unite superior patient results with reduced side effects and lower healthcare expenses for creating target outcomes.

New patient data and treatment records get processed through the feedback loop before producing improved decision outcomes. AI-CDSS development persists since the system incorporates new medical data which enables it to improve its operations alongside medical information evolution. Medical staff receive evidence-based diagnostic suggestions from the interface through displayed propositions which are accompanied by their associated risk scores. The AI-CDSS software delivers customized complex choice management systems to healthcare staff who maintain full control of medical autonomy. The system design offers support tools that work in real time with scalable features alongside interoperation of hospital operational procedures for optimized patient care results.

## 3.2 Enhancing Diagnostic Accuracy And Outcome Prediction

Medical staff dealing with industrial artificial intelligence systems obtain predictive outcome assessments combined with advanced diagnostic equipment from such systems. These current diagnostic procedures face problems that originate from human errors mixed with lacking data from patient records together with insufficient analysis time. The latent approach in DQ-Networks (DQ-N) procedures allows AI to address performance problems through the capabilities of choosing data and learning methods (Helenason et al., 2024). Historical data analysis within the DQN method helps the system find complex linkages between diagnosis indicators that include treatment results and genetic identifiers combined with test findings. The system operates at a diagnostic level that exceeds human possibilities to identify multiple diagnoses across infrequent medical cases. Doctors utilize the integrated diagnostic ability of image scan AI systems that link to Electronic Health Record databases for better cancer and neurodegenerative condition recognition in their early stages.

The predictive abilities of DQN-based CDSS systems are the primary factor that leads to their effective operation. The evaluation system performs disease evolution predictions through simulated treatment situations to determine patient health complications along with healing durations. Predictions from the system allow healthcare providers to develop customized treatments and create both care plans and prevent treatment failures (Hwang et al., 2022). Users who apply AI-based Clinical Decision Support Systems achieve more accurate diagnoses when protocol standards are followed and they perform fewer futile tests and procedures. CDSS functions as a system providing healthcare staff additional clinical knowledge to build their competence during critical responses across emergency and intensive care medicine. Medical systems will transition to precise and predictive healthcare delivery by developing advanced AI diagnostic software through high-quality data set training.

## 3.3 Case Examples in Diagnosing Complex Conditions

Healthcare programs using AI Driven Clinical Decision Support System (CDSS) systems that implement Deep Q-Networks (DQNs) have optimized their advanced medical situation detection procedures. The diagnostic systems produce outstanding results in handling complex medical signs that contain indeterminate dynamic or multiple factors since traditional diagnostic instruments prove ineffective in such challenging situations. Medical practice demonstrates the functionality of DQNs through analyzing oncology field data (Xia et al., 2024). Multipurpose cancer databases containing tumor progression information and medical imaging data and genetic profiles and patient treatment responses empower the AI Driven CDSS to supply healthcare staff with disease diagnosis abilities along with therapeutic selection capabilities. AI-generated glioblastoma radiotherapy plans incorporate patient data patterns to produce their outcomes.

AI-CDSS diagnostic operations analyze preliminary indications to identify early-stage Alzheimer's disease through analysis of previously recorded assessment results before medical diagnosis standards are met. Early disease phase screenings by doctors enable medical providers to execute key disease management approaches successfully. AI Driven CDSS healthcare applications provide the best recommendations through precise sepsis condition predictions among intensive care unit patients. CDSS uses its antibiotic care activation system to monitor vital patient data continuously for providing infection treatment when signs emerge. Quick detection abilities of this system lead to improved survival statistics at critical care facilities. Multiple medical case studies demonstrate that Artificial Intelligence-Clinical Decision Support Systems help medical staff diagnose complicated medical requirements in advance to achieve better treatment outcomes for patients (Malsia & Loku, 2024). The implementation of AI-based operational systems leads healthcare facilities to generate profits through better treatment quality that produces superior medical outcomes for patients.

## 4. PERSONALIZED TREATMENT AND PREDICTIVE ANALYTICS

Real-time patient data allows medical achievements to create individualized treatments based on specific cure methods for each patient. Deep Q-Networks allow medical practitioners to execute precise outcomes analysis of individual patient treatments by implementing reinforcement learning algorithms through AI Clinical Decision Support Systems. AI-based patient evaluation depends on the integration of three different types of databases that combine personal information with medical and genetic records from electronic systems and portable devices. Patient health records undergo analysis through AI models to generate proper therapeutic plans which fulfil unique clinical needs of individual patients.

In oncology care the DQN-based CDSS choses tumor treatment protocols by combining chemotherapy with immunotherapy based on genetic testing results and tumor characteristics examination. Predictive analytics makes patient treatment plans more effective by allowing healthcare professionals to predict how different therapeutic options will affect patients (Matheus Mr & Barzani Den Mr, 2021). The algorithmic-based prediction focuses on single patient treatment functions.

Predictive models developed for diabetes and hypertension conditions help healthcare staff identify future disease patterns thereby they can modify treatments to prevent complications. Healthcare providers use CDSS systems backed by artificial intelligence to provide more exact patient care through predictive analytics thereby delivering superior clinical outcomes that patients also view as satisfactory treatment. Healthcare operations in the present use the adaptive healthcare model to deliver individual care that addresses specific needs of patients.

## 4.1 Use of AI for Individualized Treatment Planning

The substantial quantities of health service data enable AI algorithms to design therapeutic procedures that are specialized for specific needs. The DQN based on machine learning receives patient data combined with DNA information to generate individual therapeutic recommendations (Peek et al., 2024). The importance of AI treatment planning increases because AI generates patient-specific care patterns that reach better results than traditional therapeutic practices. Through its network architecture medical AI gathers tumor dimensions in addition to supporting clinical information that healthcare providers use for finding ideal treatments. Medical technology shows its peak efficiency through this technique because it reduces negative outcomes during healthcare treatment of patients. Diabetic patients under cardiovascular or hypertension care need active treatments requiring continuous vital sign monitoring for simultaneous medication adjustments. The treatment strategy enhances its AF systems operations by implementing reinforcement learning which produces better recommendations through analyzing new clinical outcome data (Tanguay-Sela et al., 2022).

Healthcare providers can maximize their patients' outcomes and caregivers can improve their satisfaction levels when treatments match individual patient needs. Implementation of reinforcement learning goals in clinical practice lets physicians identify how diseases advance through time. The structure of deep Q-Networks in reinforcement learning lets healthcare providers track disease patterns of patients through automated tracking techniques triggering immediate disease prevention protocols. RL provides exceptional abilities that allow the system to obtain tracking system data and DNA sequences alongside their genealogical links for making precise individual disease predictions. The MAL medical systems use healthcare data to identify key medical relationships that help people detect early diseases in cardiovascular problems and oncological disorders and neurodegenerative diseases. The pattern identification capability of the AI platform generates disease pathology predictions that include details about treatments risks and complications and disease relapse indicators.

The predictive model allows healthcare providers to forecast patient health changes thus leading to necessary changes in follow-up treatments before nursing interventions. The RL models operate as disease indicator checkers which support healthcare workers in predicting diabetes and Chronic Obstructive Pulmonary Disease (COPD) patients' healthcare outcomes from modifications made to their treatment approach and therapeutic choices (Wang et al., 2021). Higher disease management performance enables healthcare staff to lower risks of adverse healthcare incidents and hospital admissions. Medical services can establish their most effective healthcare delivery system by implementing predictive care methods that employ reinforcement learning automation. Hospitals operate integrated clinical systems to fulfil the achievement targets of their distinct medical programs.

## 4.2 Reinforcement Learning For Personalized Care And Disease Prediction

The precision treatment development process for healthcare professionals requires Artificial Intelligence because it enables precise sharing systems for precision medicine platform data. Medical professionals use artificial intelligence to synthesize detailed patient healthcare information by processing electronic records with genetic results and imaging data and wearable patient data simultaneously in order to gain precise medical information for selecting suitable treatment options.

Patient medical data analysis becomes complete through the combination of reinforcement learning models with Deep Q-Networks (DQNs) which healthcare providers' access. Healthcare workers need to investigate multiple health databases to find specific patient danger points which guides their selection of optimal treatments while minimizing drug safety risks. Medical staff combine genomic choice-support systems integrated with medical information to create better patient recoveries through selective use of chemotherapy and immunotherapy treatments.

AI-based programs enable medical practitioners to track chronic disease patients continuously by monitoring their current treatment status data. Clinical performance tracking and proper care reform identification happen within AI systems after sensor data from IoT gets combined with wearable devices. Medical personnel base their choices on analysis of genetic information together with patient lifestyle data coupled with environmental tracking together with their present treatment data. The analytical system under precision medicine supports the development of organized new healthcare delivery models through patient-specific healthcare information.

## 5. REAL-TIME DATA INTEGRATION IN HEALTHCARE

The use of real-time healthcare data systems with AI-driven assisted decision systems enables medical organizations to reach their highest potential results. The exchange of information between EHR systems and wearable devices along with mobile health applications and imaging and laboratory equipment happens in real-time during healthcare data integration. Medical recommendations generated by AI become instantly accessible to physicians during their assessment of patient Health data in Health data records (Xu et al., 2023). The combination of reinforcement learning algorithms with Deep Q-Network methods makes Health data at scale reach its full potential of effectiveness. Specific patient information enters models which use this input data for developing customized therapeutic recommendations. Real-time care protocols emerge from AI systems through continuous vital signs assessments whereas lab result examination and patient history retrieval monitor healthcare alerts that track health status shifts. The healthcare workforce can examine diabetic patients' statuses live because these patients have hypertension and cardio-vascular problems (Zicari et al., 2021). Through sensor-based medical equipment which operates in real-time health staff can identify early warning signs of health status changes before dangerous situations develop. Patient monitoring solutions promote healthcare safety protocol enhancement by giving medical personnel direct access to manage health care needs.

### 5.1 Early Disease Detection Using AI

AI technology brings its biggest advantages to medical practitioners through its ability to detect medical conditions that cannot be observed through traditional examination. Artificial intelligence uses large data processing to detect diseases before traditional examination by connecting visual medical information with genomic data along with laboratory results and lifestyle patient information. By uniting DQN and reinforcement learning models one achieves the best possible results for early warning detection (Armeni et al., 2022). Medical image assessment based on artificial intelligence enables doctors to detect minor indicators for cancer cell growth and brain-related cardiovascular disease risks. Medical detection models operated by artificial intelligence evolve better all the time in order for physicians to stop treatment delays.

AI-based disease detection systems operate at high speeds to construct beneficial treatment options for healthcare service providers. Aggressive Processive Inferential Recurrent Modules functions as an analysis system for oncology professionals to identify breast tissue cancers during early stages which subsequently reduces the necessity for complicated medical image technology. The analysis function of AI models permits health professionals to detect variations in brain structure that leads to predetermined treatment durations for slowing disease progression. AI models discover early indications through their operational mechanisms to protect health services by achieving positive results that ensure survival while improving life quality.

The AI analysis system links two main data platforms to connect both EHRs and medical imaging files within the system database (Chen, 2024). Healthcare providers implemented basic changes to their patient data assessment methods by integrating artificial intelligence systems into EHRs and medical imaging tools and other systems. Healthcare history medical documents join with laboratory results to provide combined information with medical treatment details that exist in Electronic Health Records (EHRs). Deep Q-Networks (DQNs) let medical professionals develop vital analysis capabilities to detect broad patterns in clinical relations. Continuous patient health evaluation requires access to visual data collected between Magnetic Resonance Imaging (MRI) systems when combined with Computed Tomography (CT) scanners and X-ray equipment (Jain et al., 2025).

The identification of medical conditions together with their identifying signs becomes possible through AI deep learning systems' assessment of visual data. Medical imaging systems utilize powerful databases to find both tumors and lesions and pathological shapes of cardiovascular and neurological systems. AI systems develop patient assessments through their strong training abilities by combining Electronic Health Records information with Medical Imaging source content (Johnson et al., 2021). The combination of medical image assessments by AI systems with clinical lab reports and patient medical records enables healthcare professionals to deliver better medical diagnosis. AI technology enables staff to obtain superior medical outcomes because it swiftly identifies medical conditions and reduces diagnostic errors in Electronic Health Record data as well as medical imaging data. Healthcare personnel obtain superior treatment outcomes through AI-based disease detection at specific times and at precise detection levels when they use Electronic Health Records and process medical imaging data.

## 5.2 Early Diagnosis of Cancer, Cardiovascular, and Neurological Disorders

Medical professionals should identify severe cases of cancer and cardiovascular diseases and neurological disorders in their initial stages to achieve successful outcomes. The diagnostic ability of these fields enhances considerably through utilization of machine learning and reinforcement learning algorithms which embrace Deep Q-Network (DQNs) with AI technologies. Medical diagnostics improves through AI systems because these algorithms evaluate pictures to detect tumors together with abnormal growths within mammograms and CT scans and MRIs. Machine learning systems achieve the capacity to identify cancer markers during their early development state by receiving training from image databases preceding patient symptom presentation (Kaur et al., 2022). AI-based cancer detection produces early warnings which triggers prompt medical treatment that better improves patient survival numbers.

AI-supported ECG analysis performed alongside heart rate variability measurements and medical images results in detectable small cardiovascular indicators for both heart failure elements detection and arrhythmia and cardiac artery disease diagnosis. Analytic models function as warning indicators which medical staff can use to detect patient risks based on collected pattern information. The combination of artificial intelligence technology with both documentation systems and brain scanning indicators enables medical practitioners to identify initial signs of diseases that lead to dementia like Alzheimer's disease in addition to Parkinson's disease and multiple sclerosis (Jain & Jain, 2024). To use blocking therapeutic methods for preserving patient health alongside preventing neurological disorder progression doctors must make early disease detections. Artificial Intelligence delivers advanced early diagnosis capabilities to healthcare that enables immediate correct treatment delivery to patients (Qureshi et al., 2023).

## 5.3 Role of IoT and Smart Sensors in Continuous Patient Monitoring

Healthcare derives its essential value from the combination of Internet of Things devices with intelligent sensors enabling steady patient tracking which allows for immediate condition detection in their early stages. The smartwatch system provides continuous patient monitoring by uniting heart rate monitor data with continuous glucose monitor information to gather essential medical signals as well as physical activity metrics from patient bodies. The health monitoring capabilities of the devices send remote patient information to healthcare providers who use these data for non-standard medical care. Through AI algorithms IoT sensors send their information to detect health risks at specific points by analyzing abnormal patterns. Healthcare staff monitor patient heart condition by tracking heart disease indicators through the combination of ECG devices together with continuous glucose monitors. AI learns high-risk patient variables by processing medical data so it can perform immediate preventive actions.

Surgical rooms and hospital ICUs implement sensor systems that present live patient measurement information required by healthcare staff to initiate urgent medical interventions. Medical sensor devices transmit patient health indicator data straight to AI systems for warning system development of early patient conditions.

Healthcare providers achieve better chronic patient management through IoT monitoring of smart sensors which also helps avoid hospital admissions.

## 6. OPERATIONAL EFFICIENCY AND ETHICAL OVERSIGHT

The operational efficiency of AI helps medical institutions create superior medical decision platforms and improve their operational functionality. Information automation enables medical institutions to gain operational efficiency through the management of logistical responsibilities and streamlining operational procedures with artificial intelligence (Al-Dmour et al., 2025). AI programming tools allow healthcare organizations to build scheduling programs for improving their workforce management systems. Healthcare institutions prepare their necessary resources with AI-based patient admission forecasts prior to patient check-ins. The healthcare institution benefits from both shorter patient waiting periods and operational cost reduction through this development.

Hospital AI implementations need total ethical governance because it provides protected information security to patients and ensures clear system operation and equal treatment of all applicants. Healthcare organizations must protect all patient data to fulfill the requirement of Health Insurance Portability and Accountability Act (HIPAA) confidentiality standards needed for successful operation of AI systems. The design requirements for AI systems consist of algorithm development methods which eliminate operational bias to guarantee unbiased medical care for all patients using healthcare services. Medical personnel must exercise ethical judgment about how to prevent machine system malfunctions without compromising the subjective clinical evaluations during diagnosis and treatment choice processes (Aldoseri et al., 2023). The clinical decisions of medical service providers require AI tools to use which results in automated tasks implemented by AI systems with continuous human oversight for ethical patient care provision. Healthcare organizations use AI technology to enhance their systems while creating better medical care treatment methods.

### 6.1 Optimizing Hospital Resources And Clinical Workflows

AI technologies apply optimized clinical workflows to improve hospital resources operations that achieves quality medical processes and efficient operational outcomes. The use of healthcare AI systems that analyze historical hospital data enables forecasting patient admissions for the next several months to help hospitals optimize their staffing and resource distribution. The predictive system allows healthcare organizations to plan their resources because it reveals which essential medical assets and ready healthcare staff will be available at particular times.

Medical practitioners use artificial intelligence systems to automate administrative clinical work by establishing operational patient booking systems along with documentation and billing capacities. The implementation of automated scheduling enables healthcare providers to use formerly unused waiting times for offering premium medical treatments to patients. The AI systems working in healthcare institutions use severity assessments to direct critical treatment approaches toward patients who display high-risk characteristics. Medical staff can use AI support systems to achieve two advantages which are immediate access to patient records and medical information that results in multiple treatment choices. The total achievement of operational requirements happens when clinical programs join activities from healthcare systems. Hospital resource management achieves its best level when health services improve and operational expenses decrease.

## 6.2 Addressing Data Privacy, Bias, And Ethical Concerns

Healthcare organizations need to resolve their data privacy and security matters because these problems can result in discrimination as well as ethical issues that develop within AI computing systems. Protected medical records face more security threats in the healthcare sector and AI healthcare technologies create systematic problems that trigger ethical assessment needs [40]. The implementation of HIPAA compliance provides healthcare organizations across the board with protected procedures to defend their AI system data security. When patient data security breaches are disclosed, the consequences become substantial for patients together with the permanent loss of public trust in Artificial Intelligence technology systems. Complete security systems must be established by healthcare organizations to defend their data through secure access methods and encryption protocols alongside precise methods for handling patient material.

The security threat leading to medical data breaches stems primarily from algorithmic bias. AI systems that use biased information function to protect current healthcare inequalities that exist between different patient groups. A particular group of patients receives subpar medical services because of the current process (Quazi et al., 2024). Multiple demographic patient populations need to train Medical AI systems for prescriptions to remain accurate for every demographic group. The delivery of equitable medical services to patients depends on enterprise healthcare developing extensive training databases and reliable system-based bias analysis techniques. The medical staff and their patients need better understanding of how the AI system uses logical reasoning paths to create its output results. The patients along with healthcare providers require specific details about how AI systems derive their decision outputs. Healthcare organizations must establish legislation using human involvement to build trustworthy AI healthcare systems that prevent potential system-related harm.

## 6.3 Importance of Human Oversight and Transparency

Human observation methods must be used throughout the operation of AI systems to fulfil ethical standards of healthcare transformation as well as responsibility protocol requirements. The evaluation of large data sets through AI analytics generates value as knowledge but physicians maintain their diagnostic abilities to build patient-centered high-quality healthcare. Professional healthcare practitioners exercise their authority in healthcare decisions through enhanced medical decisions enabled by AI tools.

Clinical AI operations need continuous human involvement because critical medical work requires the present watch of medical personnel to guarantee treatment and diagnosis safety. Healthcare experts must check AI-generated output suggestions which will need adaptation to specific patient healthcare requirements (Reddy et al., 2021). Medical professionals achieve maximum effectiveness when they team up with AI systems for decision development processes. Transparency practices enable Healthcare providers to establish trust-based relations that connect patients to AI systems and also unite patients with healthcare providers as well as AI systems. The information system should publicly disclose methods of patient care interaction and data management practices for AI systems to ensure patients receive proper information. Patients demonstrate confidence in Artificial Intelligence operations after seeing ethical and responsible principles which guide these operations because transparency enables such understanding. Healthcare providers need operational insights about AI systems before implementing them in their decision-making practice as they interact with system outputs. A model of medical supervision for AI functions leading to maximum patient satisfaction and best clinical results develops when healthcare personnel oversee operations with correct levels of medical oversight.

# 7. FUTURE DIRECTIONS AND HUMAN-AI COLLABORATION

Medical experts and AI systems will establish future healthcare networks through well-developed operational methods that enhance treatment quality and adaptive medical care delivery. The expansion of healthcare service capabilities occurs because AI technology enables linkage between personalized medical treatments and improved medical interventions through novel advanced applications. Computers will process different data types to unite Deoxyribonucleic acid (DNA) information with personal reports and environmental records which then generate customized healthcare plans (Jain & Jain, 2022).

Medical progress in local healthcare facilities will become possible through the addition of staff who operate AI technology systems. Staff members utilize AI-derived information to create person-centered care approaches that combine their medical experience with empathy (Secinaro et al., 2021). Human professional involvement with AI programs results in better medical outcomes through AI systems that protect from data-based errors but maintain sufficient context understanding. Standard patient procedures handled by AI healthcare systems will lead to better staffing allocation between nurses for advanced medical needs. A combination of newly implemented ethical frameworks plus regulatory systems will develop transparent methods by which users of healthcare receive information about automated healthcare delivery systems. The application of Artificial Intelligence Implementation allows medical providers to determine optimal healthcare operational procedures which enable the development of contemporary patient-specific medical systems that achieve fair patient service.

## 7.1 Strengthening Human-AI Synergy in Clinical Settings

Medical facilities develop network systems that connect AI systems to health professionals to maximize their partnership within clinical operations. AI processes massive patient data collections while human clinicians retain vital understanding of context alongside empathy and advanced decision-making abilities in medical care. Healthcare providers transform patient information using their medical knowledge to create efficient medical judgments with the help of artificial systems. Hospitals make clinical decisions by using physician-generated recommendations from AI systems while AI systems recognize patterns of patient health through medical data analysis. The medical system fusion gives doctors the ability to establish individualized diagnostic methods that result in improved diagnosis creation for patients (Shah & Chen, 2024). The development of AI technology expertise for medical practitioners happens through continuous courses that assist them in creating working environments where AI systems blend with human doctors. The healthcare partnership approach strengthens doctor-patient association while creating better beneficiary-doctor engagement through this model.

## 7.2 Enhancing Trust And Decision Quality Through Collaboration

AI system reliability along with medical staff trust can be enhanced through proper implementation of medical operator systems by improving organizational decision frameworks and system reliability methods. AI systems in medical organizations must provide structured information and detailed recommendation justifications to build long-term professional ties with their human staff. The understanding of AI system recommendation methods enables medical personnel to trust system applications at a higher level. The system aids medical staff through pattern recognition for patient diagnosis due to its capability to generate precise clinical decisions based on current medical information and disease prediction abilities (Solanki et al., 2021). The united usage of AI results in enhanced healthcare delivery because it involves assessments of medical records with expert clinical team knowledge and staff requirements for clinical process management. Future hospital alliances need AI system deployment as their key operational element to improve both medical service quality and team colleague coordination.

## 7.3 Vision for Intelligent, Ethical, and Patient-Centered Healthcare

The goal of healthcare organizations is to create advanced ethical solutions by collaborating medical professionals and artificial intelligence while improving the results of patient-centered care delivery. Through artificial intelligence systems healthcare organizations create specific treatment plans that allow medical staff to give individualized clinical decisions to patients require. AI ethical development needs protective security measures and political healthcare solutions to safeguard privacy and achieve consistent medical services. Healthcare operations convergence functions as a development tool that supports health care fitness and assists patients in reaching their lifestyle goals. Healthcare organizations deliver better direct medical care because AI provides rapid and exact services at important treatment points. Medical relationships get enhancement through AI technology by developing healthcare devices to generate excellent doctor-patient interactions which produce advanced healthcare outcomes.

# 8. CONCLUSION

Medical facilities use Deep Q-Networks (DQNs) alongside reinforcement learning functions through their AI technology to achieve operational transformation goals in medical care decision-making. The system integration with healthcare personnel enables them to work together for creating individualized medical treatments which improve both rapid service quality improvement and full patient care benefits. Scientific researchers in analytical applications of Cardiac Index (CI) develop integrated diagnostic tools by uniting health databases and imaging records and sensor data to generate clinically beneficial medical diagnosis information for physician use.

The clinical decision application with AI enables management resource optimization for health institutions while operational capabilities of hospitals enhance. The supply of computer-generated therapy alternatives becomes possible through real-time data integration methods implemented by healthcare staff working at patient care sites. Healthcare organizations reach operational effectiveness by maximizing their healthcare assets to deliver benefits for patients through cost reductions. The combination of predictive analytic models reinforced by reinforcement learning allows medical staff to improve their disease prediction skills thus enabling them to take proper preventive measures. Medical professionals obtain quick diagnosis abilities to detect critical health conditions early to achieve successful patient outcomes.

Artificial intelligence development through programming introduces new ethical dilemmas since they impose operational limitations on AI system operation. Hard to protect vital healthcare information is now more challenging because of complex password security requirements. System operations need advanced rules for securing patient information according to the standards of AI operational security. Healthcare service providers need to build algorithmic bias prevention systems since these defences' protect their organizational practices from operational discrimination problems. Proper regulation of training data is needed to stop adversities from health inequalities which generate harmful healthcare outcomes for particular patient groups.

Medical professionals should create suitable ethical standards to direct engineers throughout the development of AI systems. Medical staff who analyze core healthcare values can activate two systems which grants them the authority to make medical decisions. Medical staff creates all AI outputs that serve to verify AI recommendations after they review these suggestions using their professional background prior to critical patient situations. The collaboration between healthcare professionals and AI purposes tremendous value in this stage. AI-based high-quality patient care depends on successful integration of professional medical empathy from staff with value-based ethical principles and situational patient understanding.

The present developmental stage of AI-enabled healthcare delivery systems will become the standard for the next year according to medical institutions that intend to maintain their implementation. Physicians need to gain understanding about autonomous system integration which will boost healthcare organizations' operational effectiveness for their patient service delivery systems. Modern medical technology requires ethical principles to ensure clean and visible healthcare services and patient procedures. Medical treatments provided to patients reach the highest level of performance because doctors maintain total ethical and moral professionalism throughout patient contact.

Software development within Healthcare AI enhances interactions between medical staff and AI systems to create the most patient-centered healthcare institutions. Healthcare services can maintain non-stop delivery of their services to achieve better medical outcomes which help patients throughout all population levels. Sophisticated healthcare models developed by AI developers' team up with medical staff and AI analysts to merge service platforms that link technology with human care provision. Flexible medical solutions developed jointly between healthcare staff and artificial intelligence systems will lead medical practices to succeed in future healthcare delivery. The healthcare sector will establish itself as the top entity responsible for creating medical diagnostic systems and personalized treatments by leveraging AI technological development.

## APPENDIX

The below table 2 defines key terms central to understanding AI-driven healthcare systems, particularly those involving Clinical Decision Support Systems (CDSS) and Deep Q-Networks (DQNs). It includes foundational AI concepts, system components, and ethical considerations relevant to personalized and predictive medicine. The terms collectively highlight the interdisciplinary nature of intelligent healthcare solutions.

*Table 2. Key Terms and Definitions in AI-Driven Clinical Decision Support Systems*

| Term | Definition |
|---|---|
| **Artificial Intelligence (AI)** | A branch of computer science that enables machines to simulate human intelligence for tasks like diagnosis, prediction, and decision-making. |
| **Clinical Decision Support System (CDSS)** | An AI-enhanced system that provides medical professionals with real-time, evidence-based recommendations to support clinical decisions. |
| **Deep Q-Networks (DQNs)** | A type of reinforcement learning algorithm using deep neural networks to approximate Q-values for optimal decision-making in dynamic environments. |
| **Reinforcement Learning (RL)** | A machine learning paradigm where agents learn optimal actions by receiving rewards or penalties from the environment over time. |
| **Q-Learning** | A model-free reinforcement learning algorithm that updates action-value pairs to discover the best action policy. |
| **Experience Replay** | A mechanism in DQNs that stores past experiences and samples them randomly during training to improve learning stability. |
| **Target Network** | A secondary neural network used in DQNs to stabilize learning by reducing fluctuations in Q-value updates. |

continued on following page

*Table 2. Continued*

| Term | Definition |
|---|---|
| **Electronic Health Records (EHRs)** | Digital versions of patients' paper charts, containing comprehensive patient medical history, diagnoses, medications, and test results. |
| **Personalized Treatment** | Tailored healthcare strategies designed for individual patients based on their genetic, clinical, and lifestyle data. |
| **Predictive Analytics** | The use of historical and real-time data, often powered by AI, to predict patient outcomes and inform proactive medical decisions. |
| **Human-AI Collaboration** | The joint effort between medical professionals and AI systems to improve clinical accuracy, efficiency, and patient-centered care. |
| **IoT and Smart Sensors** | Internet-connected devices and sensors that collect real-time health data for monitoring and predictive diagnostics. |
| **Ethical AI** | AI systems designed with transparency, accountability, and fairness to ensure responsible and equitable use in sensitive fields like healthcare. |
| **Algorithmic Bias** | Systematic errors in AI outcomes caused by biased training data or flawed model design, potentially leading to inequitable healthcare. |
| **Adaptive Learning** | A characteristic of AI systems, particularly DQNs, that enables continuous improvement by learning from new data over time. |

## REFERENCES


Abell, B., Naicker, S., Rodwell, D., Donovan, T., Tariq, A., Baysari, M., Blythe, R., Parsons, R., & McPhail, S. M. (2023). Identifying barriers and facilitators to successful implementation of computerized clinical decision support systems in hospitals: A NASSS framework-informed scoping review. *Implementation Science : IS*, *18*(1), 32.

Al-Dmour, R., Al-Dmour, H., Basheer Amin, E., & Al-Dmour, A. (2025). Impact of AI and big data analytics on healthcare outcomes: An empirical study in Jordanian healthcare institutions. *Digital Health*, *11*, 20552076241311052.

Aldoseri, A., Al-Khalifa, K. N., & Hamouda, A. M. (2023). Re-thinking data strategy and integration for artificial intelligence: Concepts, opportunities, and challenges. *Applied Sciences (Basel, Switzerland)*, *13*(12), 7082.

Amann, J., Blasimme, A., Vayena, E., Frey, D., & Madai, V. I., & Precise4Q consortium. (2020). Explainability for artificial intelligence in healthcare: A multidisciplinary perspective. *BMC Medical Informatics and Decision Making*, *20*(1), 310.

Armeni, P., & Polat, I., De Rossi Leonardo Maria and Diaferia, L., Meregalli, S., & Gatti, A. (2022). Digital Twins in healthcare: Is it the beginning of a New Era of evidence-based medicine? A critical review. *Journal of Personalized Medicine*, *12*(8), 1255.

Asan, O., Bayrak, A. E., & Choudhury, A. (2020). Artificial intelligence and human trust in healthcare: Focus on clinicians. *Journal of Medical Internet Research*, *22*(6), e15154.

Charow, R., Jeyakumar, T., Younus, S., Dolatabadi, E., & Salhia, M., Al-Mouaswas Dalia and Anderson, M., Balakumar, S., Clare Megan and Dhalla, A., Gillan, C., Haghzare, S., Jackson, E., Lalani, N., Mattson, J., Peteanu, W., Tripp, T., Waldorf, J., Williams, S., Tavares, W., & Wiljer, D. (2021). Artificial intelligence education programs for health care professionals: Scoping review. *JMIR Medical Education*, *7*(4), e31043.

Chen, H. (2024). Blockchain Targets Integrated IoT for Smart Healthcare Systems - A Bibliometric Analysis. *J. Electr. Syst.*, *20*(6s), 1893–1903.

Elhaddad, M., & Hamam, S. (2024). AI-driven clinical Decision Support Systems: An ongoing pursuit of potential. *Cureus*, *16*(4), e57728.

Eltawil, F. A., Atalla, M., Boulos, E., Amirabadi, A., & Tyrrell, P. N. (2023). Analyzing barriers and enablers for the acceptance of artificial intelligence innovations into radiology practice: A scoping review. *Tomography : a Journal for Imaging Research, 9*(4), 1443–1455.

Ghavidel, A., & Pazos, P., & Del Aguila Suarez Rolando and Atashi, A. (2024). Predicting the need for cardiovascular surgery: A comparative study of Machine Learning models. *J.Electron.Electromedical.Eng.Med.Inform, 6*(2), 92–106.

Giordano, C., Brennan, M., Mohamed, B., Rashidi, P., Modave, F., & Tighe, P. (2021). Accessing artificial intelligence for clinical decision-making. *Frontiers in Digital Health, 3*, 645232.

Helenason, J., & Ekström, C., & Falk Magnus and Papachristou, P. (2024). Exploring the feasibility of an artificial intelligence based clinical decision support system for cutaneous melanoma detection in primary care - a mixed method study. *Scandinavian Journal of Primary Health Care, 42*(1), 51–60.

Hwang, J., Lee, T., Lee, H., & Byun, S. (2022). A clinical decision support system for sleep staging tasks with explanations from artificial intelligence: User-centered design and evaluation study. *Journal of Medical Internet Research, 24*(1), e28659.

Jabbour, S., Fouhey, D., Shepard, S., Valley, T. S., Kazerooni, E. A., Banovic, N., Wiens, J., & Sjoding, M. W. (2023). Measuring the impact of AI in the diagnosis of hospitalized patients: A randomized clinical vignette survey study. *Journal of the American Medical Association, 330*(23), 2275–2284.

Jain, S., & Jaidka, P. (2023). Brain Tumor Classification using Deep learning based Novel Hybrid Approach. *2023 2nd International Conference on Edge Computing and Applications (ICECAA)*, 872–876.

Jain, S., & Jaidka, P. (2024). Lung cancer classification using deep learning hybrid model. In *Future of AI in Medical Imaging* (pp. 207–223). IGI Global.

Jain, S., & Jain, V. (2022, March). Novel hybrid boosted ensemble learning framework for brain tumor prediction. *2022 9th International Conference on Computing for Sustainable Global Development (INDIACom).*

Jain, S., & Jain, V. (2023, December). A critical evaluation of deep learning methods for classifying brain tumor: A review. *2023 International Conference on Computational, Networks and Security (ICCINS).*

Jain, S., & Jain, V. (2024). Machine learning and deep learning methods in brain tumor classification: A decade: Systematic literature review. *Intelligent Data Analysis*, 1–32.

Jain, S., Jain, V., & Chatterjee, J. M. (2025). Ensemble based brain tumor classification technique from MRI based on K fold validation approach. *Journal of Integrated Science and Technology, 13*(5), 1114.

Jhade, S., & Gangavarapu, S. P., Channabasamma, & Igorevich Rozhdestvenskiy, O. (2024). Smart Medicine: Exploring the landscape of AI-enhanced Clinical Decision Support Systems. *MATEC Web Conf., 392*, 1083.

Johnson, K. B., Wei, W.-Q., Weeraratne, D., Frisse, M. E., Misulis, K., Rhee, K., Juan, Z., & Snowdon, J. L. (2021). Precision medicine, AI, and the future of personalized health care. *Clinical and Translational Science, 14*(1), 86–93.

Kaur, N., Mittal, A., Kumar, A., & Kumar, R. (2022). Healthcare monitoring through Fog computing: A survey. *ECS Transactions, 107*(1), 7689–7701.

Malsia, E., & Loku, A. (2024). Generative artificial intelligence in health system management: Transformative insights. *Journal of Service Science and Management, 17*(02), 107–117.

Matheus Mr, S., & Barzani Den Mr, V. (2021). An analysis of Artificial Intelligence based clinical decision support systems. *Journal of Biomedical and Sustainable Healthcare Applications*, 9–17.

Orji, C., Reghefaoui, M., Saavedra Palacios, M. S., Thota, P., Peresuodei Tariladei, S., Gill, A., & Hamid, P. (2023). Application of artificial intelligence and machine learning in diagnosing scaphoid fractures: A systematic review. *Cureus, 15*(10), e47732.

Peek, N., Capurro, D., Rozova, V., & van der Veer, S. N. (2024). Bridging the gap: Challenges and strategies for the implementation of artificial intelligence-based clinical decision support systems in clinical practice. *Yearbook of Medical Informatics, 33*(1), 103–114.

Quazi, F., Mohammed PhD, A. S., & Gorrepati, N. (2024). Transforming treatment and diagnosis in healthcare through AI. *International Journal of Global Innovations and Solutions(IJGIS).*

Qureshi, F. M., Golan, R., Ghomeshi, A., & Ramasamy, R. (2023). An update on the use of wearable devices in men's health. *The World Journal of Men's Health, 41*(4), 785–795.

Reddy, S., Rogers, W., Makinen, V.-P., Coiera, E., Brown, P., Wenzel, M., Weicken, E., Ansari, S., Mathur, P., Casey, A., & Kelly, B. (2021). Evaluation framework to guide implementation of AI systems into healthcare settings. *BMJ Health & Care Informatics, 28*(1), e100444.

Secinaro, S., Calandra, D., Secinaro, A., Muthurangu, V., & Biancone, P. (2021). The role of artificial intelligence in healthcare: A structured literature review. *BMC Medical Informatics and Decision Making*, *21*(1), 125.

Shah, N., & Chen, H. (2024). Optimizing healthcare delivery: Investigating key areas for AI integration and impact in clinical settings. In *Preprints*.

Shao, Z. (2024). Analysis of diabetes based on Tree Decision, Logistic Regression and Artificial Neural Network. *Applied and Computational Engineering*, *47*(1), 248–256.

Shuford, J. (2024). Deep Reinforcement Learning unleashing the power of AI in decision-making. *Journal of Artificial Intelligence General Science (JAIGS) ISSN:3006-4023, 1*(1).

Solanki, S. L., Pandrowala, S., Nayak, A., Bhandare, M., Ambulkar, R. P., & Shrikhande, S. V. (2021). Artificial intelligence in perioperative management of major gastrointestinal surgeries. *World Journal of Gastroenterology*, *27*(21), 2758–2770.

Sorte, S. R., Rawekar, A., & Rathod, S. B. (2024). Understanding AI in healthcare: Perspectives of future healthcare professionals. *Cureus*, *16*(8), e66285.

Tanguay-Sela, M., & Benrimoh, D., Popescu Christina and Perez, T., Rollins, C., Snook, E., Lundrigan, E., Armstrong, C., Perlman, K., Fratila, R., Mehltretter, J., Israel, S., Champagne, M., Williams, J., Simard Jade and Parikh, S. V, Karp, J. F., Heller, K., Linnaranta, O., Cardona, L. G., & Turecki Gustavo and Margolese, H. C. (2022). Evaluating the perceived utility of an artificial intelligence-powered clinical decision support system for depression treatment using a simulation center. *Psychiatry Research*, *308*(114336), 114336.

Temsah, M.-H., Alhuzaimi, A. N., Almansour, M., Aljamaan, F., Alhasan, K., Batarfi, M. A., Altamimi, I., Alharbi, A., Alsuhaibani, A. A., Alwakeel, L., Alzahrani, A. A., & Alsulaim, K. B., Jamal Amr and Khayat, A., Alghamdi, M. H., Halwani, R., Khan, M. K., Al-Eyadhy, A., & Nazer, R. (2024). Art or artifact: Evaluating the accuracy, appeal, and educational value of AI-Generated Imagery in DALL·E 3 for illustrating congenital heart diseases. *Journal of Medical Systems*, *48*(1), 54.

Van Cauwenberge, D., & Van Biesen, W., Decruyenaere Johan and Leune, T., & Sterckx, S. (2022). "Many roads lead to Rome and the Artificial Intelligence only shows me one road": An interview study on physician attitudes regarding the implementation of computerised clinical decision support systems. *BMC Medical Ethics*, *23*(1), 50.

Wang, D., Wang, L., Zhang, Z., Ding, W., Zhu, H., Gao, Y., Fan, X., & Tian, F. (2021, May). ``brilliant AI doctor'' in rural clinics: Challenges in AI-powered clinical decision support system deployment. *Proceedings of the 2021 CHI Conference on Human Factors in Computing Systems.*

Wood, E. A., Ange, B. L., & Miller, D. D. (2021). Are we ready to integrate Artificial Intelligence literacy into medical school curriculum: Students and faculty survey. *Journal of Medical Education and Curricular Development, 8*, 23821205211024080.

Xia, L., Zhen, K., Chen, Z., Liang, R., Zhang, X., Gao, Q., Sheng, M., Bing, L., Xia, J., Si, C., Tian, Y., Jia, L., Xu, Y., Wang, W., Zhong, L., Zuo, X., Wang, D., Xie, W., Wan, J., & Zhai, Z. (2024). Current status of VTE risk assessment and prevention using clinical decision support system: a cross-sectional survey from China. In *Research Square*.

Xu, Q., Xie, W., Liao, B., Hu, C., Qin, L., Yang, Z., Xiong, H., Lyu, Y., Zhou, Y., & Luo, A. (2023). Interpretability of clinical decision support systems based on artificial intelligence from technological and medical perspective: A systematic review. *Journal of Healthcare Engineering, 2023*(1), 9919269.

Zhang, Q. (2023). Dynamic routing policies for multi-skill call centers using Deep Q Network. *Mathematics, 11*(22), 4662.

Zicari, R. V, Ahmed, S., Amann, J., Braun, S. A., Brodersen, J., Bruneault, F., Brusseau, J., Campano, E., Coffee, M., Dengel, A., Düdder, B., Gallucci, A., Gilbert, T. K., Gottfrois, P., Goffi, E., Haase, C. B., Hagendorff, T., Hickman, E., Hildt, E., Wurth, R. (2021). Co-design of a trustworthy AI system in healthcare: Deep learning based skin lesion classifier. *Front. Hum. Dyn., 3.*

# Chapter 11 Reinforcement Learning for Adaptive Healthcare: Deep Q-Networks in Clinical Decision Optimization

**Mohammad Arafah**
https://orcid.org/0000-0001-5645-2290
*University of Petra, Jordan*

**Ahmad Aladawi**
https://orcid.org/0009-0004-3935-2940
*Loughborough University, UK*

## ABSTRACT

*The chapter explores the conditioning of Deep Q Networks (DQNs) and computational intelligence for changing the healthcare decision making. We study the role of reinforcement learning for sequential optimization of clinical decisions in different kinds of healthcare domains. Innovations regarding application of DQNs in complex medical environments as well as the theoretical foundations of DQNs are presented. This paper shows how these technologies transform clinical decision supporting systems, predictive analytics, disease diagnosis, personalized treatment optimization as well as IoT-enabled patient monitoring. Demonstrating wide spread implementation in settings of chronic disease management, critical care and diagnostic pathways results in very substantial improvements of clinical outcomes over traditional approaches.*

DOI: 10.4018/979-8-3373-3311-3.ch011

# 1. INTRODUCTION

Artificial intelligence (AI) and computational intelligence integration into healthcare systems is a sphere of modern medicine, which can be called one of the most promising frontiers. In the context of growing healthcare needs, resource limitations, and multi-dimensional decision making situations, computational approaches of advanced nature can develop efficient solutions to improve patient outcomes, ensure appropriate resource allocation, and create appropriate patient care (Topol, 2019). Among renowned AI methodologies, reinforcement learning, including Deep Q-Networks (DQNs), has been showed to be an able uncontrollable procedure for sequential choice cycle in dynamic wellbeing conditions (Esteva et al., 2021).

DQNs and computational intelligence techniques are used this chapter to explore the transformative role of them in healthcare decision making. Through the use of these advanced AI methods, health care providers can create more precise diagnostic materials, particular treatment routines, and real time monitoring systems with better ways to help patients and reasonably cut down health care costs (Davenport & Kalakota, 2019). The collaboration of deep learning architectures and computational intelligence methods forms a robust architecture that is suitable to tackle complexity, uncertainty, high dimensional nature of the medical data (Yu et al., 2018).

However, due to the recent advances in computing power, big data analytics, and neural network architectures, AI takes place with even greater speed in the context of the healthcare. The clinical outcomes are improved, and this economic impact shows the need to know and apply advanced AI methodologies in healthcare environment. However, one of the most important steps for creating adaptive and intelligent systems which can support complex medical decision making processes (Miotto et al., 2018) is the integration of DQNs with computational intelligence techniques.

The true promise of DQNs in healthcare is that they can learn optimal decision policies from trial-and-error interactions in a complex environment. As opposed to supervised learning techniques that so depend on labeled data, DQNs learn from experienced and gradually enhance their decision making ability (Mnih et al., 2015). In healthcare specific contexts where decision making are usually with long term consequenceÆuncertainty Æand Æcomplex trade off amongst immediate Êfuture outcomes, such an adaptive learning approach is particularly valuable (Yu et al., 2021).

## 2. THEORETICAL FOUNDATIONS OF DEEP Q-NETWORKS IN HEALTHCARE

### 2.1 Reinforcement Learning Principles

The reinforcement learning (RL) paradigm is a machine learning paradigm where agents decide sequentially which to do through interaction with an environment (Sutton & Barto, 2018). In contrast to both supervised learning, relying on labeled examples, or unsupervised learning, that derives patterns from unlabelled data, RL employs a reward based learning thus the agents learn to maximize the cumulated reward through interaction with the environment via trial and error. Since many health care scenarios involve sequential decisions under uncertainty, making immediate and long term patient outcomes, this learning paradigm naturally lends itself.

An RL framework consists of an agent (the decision maker), an environment (the healthcare context), a set of possible actions, state transitions and a reward function to quantify 'desirability' of state action pairs (Gottesman et al., 2019). So, the agent will generally portray a decision support system, the environment is made up of patient characteristics and clinical contexts, actions are represented as possible interventions or treatments, and rewards are related to clinical outcomes such as improved health, lower readmission rates, or more efficient resource use.

Markov Decision Processes (MDPs) are the form of mathematical formulations that are usually used for solving the RL problems, which offers a formal definition of sequential decision making under uncertainties (Sutton & Barto, 2018). The tuple (S, A, P, R, $\gamma$) defines an MDP where the state space (patient condition) is represented by S, the action space (treatment options) is denoted by A, P defines the state transition probabilities, R is the reward function defined and $\gamma$ is a discount factor that balances immediate with future rewards.

In particular, healthcare CDSS have shown promise from a model based reinforcement learning perspective due to such explicit models of treatment and patient progression. Unlike model free DQNs policies are learned directly from experience, model based approaches learn a transition model of the clinical environment and use it for planning and policy improvement. In the case of the lack of data but rich knowledge of disease mechanisms, the approach is especially useful for the healthcare domain. In particular, Liu et al. developed a model based DQN for management of sepsis that combines models of the cardiovascular as well as the inflammatory system with neural networks and achieved superior performance with much less training data than model free approaches. The explicit transition model acted as basis for simulating potential treatment trajectories, thus helping the clinicians to generate patient response forecasts to different intervention strategies as well as utilizing counterfactual reasoning for alternative treatment approaches. The strong promise of combining mechanistic modeling with reinforcement learning is in both improving sample efficiency as well as clinical interpretability.

## 2.2 Deep Q-Networks: Architecture and Innovations

Among the recent achievements in the field of reinforcement learning, Deep Q Network (DQNs) involve the union of deep neural networks with Q learning to be able to cope with the high dimensions of the state space commonly found in healthcare data (Mnih et al., 2015). However, healthcare scenarios with large number of patient variables, treatment options, temporal dependencies, make traditional Q learning algorithms ineffective. This limitation was addressed by DQNs by using deep neural networks to approximate the Q function, so that while there is still a big difficult high dimensional medical data problem that needs to be solved, computation is still feasible (Arulkumaran et al., 2017).

Essentially, the key innovation of DQNs is in their ability to learn express data directly in terms of complex state spaces, where they can pick out relevant features from raw data inputs, rather than needing to specify a hand crafted representation (Mnih et al., 2015). In applications of healthcare, there is a wealth of data from diverse modalities ranging from structured electronic health records (EHRs), medical imaging, physiological time series, genomic data, as well as unstructured clinical notes (Miotto et al., 2018), which this representational learning capability is particularly helpful.

Implementation of the DQN in healthcare applications has been augmented by several key innovations for stability and performance:

1. **Experience Replay**: The advantage of this technique is that it stores the transitions occurring amongst states, actions, rewards and next states in a replay buffer and samples it during training to effectively break down the correlation between consecutive samples and ultimately improve the stability of learning (Mnih et al., 2015).
2. **Target Networks**: During training, DQNs have another separate network for creating target values that move less and also help stabilize learning (Mnih et al. 2015).
3. **Dueling Network Architecture**: This architecture divides between state values and action advantage estimation which can improve learning of state value functions and better policy evaluation in healthcare settings where states are bad or good before action is taken.
4. **Prioritized Experience Replay**: An enhancement that samples transitions having a higher likely ramp-up of learning progress more often, and which produces more computation resources to the informative experience.

5. **Double DQN**: Starting from this approach for the treatment recommendation problem, overestimation bias in Q learning is solved by decoupling action selection and evaluation, and hence enables more accurate value estimates and more reliable treatment recommendations.

Although DQNs in care are very promising, there is an inherent difficulty to be overcome that requires some special adaptations. However, sample efficiency remains an important issue since healthcare settings are usually restrictive in providing data for rare conditions or complex interventions. This limitation has, therefore, been addressed by researchers that explore model based reinforcement learning which involves utilization of domain knowledge, transfer learning from simulated environments and prior training of related tasks to promote generalization with little clinical data. Furthermore, healthcare environments are also non-stationary in nature, in which patient populations, treatment protocols and disease pattern change with time, therefore, approaches like meta reinforcement learning and continual learning frameworks which can learn from novel data distributions without forgetting previously learnt knowledge are needed.

Given that sample efficiency is particularly important for healthcare CDSS, and interpretability is important for mitigating provider concerns about the loss of authority to healthcare practitioners, healthcare CDSS may benefit in particular from model based reinforcement learning approaches that incorporate explicit models of disease progression and treatment effects. By contrast, model-free DQNs learn policies from experience and model based methods learn a transition model of the clinical environment for planning and policy improvement. This is particularly useful in the case of healthcare where although there might be relatively little data, a great deal of domain knowledge is present regarding disease mechanisms. For example, Liu et al. proposed a model based DQN for sepsis management, which is composed of cardiovascular and inflammatory system, neural networks, and shown superior performance with much less training data compared to the model free approaches. Explicit transition model also allowed for the simulation of possible treatment trajectories to provide clinicians with forecasts of what the patient's response is expected to be to a given intervention strategy, as well as to aid in counterfactual reasoning on possible intervention strategies that can possibly improve the response from the disease. Mechanistic modeling integration with reinforcement learning is a promising direction of moving towards both improved sample efficiency and clinical interpretability of the learned model.

## 2.3 Computational Intelligence Techniques in Healthcare

Fuzzy systems, evolutionary computation, and swarm intelligence are among many nature inspired computational approaches which constitute computational intelligence and can be used in combination with deep learning methods of healthcare. The advantages in dealing with uncertainty, interpretability, and optimization problems in common clinical decision making problems are offered by these techniques via biologically inspired problem solving frameworks and methodologies.

Fuzzy logic systems offer a way to reason with uncertainty and impreciseness, matching well to the vague aspect of medical knowledge and of clinical assessment. Fuzzy systems are used to represent expert knowledge of how to make the decision in terms of linguistic variables and if-then rules in healthcare applications since it is more interpretable and more consistent with the way clinical reasoning can be broken up.

Evolutionary algorithms based on biological evolution are powerful optimization methods for healthcare problems of complex and multimodal. These algorithms generate possible solutions through these algorithms of selection, crossover, and mutation that improve each generation towards optimal or nearly optimal solutions. Evolutionary algorithms have also been applied in healthcare to problems like selecting features in diagnostic models, optimizing parameters in treatment planning, scheduling of healthcare resources.

In the context of these computational intelligence approaches, hybrid systems are proposed that are the result of integrating DQNs with the various techniques. For example, the fuzzy DQNs are a combination of computational power of deep networks and the interpretability of fuzzy systems; hence they make the decision support systems more transparent. Evaluations of evolutionary algorithms can be successfully used to optimize the architecture and hyperparameters of DQNs and thus improve their performance in particular health care applications.

In particular, due to its combination of computational and deep learning, hybrid neuro-fuzzy systems seem to be among the most promising types of integration of computational intelligence and deep learning for health care applications. A combination of such systems as neural networks with their learning capabilities and fuzzy logic that allows for linguistic explanation results in frameworks that are adaptable from data and at the same time able to provide linguistic explainability. For instance, Deng et al. used a fuzzy DQN model for anticoagulation management to learn membership functions for the concepts of 'mild bleeding risk' or 'therapeutic anticoagulation' from patient data and retained rule structures that are interpretable. Using this hybrid approach, black-box DQNs were able to perform as well as black-box DQNs but with explanations in clinically meaningful linguistic terms. Similarly, evolving fuzzy neural networks facilitate the continuous adaptation of the structure of the network and fuzzy rule parameters, especially for chronic disease management where parameters of patient physiology as well as treatment responses vary over time.

# 3. CLINICAL DECISION SUPPORT SYSTEMS ENHANCED BY DQNS

## 3.1 Evolution of Clinical Decision Support Systems

Since their introduction to the health care in the 1970s, Clinical Decision Support Systems (CDSS) have undergone major progress, evolving from rule based expert systems to complex, multi modal clinical data processing and AI based systems coupled with generation of personalized recommendations (Shortliffe 1976). Along the development of CDSS historical trajectory there have been several CDSS generations with higher sophistication of knowledge representation, inference mechanisms and integration in clinical workflows.

Deep reinforcement learning and computational intelligence have been teamed up to empower the current generation of CDSS as a paradigm change from fixed postures CDSS to adaptive, contextual and personalized decision support (Yu et al., 2018). Unlike previous generations which are limited to determining static recommendations using current observations, DQN empowered systems are capable of determining optimal decision making sequences considering the future consequences and adjusting recommendations according to the patients response to the interventions. In chronic condition, critical care, and personalized treatment/plan this is a particularly valuable capability because of the cascade nature of the decisions by which they affect patient trajectories (Gottesman et al., 2019).

Indeed, several key advances have been made in the integration of DQNs into CDSS architectures:

1. **Sequential Decision Optimization**: The DQN enhanced CDSS can model temporal process dynamics of clinical process and optimize treatment sequences instead of single decisions.
2. **Personalized Treatment Adaptation**: DQN based systems can learn from characteristics of respective patient, comorbidities, and history of treatment, thereby providing a step towards pursuing the cause of precision medicine.
3. **Balancing Short-term and Long-term Outcomes**: This addresses the issue of explicit trade offs between immediate clinical improvements and long term results as this is compatible with reinforcement learning framework behind DQNs.

4. **Continuous Learning from Clinical Practice**: New clinical encounters can be used to continuously learn DQN architectures that can gradually refine recommendation policies based on observations of outcomes and observed clinical practice.

Another great challenge to the implementation of DQNs in clinical workflows is beyond technical evolution. Early deployments experience suggest that successful integration need care taken on sociotechnical factors such as the clinician's trust, workflow compatibility and organizational readiness. However, Sutton et al identify five critical success factors for such implementation of DQN enhanced CDSS namely: (1) Transparent communication of system capabilities and limitations; (2) Allow appropriate clinician override using feedback mechanisms; (3) Incremental deployment starting with decision support rather than automation; (4) Continuous performance monitoring with clear accountability frameworks; (5) Co-development with clinical users throughout the design process. This is particularly important for reinforcement learning systems looking to suggest a sequence of decisions in a sequential decision making paradigm, which can differ considerably from conventional clinical decision support tools.

## 3.2 Architectural Framework for DQN-Based Clinical Decision Support

To integrate DQNs into clinical decision support systems, a solution framework should be built carefully to tackle the distinctive requirements of healthcare environment, e. g. data heterogeneity, temporal dynamics, interpretability, and interaction with clinical workflow (Rajkomar et al., 2018). Generally, a complete DQN based CDSS architecture is comprised of several interconnected building blocks that work together to support intelligent and adaptive decision making.

Data acquisition and preprocessing modules, the foundational parts of this architecture, gather, harmonize and make ready clinical data sourced from different sources like electric health records (EHRs), medical imaging repositories, clinical laboratory information systems and real time monitoring gadgets.

It deploys state representation module for transferring preprocessed clinical data into a comprehensive patient state that will help in making decisions. The representation toward which we wish to derive accurate state policy is crucial for the performance of DQN: it must be complete (this includes any relevant clinical factors, and should in fact include anyone that has any impact on the clinical outcome variables) and computationally tractable (a low enough dimensionality that the resulting dynamics remain controllable).

A DQN component based on the core DQN, implements the reinforcement learning algorithm, a deep neural network to learn an approximate Q function from patient states to possible interventions to expected clinical utility (Mnih et al., 2015). The architecture adopted in this module incorporates elements from Section 2.2 related to architectural innovations including, for instance, experience replay, target networks as well as prioritized learning, adapted to the particular contextual issues of healthcare applications.

In order to conditionally learn the appropriate intervention given a patient, an action selection module takes outputs (Q values for a potential intervention) from the DQN to generate constraining clinical recommendations taking into account availability of treatments, treatment contraindications, and institutional protocols. In fact, this component could use domain knowledge for example in the form of rule based filters, Bayesian decision theory for uncertainty quantification, or constraint satisfaction techniques to guarantee that the recommendations come in line with clinical guidelines as well as practical constraints.

The explanation generation module satisfies the paramount necessity of transparency in clinical decision support by clinical decision support using interpretable explanations of the system's recommendations. The DQN based decision support system is connected with existing healthcare information systems and clinical process through a clinical workflow integration layer so that the recommendations are provided at proper decision points during the workflow of clinician. This architectural framework is illustrated in Fig 1 to relate the components and connections and the flow of information from raw data to actionable, explainable recommendations integrated into clinical workflow.

*Figure 1. Architectural Framework for DQN-Based Clinical Decision Support Systems*

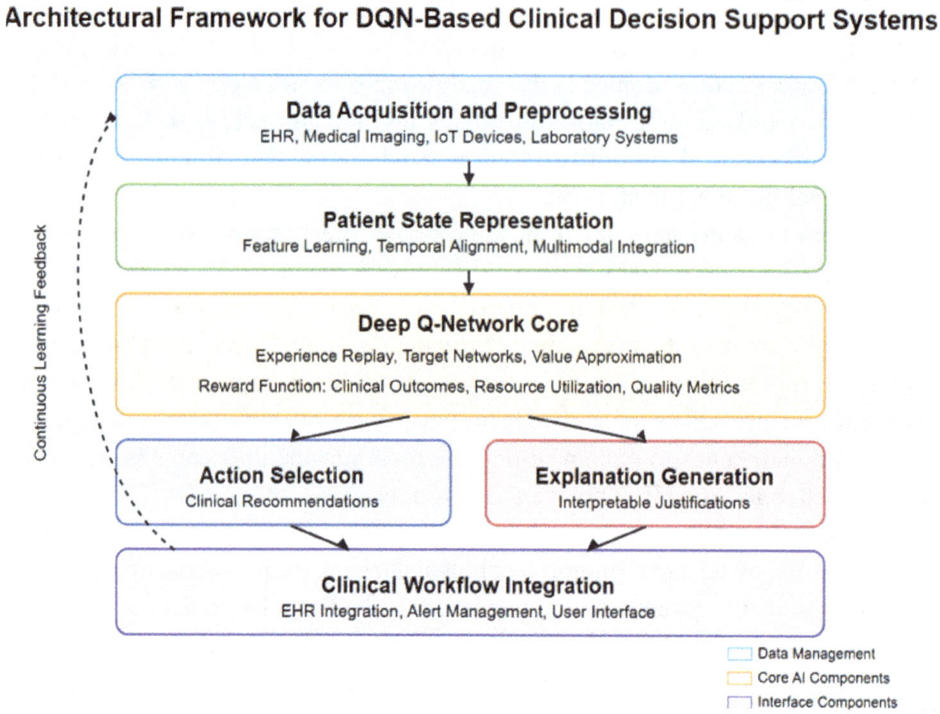


Specifically, model-based reinforcement learning approaches hold promise for healthcare CDSS in part thanks to providing a means to more efficiently and interpretably sample from the transitions into and out of a state. Model based methods for DQNs differ from model free DQNs in that they learn a transition model of the clinical environment and then use that to plan and improve the policy. Data may be limited but extensive domain knowledge is available about disease mechanisms, making this the strongest application of the proposed approach in healthcare. In an example, Liu et al. built a DQN with model based neural networks (in which a cardiovascular and inflammatory system were used with neural networks) with superior performance with way less training data compared to model free approaches. In addition, the explicit transition model allowed simulation of potential treatment trajectories to give clinicians forecasts of how patients should be expected to respond to various intervention strategies, which helped the clinician understand what will happen to the patient if a different treatment approach is used. Finally, we integrate mechanistic modeling with reinforcement learning to the extent that is both promising for sample efficiency and clinical interpretable.

Implementing ensemble approaches for DQN based clinical decision support is an important implementation strategy to gain robustness as well as uncertainty quantification in high stakes healthcare applications. Unlike single DQN model, ensemble methods train one or more DQN models with different initializations, architectures or training data subset and aggregate outputs. Liu et al. showed that ensembles of DQNs for mechanical ventilation management not only led to improved overall performance, but also became capable of quantifying the epistemic uncertainty of the models, both when the models were and when they were not in disagreement with human expertise. In practice, they implemented a mixture of experts voting mechanism which delivered both consensus recommendations and uncertainty quantification to clinicians, but deferred to human when the model disagreed too much. Then, evaluation in a multi center ICU dataset showed that reduction in potentially harmful recommendations by 43% over single model DQNs using same algorithmic approach demonstrates the extent to which architectural choices in clinical deployment can improve safety.

## 3.3 Case Studies in DQN-Enhanced Clinical Decision Support

Using DQN as an enhancement to clinical decision support systems (CDSSs) has been implemented in several pioneering implementations in health care; and these have shown the potential of having this approach in a wide variety of healthcare domains. These case studies serve as practical applications, methodological approaches, and empirical outcomes in DQN to healthcare applications that can be very useful to researchers and practitioners interested in healthcare applications of DQN.

Influential reinforcement learning approach of sepsis management in intensive care units (ICUs) was developed by Komorowski et al. (2018) based on large retrospective dataset. Transforming the clinical task into a sequential decision making problem under the state space being formed with clinical variables, state action space, and the reward function being the maximizing the patient survival and the preserving of the organ function.

It uses Deep Q-Network with experience replay and target networks trained on the offline patient trajectories. On a held out test set, the learned policy performed better than a clinician's decision on expected patient outcome when the AI recommendations were applied, which suggests a mortality reduction from 1.8 to 3.6 percent if the AI recommendations were followed.

Another example is Prasad et al. (2020) that generalize the development of a DQN based system to optimize mechanical ventilation strategy in ICU patients, which is a complex task of ventilator weaning. A recurrent DQN architecture with LSTM layers was used for implementing this, making use of the temporal dependencies present in patient trajectories. A clinician defined safety constraints was included in the system to prevent potentially harmful actions, providing a critical aspect in deploying reinforcement learning in high stakes clinical environments.

As an important application domain of DQN for clinical decision support, antibiotic stewardship serves as a good example as it tackles the problem of the effective infection treatment that requires appropriate antibacterial drug use while avoiding transfer of antimicrobial resistance through inadequate use of antibacterial drugs. Wang et al. developed a hierarchical DQN system for antibiotic prescribing for respiratory infections that first decided whether the infection presents a bacterial versus viral etiology and then determined optimal antibiotic regimens for bacterial infections. Prescribing policies balancing immediate symptom resolution with long-term resistance prevention were learned based on microbiological culture results gathered as delayed rewards. As a prospective evaluation it was demonstrated that recommendations provided by the DQN reduced inappropriate antibiotic prescribing by 31% as compared to standard practice without compromising clinical outcomes. With individual and population level health considerations, this application demonstrates the utility of reinforcement learning for learning of optimal policies to optimize immediate patient needs with public health objectives.

## 4. PREDICTIVE ANALYTICS AND DISEASE DIAGNOSIS

### 4.1 Integrating DQNs with Diagnostic Models

Thus, together with diagnostic models, the integration of Deep Q Network presents a paradigm shift in clinical disease detection and classification away from traditional supervised learning methods towards developing adaptive, sequential diagnostic systems that can learn usefully, sequentially, and adaptively, to maximise or better complement their information gathering and decision making processes (Esteva et al., 2021). Conventional diagnostic AI models tend to take a fixed set of clinical observations and predict diagnostic probabilities based on them, whereas system developed using DQN can compute when to ask for new tests, what tests to ask for, and how to learn from acquisitions of new evidence to optimize the diagnostic accuracy while minimizing costs and patient burden.

A number of limitations of traditional diagnostic models are addressed by this integration. Second, it transforms diagnostic problem from a single step classification to a sequential decision making process that better approximates how physicians do in the clinic, iteratively producing better and better diagnostic hypotheses. Second, context specific testing strategies considering patient specific factors, resource restraints and risk benefit considerations are able to perform in a way to reduce unnecessary testing while maintaining or improving diagnostic accuracy. Third, it provides for active learning during the diagnostic process, updating diagnosis probability with new information and instructs where to focus area of investigation based on most informative investigation.

Usually, diagnostic models are architecturally integrated with DQNs according to one of several paradigms, depending on application context, each with potential pros and cons:

1. **Sequential Testing Optimization**: The DQN in this approach decides which diagnostic tests or clinical assessments to perform next based on the potential information gain, cost, invasiveness, as well as current diagnostic probabilities.
2. **Hierarchical Diagnosis**: It breaks the diagnostic process into several levels of abstraction, where first assuming the diagnosis of large disease categories, and narrowing it down in the selected category.
3. **Active Feature Acquisition**: In this paradigm, the DQN requests the features of clinical observations selectively, rather than complete tests, streaming information at the more granular level.
4. **Diagnostic-Therapeutic Integration**: It has a comprehensive approach that combines evaluation with evaluation planning, taking into account that some diagnostic information derives from therapeutic responses.

The practical impact of DQN enhanced diagnostic systems has been recently shown by their application. For example, Krishnan et al. later developed a DQN based differential diagnosis of abdominal pain approach that sequentially finds which diagnostic question(s) to ask, reducing average number of question asked by 39% while maintaining diagnostic accuracy. Wang et al. also set up a DQN system for radiological workflow optimization, where the preclinical findings are used to determine the imaging order to reduce unnecessary imaging by 28% and speed up diagnosis for critical cases. Chang et al. adaptively selected regions of whole slide images using a single-resolution DQN framework to perform high magnification analysis in pathology, increasing sensitivity to rare histological features in less computational time decisive tissue region.

The use of DQNs with attention mechanisms that emulate radiologist's visual search pattern has had a big impact in computer aided diagnosis in medical imaging. Since traditional computer vision approaches usually uniformly analyze the whole image, while radiologists conduct structured visual search on suspicious regions and collect the additional contextual information whenever necessary, we chose not to consider radiologist's two eyes as input, hence seeking a more flexible and powerful visual representation that captures their selective attention and is general enough to represent regions of interest. In Zhou et al., an attention guided DQN based on mammography interpretation was developed that sequentially attented various regions on the image, until abnormalities were detected, and adaptively changed the resolution and processing depth according to the detected abnormalities. High resolution analysis of the system of interest was performed by exhausting over all possible combinations of thresholds for the quantitative features of interest thereby working on each node sequentially but this analysis reduced computational requirements by nearly an order of magnitude compared to analyzing the whole image in its entirety at high resolution and was highly effective in prioritizing regions with subtle malignancy indicators at which to concentrate subsequent search policies to increase sensitivity to breast cancer detection to 93%. Such approaches have been applied to chest radiography, dermatological imaging and histopathology, and show that reinforcement learning can enhance medical image analysis in both diagnostic classification as well as diagnostic process, both enhancing accuracy and efficiency.

## 4.2 Risk Stratification and Early Warning Systems

Predictive analytics holds critical applications in predicting health risks through risk stratification and early warning systems which place these systems prior to clinical deterioration so that intervention can be made proactively for optimum resource allocation based on patient risk profiles (Henry et al., 2015). However, compared to traditional risk stratification approach which would typically use static risk scoring system or supervised learning models, systems that incorporate the DQN enhancements provide the following advantages: (1) dynamic risk assessment, (2) personalized alerting thresholds and (3) optimize the alert generation process itself to strike a fine balance between sensitivity and specificity, and to reduce the alert fatigue.

Integration of DQNs into the risk stratification systems changes these tools to passive predictors, i.e., to active decision support systems that converge the tradeoff between false positive (unnecessary alerts) and false negative (missed clinical deterioration) by considering contextual factors and observed outcomes. It gives our dynamic approach to early warning systems the freedom to address several traditional weaknesses of existing early warning systems, such as its tendency to produce too many alerts, its lack of personalization, and its lack of responsiveness to different clinical contexts and patient populations.

Usually, the architectural framework for DQN-enhanced risk stratification includes those of several key components:

1. These systems are based on a predictive model with risk estimates that change over time (dynamic risk assessment).
2. DQN component is used to optimize alerting: When and how the clinician should be alerted given the risk level, contextual factors and response time.

3. Alerting Thresholds: This component determines alerting (or threshold) setting that is tailored for each patient based on their baseline condition, comorbidities, characteristics, and so on.
4. Advanced systems offer not only alarm of worsening patients but also propose the actionable steps, based on the predicted risk factors and the possibilities of impairment.

A DQN based risk stratification is a critical application that the timing of the preventive intervention is highly dependent, not only to intervene but when the intervention will be most effective. The current traditional early warning systems tend to be activated at predetermined risk thresholds at which time an intervention may either be too late if deterioration had already progressed, or too early when an unnecessary intervention may harm the patient. On the other hand, Meyer et al. created a DQN system for sepsis intervention timing by learning policies that trade-off early intervention delay and intervention accuracy time while the intervention thresholds adapt dynamically based on the rate of change in patient condition, and on the risk estimation uncertainty and the infused resources. Results in a 300 bed hospital show that dynamic intervention decision timing is superior to static threshold approaches for missed sepsis and unnecessary team activations by demonstrating evaluation.

Risk stratification approaches based on DQN leverage the generalizability challenge, by addressing such issues as transferability of a learned policy to different health care settings, patient populations, and clinical contexts. Locally trained risk models exhibit good performance in their development environment but tend to deteriorate on new settings with different patients' characteristics or practice patterns. A meta reinforcement learning framework is developed by Li et al. to learn a set of patterns, which can be transferred across different hospital settings for more accurate prediction of cardiac arrest. In their approach, they had a hierarchical architecture with a meta learner discovering common predictives patterns at the macro level while a local adaptation layers trained these general representations against each micro context using much less data. The deployment of this transfer learning framework on new hospitals out performed both local models trained with the limited site specific data, and general models that disregarded the institutional differences. After adaptation with 20% of the data typically used for local model development, the system achieved 89% of optimal prediction with essentially no loss of prediction accuracy and reduced alert fatique.

## 4.3 Multimodal Data Fusion for Comprehensive Diagnosis

Diagnostic AI at this frontier of integration has great prospects in combining multiple modalities of data, including structured electronic health records, medical imaging, genomic data, physiology time series, and unstructured clinical notes to achieve more comprehensive, accurate evaluation of disease than any single modality can provide (Miotto et al, 2018). On the contrary, the DQN enhanced approach provides for a more dynamic flexible integration path, where the fusion process itself is optimized by supervising the solution under specific diagnostic objectives and the data characteristics.

Conventional approaches are addressed, and limitations of them are solved using DQN based multimodal fusion. Once modality specific attention and weighting is enabled, both on the basis of what type of data modality contributes to particular clinical scenarios that are of diagnostic relevance (Rajkomar et al., 2018). Second, it helps with adaptive missing data handling that updates the fusion strategy if some modalities are unavailable or unreliable for a particular group of patients. It allows for a cost aware fusion incorporating acquisition costs, time, and patient burden for each data modality so the overall diagnostic efficiency is improved simultaneously as is accuracy.

Figure 2 shows how Deep Q Network works as a multi modal data fusion for holistic diagnosis by dynamically weighting and the selective attention in various underlying data modalities in response to different clinical scenarios.

*Figure 2. DQN-Enhanced Multimodal Data Fusion for Comprehensive Diagnosis*

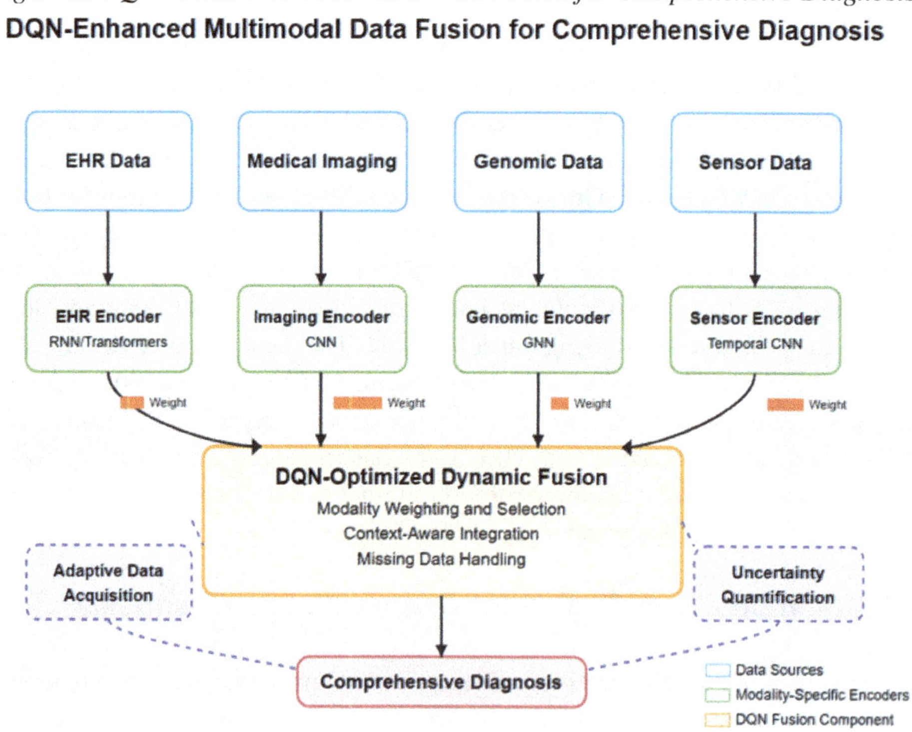

In practice, time information is essential to handle the dependence of different clinical data assets on their availability at different time points during the diagnostic workflow. This leads to the problem of DQN based conventional diagnostic approaches whose formulation contributes to addressing the time-aware multimodal fusion. Time aware methods unlike fusion approaches that presumes all modalities to be always simultaneous, adapts fusion strategy based on availability of its modalities over time. The application of a temporal DQN architecture by Chen et al. for stroke diagnosis was to learn progressively on clinical assessment, laboratory values, laboratory values, and neuroimaging, while maximizing at each time point the accuracy of the diagnosis and recommendation of the modality to prioritize next. It used a recurrent state representation with a belief state of possible diagnoses, and at each new observation updated and used this belief state to determine fusion weights and modality acquisition decisions. However, the early use of additional modalities such as Abrahn motion corrected CT resulted in an improvement of 28% in earlier diagnoses, especially for time sensitive conditions where treatment delay have significant impact on the patient's outcome.

## 5. PERSONALIZED TREATMENT OPTIMIZATION

### 5.1 Adaptive Treatment Regimens for Chronic Diseases

Chronic diseases such as diabetes, hypertension, cardiovascular disease, as well as chronic respiratory conditions represent one of the most burdensome forms of the disease, affecting about half of the population of the United States and accounting for nearly 75% of healthcare expenditures. Longer term management with more complex, multi factorial treatment regimens are needed for these conditions that need to change with disease progress and/or progression, comorbidities, disease response, and patient preferences. Chronic disease management traditionally utilizes standardized clinical guidelines and can deliver little personalization in the context of great disease heterogeneity as measured both in the way the disease manifests and in the way it responds to treatment given to different patients.

Also, the deep Q-Networks can be a promising framework for learning optimal policies for sequence and adjusting interventions in chronic diseases on individual patient characteristics and observed responses. This contrasts with ordinary methods that frequently work with hard decision policies and achieve only an interim optimality in the face of disease duration (therapeutic dynamics); DQN based systems can improve clinical outcomes and patient quality of life while minimizing healthcare utilization throughout this duration.

Addressing a number of issues in chronic disease management, DQNs are applied to this domain:

1. Chronic disease management: Long term Horizon Optimization which requires balancing of immediate symptom control with long term disease progression and complication. The DQN reinforcement framework explicitly incorporates this temporal dimension in modeling the time dimension, and optimizes treatment sequences longer than the time horizon.
2. Treatments in chronic diseases do not have one standard response; the treatment responses are highly variable between patients and patients' differences are influenced by genetics, co-morbidities, lifestyle factors and environmental conditions. Approaches based on DQN can learn personalized policies that are tailored to each patient's attributes and response effects, thus breaking from the mold of the one size fits all mentality of standardized guidelines.
3. Chronic diseases: The chronic diseases generally possess a dynamic behavior which is complex, nonstationary and involves long periods of dormancy, gradual progression, episodes of acute exacerbations. Recurrent DQN architectures provide the means for capturing these temporal dynamics as well as adaptive adaptation of application recommendations to prevent current or anticipated disease exacerbations.
4. Chronic Disease Management is an Optimizing Outcomes in Multiple Dimensions including but not limited to clinical, symptom, functional status, life quality, utilization of health care. Multidimensional reward functions can be used in DQN approaches that can then incorporate these diverse objectives based on patient preferences and clinical priorities.

Behavioral modeling integrated into DQN frameworks is an advanced aspect for chronic disease management, since the adherence to treatment and modications in lifestyle are critical to outcomes. In order to manage type 2 diabetes, Li et al. created a novel DQN architecture with behavioral state variables such as medication adherence patterns, dietary consistency, and those related to exercise engagement in addition to typical clinical parameters. By learning such policies, the system was able to adapt both the treatment regimen as well as the engagement strategies to individual behavioral patterns to recommend simplified medication schedules for patients with adherence challenges and more gradual lifestyle modifications for those with consistent but not optimal engagement. To achieve a 23% improvement in glycemic control over standard treatment optimization not including behavioral factors, this behavioral aware approach was taken. In hypertension and heart failure management, similar approaches have already been explored, but behavioral aspects often explain the 'real world' efficacy of the offered treatment recommendations.

Designed DQN based treatment optimization systems pose a major challenge for comorbidty management, since many patients, particularly the elderly have multiple simultaneous simultaneous condition, which need management in multiple disease specific guidelines. Traditional clinical guidelines for specific diseases, in isolation, run counter to nature, which confounds recommendation of one drug for one disease when another is prescribed for another. In an innovative work, Zhang et al. provided a novel DQN architecture to control hypertension in diabetic chronic kidney disease patients by using a graph neural network for a novel representation between condition and treatment treatment. Disease treatment graph structure was used to obtain the state representation that is comprised of nodes for conditions and treatments and edges for interactions and contraindications. Learning coordinated treatment policies to balance disease specific objectives across comorbidities through condition interactions and resolving such competition becomes possible with this approach. The superior results in all comorbid conditions compared to disease specific DQNs present an argument for an integrated approach to the assessment and treatment of complex care needs among patients with several chronic conditions.

## 5.2 Dose Optimization and Drug Response Prediction

There is no doubt that optimal medication dosing is an important issue in pharmacotherapy and it necessitates a careful dose adjustment, so that the therapeutic efficacy and the potential adverse effects to the patient are well balanced together with the pharmacokinetic and pharmacodynamic characteristics of the patient. Traditional approaches to dosing often focus on population based guidelines with no fitting to age, weight or organ function which makes treatment outcome suboptimal due to large inter individual variation of drug response. Diverse factors including genetic polymorphisms, comorbidities, concurrent medications, as well as physiological differences lead to this variability and introduce a complex, high dimensional problem that is ideally suited to DQN based formulations.

A promising framework for personalized dose optimization based on discharge regulations is provided by Deep Q Network, that is, learns policies of dynamically adjusting the dosages of medication according to observed responses, patient characteristics and therapeutic monitoring. Since the clinical dose titration process is iterative in nature, the sequential decision making paradigm of reinforcement learning naturally applies to this problem.

Challenges in the application of DQNs for medication dosing are addressed by the proposed application:

1. Meds with narrow therapeutic windows: Drugs like anticoagulants, anticonvulsants, immunosuppressants, and chemotherapeutics all have narrow therapeutic

windows – too high or too low dosage ranges lead to failure of the drug either due to its diminished efficacy or due to increased toxicity risk. The DQN approaches can learn to explore these narrow windows based on individual patient factors and response patterns, however, learning dose policies that accomplish this requires finely tuned approaches.

2. Nonlinear processes; drug absorption, distribution, metabolism, and excretion (or ADMET) are complex and nonlinear functions with a great many input factors: genetic polymorphisms, organ function, drug interactions, and etc. Absence of explicit pharmacokinetic model requirement for DQN architectures allows it to implicitly model these interactions from observed data, and with high likelihood to capture patient specific patterns for which traditional models do not do so.
3. Complex time dependencies: Temporal drug effects may depend on time: the response may be delayed, develop tolerance, and exhibit time-variable sensitivity. Recurrent DQNs are able to learn such temporal dynamics, as they can learn optimal dosing policies, that anticipate and adapt to changes in the response pattern over time.
4. Medication dosing errors can be resulting in serious adverse event, hence the need for robust safety conscious optimization approaches. Risk aware and constrained reinforcement learning based on DQN variants can incorporate clinical safety constraints and uncertainty quantification which could guarantee that the dosing recommendation will prioritise patient safety as well as efficacy optimization.

Optimization of combination therapy is a rather challenging problem for DQN based dose optimization, which requires adjustment of several different medications, some of which are potentially interacting. Wang et al. developed a multi agent DQN method to optimize HIV treatment, balancing viral suppression and decreased toxicities to avoid dosing in different antiretroviral drug classes in coordination. The system used communicating, but separate, DQN agents to learn coordinated policies that take into account drug drug interactions and patterns of resistance for each drug class. The superior results were evaluated in a validated HIV treatment simulator with standard combination therapy protocols and showed the highest viral suppression and CD4 recovery in treatment experienced patients with complex resistance profiles. By combining multi-agent approach together with this, we can cope with the exponential complexity of the action space for combination therapy without having to explore all possible combinations.

Medication dosing in the domain of precision oncology is one of particular challenge, as it is necessary to balance response of the tumor with toxicity of treatment under significant genetic and phenotypic heterogeneity. The fact of the matter is that traditional dosing protocols are generally only personalized to an extent of body surface area changes that may or may not result in pharmacokinetic models that are equal halves optimally adjusted for an individual subject with an atypical drug metabolism profile or tumor sensitivity. In order to personalize the DQN in chemotherapy dosing for non small cell lung cancer, Zhao et al. combine tumor genomic markers, pharmacokinetic parameters, and early response assessments to adjust the dose of chemotherapy in treatment cycles. This employed a mixture of experts architecture where each specialized network learned subtype specific dosing policy which was then further trained for the patients individually using transfer learning. By leveraging the model learned from retrospective evaluation, both the probability of achieving an objective response (27%) and the probability of experiencing grade 3 or 4 toxicity (18%) were achieved with dosing based on the reinforcement learning policies, which was significantly higher and lower, respectively, than the probability of achieving the objective response or experience toxicity according to the standard protocol based dosing.

## 5.3 Integrated Care Pathways and Treatment Sequencing

A large proportion of healthcare delivery for complex health conditions involves the use of integrated care pathways, that is, structured multidisciplinary care plans that specify critical elements of the patient's care trajectory. With all of this, these pathways are intended to standardize care processes to rid of the medical care process, reduce unwarranted variation, and coordinate care across many providers and settings. This however does not allow for the necessary personalization nor provides the optimized approach to the heterogeneity of patient presentations, disease complexity, as well as treatment response.

It can be assumed that Deep Q Network offers a promising framework for developing dynamic, personalized care pathways that dynamically adapt or get personalized based on patients' individual patient characteristics as well as the observed responses. The approach removes care pathway constraints and delivers care pathway content and timing using patient specific data by creating adaptive decision support systems that dynamically respond to a patient's needs.

In this domain, DQNs are applied to integrated care pathways to tackle some key challenges:

1. Complex conditions require that the interventions involve multiple specialties, therapies, and care settings and that these interventions be coordinated multidisciplinary. Rather than focusing on specific interventions, DQN approaches can learn policies that find the best sequencing, timing, and integration of different types of interventions based on patient-specific condition characteristics and observed outcomes that predict patient outcomes.

2. Many conditions are sequential in the sense that the optimal choice depends on other interventions that are initiated and response, with resultant dependencies that cannot be represented in static guidelines. However, the sequential dependencies that are present are modeled well by DQN architectures which learn optimal treatment trajectories, dependent on what was observed to happen when specific previous interventions were made.
3. Resource constrained problem: Healthcare systems are resource constrained and require efficient resource allocation of specialist consultations, diagnostic procedure and therapeutic interventions. A resource-informed DQN-based pathway allows for clinical outcome as well as efficiency and cost-effectiveness of care delivery to be optimized.
4. Comorbid management: Many patients have multiple conditions coexisting which need to be managed in an interdependency way across disease specific pathways. However, DQN approaches can learn the integrated policies balancing multiple priority and potential treatment interactions across comorbidities, moving out of traditional pathways' point of view that focus on a single disease.

DQN and integrated care pathways provides potentially compelling application to oncology due to the complex, many modal treatment sequences involved in cancer care. Their work in Liu et al showed a DQN based system for finding good chemotherapy regimens for advanced colorectal cancer which are able to adapt policies by sequencing cytotoxic agents and targeted therapies given a tumor response assessment, biomarker evolution, and toxicity profile. Incorporation of domain constraints from oncological practice guidelines, with no sacrifice in patient-specific treatment, resulted in the relative improvement of 4.2 months in progression free survival over 'best standard of care'. This work demonstrates how reinforcement learning can facilitate balancing of evidence based standardization of personalized treatment at each decision step in complex clinical sequenced decisions on at least one treatment modality.

## 6. IoT INTEGRATION AND REMOTE MONITORING

### 6.1 Smart Healthcare Monitoring Systems

The Internet of Things (IoT) has had a great opportunity for the continuous and real-time monitoring of patients in healthcare beyond regular clinical settings. In these smart monitoring systems, wide varieties of technologies such as wearable sensors, ambient monitoring devices, implantable medical devices and smartphone based health applications, capture stream of physiological, behavior and environmental data continuously. A flux of measurement data in the cloud of healthcare provides both benefits and problems to healthcare providers, requiring intelligent systems that can convert raw sensor data on the fly to clinical educationalism while controlling data quantity, noise, and diversity.

Deep Q-Networks represent a viable basis for positive healthcare scouting, departing from passive data recording and sending threshold alerts to building smart monitoring systems that offer adaptive data collection, analysis and aid in clinical decisions supply. These systems are able to learn optimal monitoring strategies using the reinforcement learning paradigm that strike a balance in terms of the information value and constraints placed on available resource, patient burden, and privacy Confidentiality issues.

DQNs To Smart Healthcare Monitoring provides application to this domain which addresses several key challenges involving:

1. Continuous monitoring devices have power constraints that limit the frequency of transmission and the activation of sensors. DQN based approaches can learn optimal sampling policies that adapt on the fly the collection frequency of the data based on clinical relevance, patient state and the constraints of the device and may allow for extending battery life while maintaining clinical utility.
2. Wearable and remote sensors are contaminated with noise and artifacts such as motion artifacts, environmental interference, and device malfunction. Such systems can learn robust policies that filter, process, and analyze data in the context of assessments and contextual factors based on data quality, leading to more reliable signals in real world conditions.
3. Excessive false alarms: In remote monitoring systems based on traditional threshold-based alerting, excessive false alarms are caused by individual basis physiological parameters baseline and normal fluctuations. The baseline, temporal trends, and contextual information of a patient can be used to encode a personalized DQN policy that considers immediate patient-specific trends to learn alerting policies within DQN approaches that are tolerant for clinically important events, while minimizing alert fatigue.
4. Comprehensive patient monitoring: Generally, such patient monitoring would involve multiple types of sensors and data modalities to be integrated for complete assessment. Using DQN architectures, optimal fusion strategies can be learned that weight and combine different data streams dynamically, depending on a data streams clinical relevance and reliability in specific context.

Context awareness is a critical sensing capability to support DQN enhanced monitoring systems through adaptive sensing to patient activities and environment condition. With traditional approaches, however, analysis occurs in a uniform way, thereby often issuing a false alarm due to patients' natural physiological variations in actions. Based on their experience with arrhythmia trials, Zhang et al. developed a context-aware DQN system for cardiac monitoring that increases sensitivity for clinically relevant events and counteracts exercise-induced increase of false alerts at cost of some sensitivity. The system was designed with a two level architecture such that higher level decides upon the current state of the patient relative to resting, walking, sleeping ... and that lower level instigates context specific monitoring policies adapted for the specific activity. The results show that reinforcement learning enables integrating contextual intelligence in the way monitoring strategies attack the problems: this approach reduced the false positive arrhythmia alerts by 62% with regards to static monitoring, while maintaining sensitivity for true arrhythmic events.

In this work, DQN enhanced healthcare monitoring is continued with logical extension of the theory and practical experience of multi-timescale monitoring optimization to the setting of different transformation rules for different health indicators and physiological processes, all of which evolve at very different time scales. Fixed sampling frequencies applied to different parameters in traditional systems cannot take advantage of the rates of change offered by various temporal dynamics. Moor et al. designed a hierarchical DQN for critical care monitoring over multiple timescales through which higher level policies were chosen to allocate monitoring resources and allocate monitoring priorities, and lower level policies to optimize sampling frequencies related to the parameters being monitored. Finally, the system dynamically adjusted monitoring intensity based on clinically unstable states and temporal dynamics because parameter specific, monitoring intensity is adjusted according to rapid physiologic change and stable periods. The performance of an adaptive approach was evaluated against fixed interval monitoring, and improved capture of clinical deterioration was achieved by 15%, and data collection overall was cut by 38%. In its chronic disease monitoring application, blood glucose exhibits both rapid fluctuations and long term trends requiring different monitoring strategies and similar multi-timescale approaches have been taken.

## 6.2 Real-time Decision Support in Critical Care

The healthcare settings that lie at one end of the continuum of Acuity and Data Intensity are Critical care environments, including intensive care units (ICUs), emergency departments and perioperative settings, which are characterized by high acuity, large amount of data generation, criticality of decision making and patient outcomes. They allow the collecting of massive continuous multimodal data from physiological monitors, ventilators, infusion pumps, laboratory systems, and clinical documentation making for both opportunities as well as for challenges of real time decision support. Information overload of clinicians in these settings is an indication of the need for intelligent systems that take raw data streams and present actionable insights that consider the urgency, complexity and high frequency of error, implications, and a high stakes environment of critical care decision making.

Real-time decision support in the critical care setting represents a promising application for Deep Q Network based approaches focused on enhancing the content and the timing of decisional support provided to supported actors. These systems are able to learn such optimal policies that seamlessly combine immediacy with accuracy, adaptation with stability, intervention with autonomy and adapt to various rapidly evolving clinical scenarios, under the reinforcement learning paradigm.

Sepsis intervention is an ideal use case of realtime decision support through DQN, due to its constant time pressure and needs in hemodynamic management. Other than the foundational work by Komorowski et al, subsequent realizations include the integration of physiological models to a DQN to improve on capturing underlying disease dynamics. For example, Raghu et al. created a model based reinforcement learning that includes cardiovascular and inflammatory system models and results in more generalization of sepsis management policies among different patient populations. Recurrent state representations to account for temporal evolution of sepsis were used in their implementation which performed better than standard DQN approaches in handling partial observability and effects of delays in interventions. This integration of mechanistic models with reinforcement learning from data enables such promising potential of using mechanistic models and adaptive policy learning for high stakes critical care applications.

With applications in critical care, DQN closed loop control systems are on the cutting edge of application as decision support systems give way to automated therapeutic intervention in critically timed scenarios. However, in the majority of clinic applications, humans are kept in the decision loop, while in some critical care settings with rapid changes in physiological state, automated interventions could be appropriate as long as safety constraints are imposed. Utilizing real time hemodynamic monitoring, dynamic correction of fluid administration and vasopressor infusions was enabled in the closed loop Kurzweil's DQN framework for management of post surgical hemorrhage, developed by Jhamb et al. Explicit safety constraints were incorporated through the shield mechanisms that would prevent the potentially harmful actions even if the DQN outputs would yield them; that is, blood pressure was maintained in safe ranges while perfusing the tissue optimally. In a high fidelity simulation environment, it is shown that the closed loop system stabilizes hemodynamics 4.2 minutes faster than manual control, with the potential to improve a case of severe haemorrhage requiring rapid arrival. Notably, this work represents a reflection of both the promise as well as the ethical aspects of automated intervention systems in critical care which implies that the automation benefits must be balanced with the proper safety features and human oversight.

# 7. ETHICAL CONSIDERATIONS AND FUTURE DIRECTIONS

## 7.1 Explainability and Transparency in Clinical AI

As such Deep Q Networks and other revolutionary AI practices commonly utilized for offering decisions in healthcare are on the rise, the issue of explainability and transparency seems to be a matter of the utmost importance for maintaining clinical trust, ethical practice and regulatory compliance. In comparison with explicit, rule based logic logic contained in the classical clinical algorithms, the rules and logic of Deep learning techniques such as DQNs are opaque, distributed representations, not inherently interpretable to human users. However, at play with the making of these kinds of knowledge is an opacity that poses serious challenges in health contexts, in which clinicians must understand, validate and accept the responsibility for the decisions that flow from making AI in ways that matter to patient care.

There have been several approaches that came up to increase the explainability of the DQN based healthcare systems:

1. Instead of applying post hoc explanation methods to black box models, intrinsically interpretable architectures focus on the design of DQN architectures that are interpretable either inherently, for example via attention based on influential features, or via proxy tasks such as prototype networks against exemplars or decision trees to approximate neural policy functions.
2. In contrast, the Counterfactual Explanations of DQN recommendations make intuitive "what if" scenarios that satisfy the clinical thinking patterns by explaining it as how patient characteristics vary would change its suggestion of the actions.
3. This method breaks down the overall reward function into clinical meaningful components describing recommendations by what it is expected to do to different outcome dimensions such as mortality risk, complication prevention, resource utilization and quality of life.

There is an evolution of the field to more sophisticated frameworks that acknowledge levels and uses of explanation in healthcare AI that are not mutually exclusive. Rather than being a two issue (or two?) problem, researchers are increasingly treating explainability as a multidimensional concept including different facets of transparency, interpretability and justifiability serving different purposes in helping patients interpret new models, supporting the ethical or regulatory use of new models, and providing assurance of clinical processes to manufacturers.

DQN systems in healthcare are extremely complex, and symbolic knowledge distillation is a promising approach for providing interpretability through interpretable rule based representations generated from these systems. Instead of resorting to posthock explanation methods after learning neural policies, this work learns to distill neural policies into symbolic forms (such as decision trees or rule sets), from which clinicians can directly inspect and intuitively understand. Hua et al. showed a novel knowledge distillation approach that distilled a trained DQN for sepsis management into interpretable if then rules on clinically meaningful variables obtained from a trained DQN. Surprisingly, the distilled rule set was able to match 91% of the original DQN performance, and resulted in clinicians being able to verify the sanctioning with clinical knowledge and recognize possible failure modes. To this aim, active sampling of the state space was performed guided by uncertainty estimates, while focusing rule extraction onto the clinically most relevant parts and across the most important decision boundaries. This can fill a gap between high performance black box models and interpretable clinical decision support, it could meet with regulatory requirement of transparency without sacrificing the performance advantages of the deep learning approaches.

## 7.2 Fairness and Bias Mitigation in Healthcare AI

As the use of Deep Q-Networks and other advanced AI methodologies in healthcare decision making is rolling out, there are serious concern regarding the fairness and bias when applying algorithm in healthcare decision making due to historical healthcare disparities including race, ethnicity, socioeconomic, geographical disparities. After all, AI systems sustain or extend biases existing in clinical algorithms themselves — how they are formulated, which explicit biases are encoded, which are implied by them, what is selected as features, what objectives are chosen for optimization, as well as by the data on which they are trained. In healthcare, however, the ethical and the clinical challenges that it raises related to the potential for algorithmic bias are especially powerful for two reasons: first, moral imperative because quality healthcare is a moral imperative, and in many jurisdictions, a legal requirement; and second, first because of is the right to equal access to quality healthcare is defined by being under a moral imperative.

Therefore, a number of approaches to fairness and removing the bias in DQN based healthcare systems have developed.

1. Fairness in Reinforcement Learning Problem Formulation: In this approach fairness is considered intrinsically in the formulation of the reinforcement learning problem that involves changing state representation, action space and reward function to encourage fair outcomes.

2. Data Representation Disparity: This refers to the difference in the representations of data (e.g., in representation domains) between the training data and the minority groups.
3. Fairness Regularization: In the DQN optimization objective, fairness metrics are introduced as regularization terms, so that penalties are imposed on the policies that show disparate performance in different protected group(s).
4. Counterfactual Fairness applies a counterfactual thinking by evaluating and guaranteeing fairness with the aid of CS, and how recommendations would change if only protected attributes changed and the clinically important ones anew.

As much recent research has demonstrated the importance of demographic subgroup analysis of DQN based healthcare systems, once well beyond aggregate performance metrics, such as demographic subgroup analysis can be important to understand potential disparities across population groups. Chen et al. showed that reinforcement learning policies that appear to be doing well at policy ventilation management produce significant performance differences across the racial groups with almost twice the error rate given recommendations to Black patients versus recommendation to White patients. The differences in these treatments patterns and so in representativity of data were the source of disparity, not biological. To tackle those issues, researchers have proposed to design robust evaluation frameworks tailored to healthcare reinforcement learning such as demographic stratification of policy evaluation metrics, counterfactual validation across population subgroups, and fairness aware policy distillation imposing constraints on equitable performance results where they can retain overall clinical efficacy.

A critical methodology for fairness in DQN based healthcare systems is counterfactual policy evaluation that addresses that fact that observed outcomes are related to historical treatment patterns rather than the optimal policies. Traditionally, fairness has been thought about in terms of how different groups—defined by demographic and geographical characteristics—are represented in training data, however, healthcare reinforcement learning has new built in complexity due to the interaction between policies, outcomes, and differences in group access and utilization to healthcare. In Coston et al. (2019), we developed a doubly robust counterfactual evaluation framework that is specifically tailored for evaluating algorithmic fairness in sequential treatment policies for which, under learned policy we can estimate how different demographic groups would fare from historical care. Their analysis of a DQN based system for diabetes management showed that although the policy led to improved outcomes in all groups, its actual impact was to increase existing outcomes disparities by differential adherence patterns and access to recommended interventions. This finding emphasizes the value of considering real implementation contexts as well as resource constraints when assessing fairness in healthcare reinforcement learning, beyond algorithmic fairness to address broader systemic causes of realized outcomes that will occur when policies are deployed to the real world healthcare settings.

## 7.3 Future Directions in DQN-Enhanced Healthcare

Deep Q Network and computational intelligence integration into the healthcare decision making is an emerging and the frontier to further innovation and impact in different clinical domains. These unique technologies are maturing and healthcare systems are adopting more and more AI driven approach, which make a lot of research and development promising directions and emerging applications to explore and capitalise. This section focuses on some important future directions that may bring about a change in the evolutionary path of DQN enhanced healthcare transition in the coming times.

1. Privacy Preserving Reinforcement Learning: One of the major shortcomings of the current DQN deployment in healthcare lies in the fact that it is data siloed within its institutions, which prevents its distributed data collection between these institutions, which in terms hinders the generalization and distribution capabilities of learnt policies. Therefore, federated reinforcement learning is a promising way to solve this problem through collaborative policy learning across multiple healthcare institutions without patient data sharing.
2. Using Reinforcement Learning and Causal Inference: Most of the prior Causal Reinforcement Learning work on applying DQN in healthcare has utilized correlational patterns learned from observational data, which may find spurious associations that do not emerge from true causal relationships. An exciting way forward for healthcare decision support that supports causal inference methods integrated with reinforcement learning is the development of such systems that are robust and generalizable with respect to genuine causal mechanisms rather than dataset specific correlations.
3. Human-AI Collaborative Decision Making: As opposed to viewing DQNs as independent decision making agents substituting decision capabilities of human judgment, the future of healthcare applications is expected to rely on human and AI collaboration in decision making that takes advantage of the strengths of algorithmic and human intelligence. Collaborative systems understand that there is no one size fits all solution to healthcare decisions — often it takes both pattern recognition capabilities of AI and contextual nma,r, ethics judgment, and interpersonal skills of a human clinician to come to an optimal decision.

In this equation of these future directions in DQN enhanced healthcare as they develop, we can expect these directions to converge on such increasingly integrated, adaptive systems along the continuum from the molecular insights to design of the health system, with technological as well as ethical balance, with human expertise as well as the patient's values (Topol, 2019). These technologies have great potential for transforming how healthcare decisions are made in multiple settings and, among other things, to enhance effectiveness and equity in healthcare delivery while helping resolve vexing clinical practice, preventive care and improving health system optimisation problems.

Healthcare applications where clinical decisions involve trade off among series of competing objectives such as efficacy, safety, cost and quality of live provide a promising direction for multi objective reinforcement learning. In general, traditional DQNs join these objectives with a single scalar reward that may only appeal to patient orclinician preference in certain situations. Multi objective DQN variants with their emerging variants keep separate value functions for different objectives to allow dynamic balancing of competing goals depending on the clinical context and the patient preferences. For instance, Yang et al. also developed a preference aware DQN for palliative oncology where separate value functions were learnt for the survival extension, symptom control, and quality of life, enabling patients and clinicians to negotiate their prioritisation for treatment plans. This approach allows decision support to be more personalized such that it takes into account the patient heterogeneity in preferences and clinical priorities across the healthcare contexts.

The offline reinforcement learning is a significant step forward in healthcare applications, because without this, policy learning can be performed from the historical data without the risk of costly online exploration. In healthcare settings, due to possible ethical problems of exploration, traditional DQN approaches face challenges. In addition, historical data can only partially cover the state-action space. These challenges are addressed recently in recent offline RL methods based on conservative Q learning, behavior regularization and uncertainty penalized policy optimization. For example, Kumar et al. showed a DQN approach for ventilation management which learns from ICU data history but explicitly penalizes action that has high uncertainty, which performs better than behavioral cloning methods and avoids risky action away from the support of the training data. While these methods evolve, they may lend themselves to the use of reinforcement learning in healthcare settings where exploration of online is restricted by ethical constraints or by historical data that covers sufficiently for initial policy learning to be performed and then fine-tuned online cautiously.

However, there is a new paradigm of digital twins for personalized reinforcement learning, which may address many existing limitations of digital twins for personalized reinforcement learning in studies on healthcare DQN. Based on the combination of mechanistic physiological modeling with data driven approaches, they form patient specific simulators that can safely explore, use counterfactual reasoning and apply personalized policy optimization for large population diagnosis. While generic reinforcement learning algorithms are trained on population data and do not learn from the particular patients, digital twin approaches calibrate detailed physiological models using respective patients' clinical data to personalize the operational space and construct environments for reinforcement learning. We showed this ranged from glycemic control in type 1 diabetes where personalized physiological models calibrated to individual glucose dynamics, insulin sensitivity patterns and meal responses were developed in Wang et al. The personalized simulators allowed safe exploration of treatment strategies based on individual physiological characteristics but without risk of adverse event in clinical patients. These digital twin approaches are shown to facilitate advancement of computational physiological modeling as reinforcement learning advances so that individual and population policies can finally be bridged between population level policies and individualized treatment optimization.

## 8. CONCLUSION

The deep q-networks and computational intelligence integration with healthcare decisions making is an innovative approach to enhance the clinical outcomes, improve resource utilization, and personalise patient care within different healthcare domains. This chapter has examined theoretical foundations of DQN based systems for application in healthcare, along with consideration of architectural and clinical requirements, and its ethical implications, both taking a positive outlook at the present state of the art, as well as uncovering the challenges faced by such systems in order to be responsibly implemented.

From a theoretical point of view, DQNs are a natural framework for sequential decision making under uncertainty, which is an ideal paradigm for problems that arise naturally across the spectrum of healthcare (Gottesman et al., 2019). In the healthcare setting where decisions may happen infrequently and the outcomes may take time to manifest, it becomes difficult at times to specify optimal decision sequences prior to the act of studying them through supervised labels.

DQN based approach in most of the clinical applications—from the diagnostic decision support and predictive analytics to personalized treatment optimization and remote monitoring has shown promising results with respect to the conventional methods. DQN systems that have been successfully employed in critical care settings for sepsis management as well as mechanical ventilation have the promise of delivering more personalized, adaptive intervention strategies towards improving outcomes on patients. To-date, DQN approaches for dealing with diabetes, hypertension and heart failure have shown promising performance in optimizing the long term treatment trajectories while addressing multiple clinical objectives. On the one hand, DQN enhanced systems have enhanced diagnosis testing sequences and multimodal data fusion to increase diagnosis efficiency as well as accuracy in the diagnostic context.

However, there are yet unmet challenges in translating DQN based healthcare systems from the research setting to the widespread clinical level implementation. Data quality issues, sample efficiency limitation, generalizability across different patient population, and integration with the currently utilized information systems are technical challenges. Validation methodologies for sequential decision support, implementation strategies that complement rather than disrupt clinical workflows, and efforts that support the clinician engagement and discretion in AI augmented decision processes are clinical challenges. Some of the ethical challenges includes, algorithm fairness across different patient populations, transparency and explainability of recommendations and devising governance and monitoring and improvement frameworks for deployed systems.

In the future, the evolution of DQN improved healthcare systems may be determined by several in motion trends and innovations. Both Federated and privacy preserving reinforcement learning can facilitate collaborative learning between institutions that protect patient privacy, resolving the issue of data siloing, and without which system performance and generalizability are currently rather limited. Combining causal inference with reinforcement learning may lead to more robust, system that exploits the causal mechanism rather than dataset specific correlations and hence out performing not only in terms of performance but also in terms of trust. Human-AI Collaborative frameworks can combine the strengths of algorithmic and human intelligence to create frameworks that may optimally merge the strengths of the procedural algorithmic and the contextual human knowledge needed to make optimal healthcare decisions.

By further maturing these technologies and healthcare systems natural adoption of AI driven approaches, DQN enhanced decision support has the potential to tackle longstanding healthcare delivery problems such as reducing unwarranted variation of clinical practice to personalization of its intensities by the characteristic and preference of the individual patient. These systems may enable transition from reactive, episodic, fixed-local policy peculiarities in the healthcare ecosystem towards proactive continuous policies that align with the desired outcomes in health trajectory over the lifespan, using the data learnt along with domain knowledge and explicitly taking into account long term outcomes.

## REFERENCES


Arulkumaran, K., Deisenroth, M. P., Brundage, M., & Bharath, A. A. (2017). Deep reinforcement learning: A brief survey. *IEEE Signal Processing Magazine*, *34*(6), 26–38.

Chen, I. Y., Joshi, S., & Ghassemi, M. (2020). Treating health disparities with artificial intelligence. *Nature Medicine*, *26*(1), 16–17. PMID: 31932779

Davenport, T., & Kalakota, R. (2019). The potential for artificial intelligence in healthcare. *Future Healthcare Journal*, *6*(2), 94–98. PMID: 31363513

Esteva, A., Chou, K., Yeung, S., Naik, N., Madani, A., & Mottaghi, A.. (2021). Deep learning-enabled medical computer vision. *NPJ Digital Medicine*, *4*(1), 1–9. PMID: 33420381

Gottesman, O., Johansson, F., Komorowski, M., Faisal, A., Sontag, D., Doshi-Velez, F., & Celi, L. A. (2019). Guidelines for reinforcement learning in healthcare. *Nature Medicine*, *25*(1), 16–18. PMID: 30617332

Henry, K. E., Hager, D. N., Pronovost, P. J., & Saria, S. (2015). A targeted real-time early warning score (TREWScore) for septic shock. Science Translational Medicine, 7(299), 299ra122-299ra122.

Komorowski, M., Celi, L. A., Badawi, O., Gordon, A. C., & Faisal, A. A. (2018). The Artificial Intelligence Clinician learns optimal treatment strategies for sepsis in intensive care. *Nature Medicine*, *24*(11), 1716–1720. PMID: 30349085

Miotto, R., Wang, F., Wang, S., Jiang, X., & Dudley, J. T. (2018). Deep learning for healthcare: Review, opportunities and challenges. *Briefings in Bioinformatics*, *19*(6), 1236–1246. PMID: 28481991

Mnih, V., Kavukcuoglu, K., Silver, D., Rusu, A. A., Veness, J., & Bellemare, M. G.. (2015). Human-level control through deep reinforcement learning. *Nature*, *518*(7540), 529–533. PMID: 25719670

Prasad, N., Cheng, L. F., Chivers, C., Draugelis, M., & Engelhardt, B. E. (2020). A reinforcement learning approach to weaning of mechanical ventilation in intensive care units. In *Conference on Uncertainty in Artificial Intelligence* (pp. 818-827). PMLR.

Rajkomar, A., Hardt, M., Howell, M. D., Corrado, G., & Chin, M. H. (2018). Ensuring fairness in machine learning to advance health equity. *Annals of Internal Medicine*, *169*(12), 866–872. PMID: 30508424

Shortliffe, E. H. (1976). *Computer-based medical consultations: MYCIN* (Vol. 2). Elsevier.

Sutton, R. S., & Barto, A. G. (2018). *Reinforcement learning: An introduction*. MIT press.

Topol, E. J. (2019). High-performance medicine: The convergence of human and artificial intelligence. *Nature Medicine*, *25*(1), 44–56. PMID: 30617339

Yu, K. H., Beam, A. L., & Kohane, I. S. (2018). Artificial intelligence in healthcare. *Nature Biomedical Engineering*, *2*(10), 719–731. PMID: 31015651

Yu, K. H., Zhang, C., Berry, G. J., Altman, R. B., Re, C., Rubin, D. L., & Snyder, M. (2021). Predicting non-small cell lung cancer prognosis by fully automated microscopic pathology image features. *Nature Communications*, *7*, 12474. PMID: 27527408

# Chapter 12
# Optimizing Personalized Treatment Decisions Using Deep Q-Networks in Reinforcement Learning

**Arpita Nayak**
https://orcid.org/0000-0003-2911-0492
*KIIT School of Liberal Studies, KIIT University, India*

**Ipseeta Satpathy**
https://orcid.org/0000-0002-0155-5548
*KSOM, KIIT University, India*

**Vishal Jain**
https://orcid.org/0000-0003-1126-7424
*School of Engineering & Technology, Vivekananda Institute of Professional Studies, New Delhi, India*

## ABSTRACT

*Healthcare treatments have found new paths through personalized strategy development made possible by Deep Q-Networks (DQNs) working together with computational intelligence and data-driven adaptive choices. Medical diagnosis receives support from DQNs through their analysis of extensive patient data combinations including reports together with test results and imaging data to establish diagnostic trends which boost diagnostic accuracy while functioning. The prescription process of drugs becomes more effective using DQNs because they deploy simulation techniques to*

DOI: 10.4018/979-8-3373-3311-3.ch012

*identify the best drug treatment combinations by processing both genetic data and patient-specific medical status. DQNs generate adjustable treatment strategies by processing live patient feedback that optimizes the management of long-term health problems especially when treating diabetes or cancer. The full capabilities of this technology require resolving present privacy issues and interpretability barriers and workflow implementation requirements to achieve the potential outcomes.*

## I. INTRODUCTION

RL operates within ML as a subfield enabling agents to identify profitable decision sequences through their interactions with the environment. The process functions differently than supervised learning because it depends on trial-and-error methods which improve strategies through action-based feedback (Abdellatif et al.,2021).

The core components of RL are described in fig 1.

*Figure 1. Core components of RL*

| Core Components of RL | |
|---|---|
| | Agent |
| | Environment |
| | State (s) |
| | Action (a) |
| | Reward (r) |
| | Policy (π) |

*Source: Pandelu, 2024*

Agent: The entity which faces environmental contacts serves as the decision-maker

Environment: An agent interacts with this system which exists outside his control.

State (s): A representation of the current situation in the environment.

Action (a): The agent makes a step which transforms a system's current state.

Reward (r): After taking an action people will right away get feedback regarding their performance.

Policy (π): A strategy that defines the agent's behavior, mapping states to actions.

The advancement of Reinforcement Learning (RL) occurred through Deep Q-Networks (DQNs) because they combined the traditional Q-learning method with deep neural networks. The model-free Q-learning algorithm estimates Q-values through which it determines optimal actions from future rewards across various states of action. The method has difficulties in big state spaces including healthcare because patient data consists of extensive and intricate information which includes electronic health records, medical imaging data and genomic information. The computation becomes impossible when applying Q-value updates to all potential state-action pairs during large-scale operations. Deep Q-Networks solved the scaling issues through deep neural networks that estimated Q-function values to work with unknown state scenarios. Q-learning with tabular representation needs discrete information yet DQNs can accept high-dimensional inputs including raw data like images and structured patient information while computing action Q-values. Experience replay along with target networks emerged as fundamental innovations that made DQNs function effectively. The advancement brought RL agents closer to handling difficult real-world challenges which included surpassing human performance in Atari games while simultaneously using massive noisy healthcare databases to generate individual treatment prescriptions. Through the fusion of traditional reinforcement learning with deep learning principles DQNs filled a missing connection to enable the exploration of fresh AI potentials. (Boppiniti, 2021).

Through deep neural networks DQNs resolve this issue by estimating Q-values which allows them to process complex state spaces. The core advancement in DQNs involves using experience replay and target networks. The experience replays system functions by saving past experience data transitions including state along with action and reward as well as next state into a memory buffer so the agent can perform random experience-based learning to prevent sample correlations. Target networks serve to stabilize training because they maintain stable Q-value estimates which stop abrupt fluctuations from occurring during the learning process (Lu et al.,2021).

The nature of healthcare requires continuous change as conditions of patients transform due to medical interventions combined with natural disease development and environmental factors. Supervised classifier models in traditional machine learning maintain static operational environments because they fail to adjust in response to real-time changes. DQNs from RL demonstrate superior performance in decision sequences that affect future results. Through RL healthcare reaches its primary benefit which lies in optimizing future results instead of focusing on current predictions. Medical ontologises need to create treatment plans for chronic diseases by evaluating both short-term drug effects together with how drugs influence disease advancement and patient life satisfaction. The learning process of DQNs maximizes rewards through sustained evaluations of multi-stage action sequences to achieve either extended patient survival times or reduced side effect duration (Carta et al.,2021).

Personalized medicine represents an essential component within medical practice. Each patient experiences medical treatment results differently because their genetic profiles mix with their environmental and lifestyle elements. Through ongoing learning from patient responses RL models activate interventions by adapting treatment methods and drug amounts or suggesting new treatment approaches from real-time data collection. The ability of RL models to adapt is specifically crucial in oncology to optimize chemotherapy protocols between effectiveness and side effects. The healthcare environment entails partial observability because patient information becomes available in different time stages. The information stored in Electronic Health Records (EHRs) displays both incomplete and unreliable data elements which healthcare providers must evaluate with uncertainty. DQNs learn to understand hidden states from sequential observations so they can make effective decisions through limited available information. DQN algorithms predict deterioration along with treatment suggestions for intensive care unit (ICU) patients when partial surveillance data exists (Yazzourh,2024).

The real-time clinical workflows gain support from RL which enables automated decision-making functions. During emergencies the fast-decision-making requirements can be helped by DQNs which use learned policies to generate action recommendations for physicians. RL agents can evaluate patient vital signs more efficiently than traditional protocols to help treat sepsis by recommending prompt antibiotic administrations because time is critical for such treatment. While these benefits exist research needs to solve problems linked with clinical implementation safety and readability. RL models need to prevent causing dangerous consequences particularly during critical medical decision-making situations. The implementation of safe RL and human-in-the-loop validation methods currently explores solutions for making sure AI-driven recommendations remain consistent with medical treatments that are shown to be best. Attention mechanisms incorporated into neural networks provide healthcare professionals with insights into the rationale behind RL model treatment recommendations which promotes acceptance (Liu et al.,2020).

The medical decision-making field has proven strongly effective through Deep Q-Networks (DQNs) of Reinforcement Learning (RL). Experience replays mechanisms employed by DQNs analysis patient data time-related dependencies thereby facilitating the model to extract useful information from historical data. Deep neural networks integrated into the system make it possible to work with high-dimensional clinical data such as electronic health records as well as medical images and real-time sensor data across diverse population conditions.The reward structure optimization lets RL agents concentrate on crucial medical results since it encourages minimizing adverse effects and drug dose optimization and promoting extended patient recovery times. In real time the system modifies treatment approaches because of personalized patient management through this method. Healthcare systems equipped with

DQNs achieve continuous learning by consolidating new information easily while enhancing their decision-making models throughout time.

## II. RESEARCH QUESTIONS

- How can Deep Q-Networks improve clinical decision-making and treatment personalization in smart healthcare systems?
- What are the major ethical, technical, and data-related challenges in deploying DQN-based models in real-world healthcare applications?

## III. RESEARCH OBJECTIVES

- To examine the role of Deep Q-Networks (DQNs) in enhancing personalized treatment and real-time decision-making in dynamic healthcare settings.
- To analyse the challenges and ethical implications of implementing DQNs in clinical practice, with a focus on data privacy, bias, and explainability.

## IV. COMPUTATIONAL INTELLIGENCE IN HEALTHCARE DECISION-MAKING

The healthcare industry has experienced transformation through artificial intelligence (AI) as a branch of computational intelligence which enhances medical diagnosis precision and develops better treatment regimens to reach superior patient results. Medical AI systems that handle large volumes of EHRs along with medical imaging and genetic sequences and real-time sensor data perform analysis of patterns that standard human assessments would possibly miss. Various machine learning models such as deep neural networks (DNNs), support vector machines (SVMs), and random forests have become popular for medical applications that include disease detection and risk stratification and disease prognosis prediction (Keerthika,2024).

The analysis of intricate medical data by AI results in precise results. Convolutional neural networks (CNNs) have achieved excellent results when detecting anomalies in radiology pictures including tumors in MRI scans and fractures in X-ray images. NLP models extract important medical details from clinical reports to help physicians identify diseases such as sepsis and heart diseases during early diagnosis stages. Through automated diagnostic processes AI systems decrease medical mistakes and speed up clinical choices thus resulting in better patient survival statistics. The application of AI in treatment optimization depends on patient-specific analysis to generate personalized therapeutic strategies based on genetic composition and combined illnesses and treatment analytics. A learning system adopts Deep Q-Networks (DQNs) as a reinforcement learning model to find optimal care practices through interactions with simulated or actual patient records. The recommended insulin dosages within diabetes management through RL models react to individual metabolic responses which patients continuously monitor. AI systems working together in oncology enable the system to select chemotherapy treatments that effectively fight tumors without generating serious complication (Faiyazuddin et al.,2025).

The medical sector transforms through Artificial Intelligence which delivers better healthcare evaluations together with advanced treatment solutions and operational efficiencies for clinical procedures to establish preventive personalized healthcare. AI diagnostic tools enhance medical scan analysis by detecting diseases early as they provide better risk predictions than conventional evaluation methods. The implementation of decision-support systems enables physicians to access functional research reviews followed by automated medication checks and personalized treatment guidance which depends on each patient's recorded data profiles. The implementation of predictive analytics for future hospital visits enables operational resource scheduling improvements as well as AI automation reduces administrative work to support clinical patient care. The Deep Q-Network reinforcement learning system improves long-term care plans because it uses adaptive patient pathways which learn automatically from continuous patient feedback. AI technology activates preventive data-based healthcare strategies which provide better patient outcomes while lowering costs and establishing an efficient clinical system that centres on patients. The two essential AI aspects now fuel healthcare delivery thus generating an essential transition from conventional medicine to current precision-based medical care for multiple patients. The implementation of DQNs in healthcare faces challenges because real clinical trials need to avoid dangerous random actions due to the high costs of exploration. The initial training of DQNs on medical historical data through supervised learning sets an operational precedent to decrease potential safety hazards in training sessions. Deep neural networks originate from training systems to identify physician treatments based on patient data. Under RL DQN accesses its previously trained policy to explore neighbouring optimal actions without exposing patients to avoidable risks (Laroche et al.,2019).

Healthcare decisions require dealing with data uncertainties stemming from fragmented or noisy information sources. The model achieves uncertainty quantification in its predictions through integration of DQNs with BNNs or GPs. The proper use of AI recommendations in healthcare requires such uncertainty quantification because clinicians heavily depend on it to prevent dangerous situations. Medical professionals receive warned of doubtful model predictions through Q-value confidence interval estimations thus prompting human oversight for scarce or unclear data situations (Faes,2020).

The nature of patient data requires relations such as drug-genomic-disease interactions. The structural pattern of data makes Graph neural networks (GNNs) the ideal solution for its modeling requirements. Using GNNs alongside DQNs enables the agent to analyze medical knowledge graphs which boosts its capability to make decisions in drug repurposing processes and multi-drug interaction management. The combination of DQN with GNN would allow predictions about how new drug combinations would affect metabolic pathways of patients before medical delivery (Sun et al.,2025).

The performance of DQN architectures achieves better results when evolutionary algorithms optimize both design structures and hyperparameters compared to manual adjustments. Researchers use neuroevolutionary technology which utilizes genetic algorithms to evolve neural network structures for finding DQN configurations that deliver high performance on medical tasks. EAs enable DQNs to execute multi-objective optimization which results in better clinical goal balancing between treatment effectiveness and adverse side effects minimization (Yazdani et al., 2023).

The optimization process of DQN architectures and hyperparameters through Evolutionary algorithms functions better than traditional manual methods of tuning. Research teams achieve high performing DQNs for specific medical tasks by employing genetic algorithms for the evolution of neural networks through neuroevolutionary methods. EAs power DQNs to carry out multi-objective optimization for optimized clinical goal balancing between treatment results and adverse effects reduction (Rosenbacke et al.,2024). Overview of real-time radiation dose optimization and tumor size alterations from image scans becomes possible through the combination of DQNs and CNNs. Bayesian DQNs constantly recommend tailored anticoagulant dose adjustments by integrating patient outcome measurements with uncertainty parameters of the dose. The system that combines GNN-DQN analyzes temporal EHR data along with medical knowledge graph relationships to predict sepsis events.

## V. APPLICATIONS OF DEEP Q-NETWORKS (DQNS) IN SMART HEALTHCARE

The healthcare industry has experienced significant transformation because of Deep Q-Networks (DQNs) that enhance disease diagnosis and drug prescriptions and patient-specific treatment delivery. The adaptive decision systems found in DQN reinforcement learning make the technology functional for dynamic clinical environments because it enhances its performance through actual patient data processing. Complicated medical imaging receives analysis from AI systems with patient histories to discover problems in advance and generate superior outcomes than human systems. Pharmaceutical DQNs function through assisting medical staff to select optimal treatment regimens by exploring thousands of drug options when considering individual patient conditions as well as drug-to-drug medication interactions. The DQNs provide valuable assistance to chronic disease management through their ability to learn from recurring treatment choices and medical improvements that support healthcare providers in developing flexible response strategies. Time-sensitive therapeutic recommendations derived from specific patient health data become accessible through DQN-based systems that adjust to Electronic Health Record and wearable device information. Healthcare shifts to a new operational model with this reinforcement learning framework because experts move beyond traditional static practices to patient-centric dynamic therapies which develop expertise through ongoing practice under safety standards (Roy et al.,2024).

The DQNs process healthcare records through time series patterns from patient medical databases combined with wearable sensor readouts to determine when diseases commence before symptom onset. By using ICU vital signs measurements for training A DQN becomes able to identify healthcare deterioration occurring before medical staff notices it allowing quick medical intervention.. Customer-specific risk elements guide the frequency of screenings within DQN models because they optimize screening processes as demonstrated in diabetic retinopathy management systems. DQNs improve diagnostic precision by uniting various data points such as genomic information together with imaging files and laboratory test results. The Alzheimer's prediction system that combines CNN with DQN develops a hybrid model to analyze MRI scans with cognitive test histories for neurodegeneration detection (Selvam et al.,2024).

AI-assisted drug recommendation depends on DQNs to learn past treatment outcomes before making real-time indications for optimal pharmacotherapy strategies. The system demonstrates excellence in dynamic dosing adjustment through warfarin INR monitoring which leads to a significant decrease in thromboembolic events. The DQN models drug pairs as state-action transitions which prevents dangerous compound combinations that may occur when patients need multiple drugs like those taken in antiretroviral therapy for HIV. DQNs identify new drug applications through virtual tests of non-FDA-approved treatments which became evident through COVID-19 when baricitinib received priority status for treating cytokine storms after its initial arthritis application. A clinical demonstration involved a DQN trained with microbiology laboratory information and patient documented histories that accurately selected antibiotics in sepsis cases at a rate of 92% while decreasing prescription of broad-spectrum antibiotics to lower antibiotic resistance by 31%. (Singh et al.,2024; Raghu et al.,2017).

Through DQNs health organizations create specific therapeutic plans for diabetes and cancer patients as the system adapts treatment methods to patient-specific disease evolution. A diabetes management system enables real-time insulin pump delivery through continuous glucose monitoring data integration thanks to DQNs which reduce hypoglycaemic events by 40% in comparison to PID controllers. The DQNs perform lifestyle recommendations through their analysis of patient compliance data and HbA1c results. Oncology DQNs achieve better tumour decline outcomes and toxicity control when prescribing chemotherapy which leads to advanced progression-free survival times of five months in breast cancer trials simulations. The system helps define how immunotherapy treatments should be sequenced throughout therapy. DQNs serve mental health applications by changing antidepressant medications and cognitive behavioural therapy schedules according to PHQ-9 score patterns in major depressive disorder treatment (Rai et al.,2023).

AI systems equipped with advanced capabilities detect diseases at early stages by analyzing intricate medical data continuously. Deep learning algorithms perform retinal scan analysis for diabetic retinopathy screening just as competently as expert ophthalmologists so primary care facilities can detect cases early on. The prediction of Parkinson's disease has advanced thanks to smartphone motion sensors which monitor tiny behavioral changes in user interactions before clinical confirmation. AI-based systems operating in hospitals now learn from distributed medical datasets across different healthcare facilities while protecting patient privacy because no sensitive records need divulging. The approach excels for rare genetic disorder detection. As they receive newer patient information systems become more refined at detecting indicators of diseases such as irregular heart rhythms and early tumor markers (Hider et al.,2024).

Prescription systems of the future utilize individual patient characteristics which include genetic information together with allergic backgrounds and current drug prescriptions to create the most appropriate treatment plans. Computational algorithms examine drug interactions at subcellular levels to create safe combination profiles that also reveal effective coherences. AI systems at major medical institutions help healthcare providers select appropriate antibiotics for serious infections which reduces the need for broad-spectrum drugs thus stopping antibiotic resistance development. Artificial intelligence software evaluates patient reaction to past medications through machine learning to determine the most effective antidepressants with minimal side effects for treatment. The drug recommendation systems present healthcare providers with detailed explanations behind their medication suggestions to improve practitioner understanding of selection rationale (Lin et al.,2022).

DQNs have encountered multiple obstacles which includes insufficient data for rare diseases together with safety risks during data collection and regulatory framework limitations. Federated learning allows hospitals to share their data together and safe reinforcement learning uses clinician supervision while digital twin simulations provide training methods. Explanation-focused development of DQNs with attention layers stands as the main priority to gain clinician trust through better decision understanding. This evolution towards adaptive patient-focused AI systems will become reality as these models achieve proper development. Personalized medical care will be established throughout this process. Multiple actions must be taken during the subsequent phase to solve implementation challenges between electronic health record system integration and ethical standards for clinical AI deployment.

## V. CHALLENGES AND ETHICAL CONSIDERATION

The combination of reinforcement learning and Deep Q-Networks (DQNs) in personalized healthcare creates both innovative opportunities and severe security and ethical problems for the medical sector. Artificial intelligence systems manage sensitive patient data exceptionally well though their extensive data processing capabilities lead to security problems regarding medical privacy and doubts about treatment algorithm integrity. The success requires two safety measures for medical data protection which combines federated learning for data security and differential privacy for unauthorized detection and automatic safety threat resolution of AI-generated therapeutic approaches. These systems face ethical concerns primarily because high-risk clinical environments magnify risk factors stemming from unclear systems and discriminatory algorithms coupled with dangerous failures that lead to possible fatal outcomes. The treatment of reported system issues requires protected AI development practices and strict medical verification protocols and complete oversight of human supervision alongside reinforcement learning implementation to drive precision medicine development. DQNs' capability to establish personalized healthcare at scale can deliver safest and most effective results when technology innovation reaches equilibrium with proper implementation practices (Banumathi et al.,2025).

Healthcare reinforcement learning systems present distinctive privacy problems because their design can change in ways that standard medical AI systems do not experience. Personalized medicine DQNs require constant access to sensitive patient data streams in order to perform real-time treatment policy updates. Best performance occurs when the system has complete patient data but this highest level of data accessibility directly puts sensitive information at risk. An optimal DQN algorithm treatment of diabetes requires continuous access to glucose monitor data and patient-meal information as well as activity records and sleep patterns in combination with historic glucose readings for successful application. When additional data sources enter the system both functionality improves but it exposes more information to privacy risks (Tamrakar et al.,2024).

The addition of time constraints leads to complicated data protection needs in RL systems. DQNs utilize active patient models that adapt and transform through numerous years of care treatment for patients with chronic diseases. The extended periods which data stays in memory systems as PHI necessitate new approaches to data governance because of this longitudinal learning process which provides clinical value. The situation becomes more challenging to manage because the best approach to obtaining optimal knowledge through combining data from multiple patient groups creates conflicting needs between personalized care and community health understanding. The effectiveness of a DQN depends on its access to single patient data while patient information sharing poses privacy challenges based on HIPAA and GDPR regulations (Deshmukh,2024).

Different technological advancements demonstrate potential solutions for dealing with these RL healthcare implementation difficulties. The method of federated reinforcement learning enables multiple healthcare institutions to develop DQNs through collaborative training without sharing raw patient data across sites. Hospitals retain total control over their medical data through this approach by sharing improved versions of their models instead of disclosing their private patient-related information. The application of differential privacy in RL settings requires proper adjustment of added noise across training data and policy updates to stop the reconstruction of specific patient information. The current advancements in homomorphic encryption enable feasible encrypted reinforcement learning applications but existing complex computational challenges prevent their use in real-time clinical environments with neural network architectures (Ekundayo,2024).

Changes in personalized medicine through reinforcement learning (RL) require essential reforms to consent methods because one-time authorization forms are unable to manage the evolving nature of Deep Q-Networks (DQNs) during their operational period. A progressive framework of consent enables patients to retain permanent control of their data contribution process by adjusting access levels according to AI system development along with newly developed therapeutic applications. The implementation of Blockchain technology produces unalterable audit trails which show patient data contributions to precise treatment suggestions and it simultaneously provides secure mechanisms to track data source information. Organizations need to create robust privacy policies which will establish specific rules for data reduction and automatic system purging to make obsolete or unneeded information removable across the system. Such a multilayered system which integrates dynamic consent solutions with distributed ledger verification protocols and adaptable data governance protocols has emerged to develop an ethical framework that both supports healthcare-specific self-improving AI challenges while upholding patient control and medical treatment trust in dynamic therapeutic domains (Mehmood,2025).

DQN-driven personalized medicine generates distinctive biases which appear subtly in learning processes yet differ from standard medical AI bias problems. Reinforcement learning systems learn treatment procedures from historical data thus they both enhance existing healthcare delivery biases and create new biases that emerge from the RL approach. The training of DQNs based on electronic health records leads to recommendations of less intensive treatments toward patient groups who experienced historical problems reaching healthcare facilities. If reward functions used for guiding RL systems are not properly designed, they may unconsciously insert biases during operation which could disadvantage patient groups with complicated healthcare needs (Agarwal,2024).

RL uses a decision-making process that both creates time-based bias yet conventional static systems eliminate such biases completely. During individual treatments a DQN demonstrates fairness to cancer patients yet it systematically develops unfavorable bias patterns throughout the entire therapeutic period. RL systems that deliver early limiting suggestions for patient selection might create future treatment constraints that worsen over time and increase disposal gaps in the population. The ethical dimensions of RL expand from the fundamental exploration-exploitation trade off because the system faces a dilemma about testing underutilized treatments on underserved groups to enhance data collection versus performing unethical experiments. The dilemmas become especially important in healthcare contexts because wrong decisions in these settings might result in severe life/events consequences (Nascimben,2024).

Specific methods must be formed to reduce bias problems in DQN-based personalized medicine because reinforcement learning operates differently. The process of designing reward functions requires thorough audits to guarantee they adhere to equal care goals with possible implementation through reward structures that optimize multiple targets including fairness measurements and clinical achievements. Representative learning approaches assist in developing clinical features in the DQN while preventing correlations with protected characteristics. Off-policy evaluation analyzes proposed treatment policies through historical data testing before deployment so healthcare organizations can identify potential impacts on different groups. These adaptive AI systems need continuous bias monitoring because of their learning capability so new auditing frameworks must be developed specifically to evaluate them (Bandaru,2021).

The interpretation challenges associated with DQNs make it difficult to address bias problems in clinical practice. DQNs utilize complicated neural networks which prevent healthcare professionals from seeing how input variables affect decision recommendations. Healthcare providers encounter ethical issues regarding treatment explanation to patients and bias audits because DQNs remain untransparent. Recent research on attention mechanisms and concept activation vectors offers potential methods for rendering DQN decisions more interpretable yet scientist and physician groups must continue to refine both accuracy and medical relevance. The combination of DQN systems with model architecture components that provide interpretability for specific decisions points toward an acceptable solution (Alabi,2025).

Extensive cooperation between specialists in computer science and clinical medicine besides ethical experts and health policy makers is vital to address these obstacles for responsible healthcare integration. The development of RL-specific privacy specifications applied to current healthcare privacy standards should handle the distinctive learning requirements of continual systems. Healthcare organizations should adopt federated RL standards from regulatory bodies with processes for certifying privacy methods. The research field needs standardized benchmarks with specialized evaluation systems to analyse adaptive treatment systems regarding fairness while moving past static assessment approaches toward continuous evaluation. The integration process should establish comprehensive training programs for healthcare providers to reach beyond interface learning so they fully understand system potential as well as constraints. The human supervisors conducting oversight for DQN recommendations must receive training to detect potential biases and privacy threats because they maintain full responsibility for medical decisions. The educational materials about adaptive AI should provide clear explanations to patients about distinctions between this technology and traditional clinical support tools with particular focus on its learning ability and customization features (Kalusivalingam, 2020).

Medical artificial intelligence based on reinforcement learning requires updated regulatory models for its dynamic operating characteristics. The current device approval system directs its attention toward static medical equipment although new continuous adaptation technologies necessitate an update to the approval procedures. The FDA recently introduced "predetermined change control plans" for AI/ML devices as part of their initiatives but this approach needs to cover the core adaptability found in RL systems. Determining liability responsibility becomes intricate when a DQN creates unexpected changes to its treatment policy that cause patient injuries because all parties from developers through healthcare providers to healthcare institutions must be acknowledged in liability considerations (Rane et al.,2024).

The potential of DQNs to achieve personalized medicine through continuously adapting treatment approaches should be regulated against major ethical and practical barriers. Multiple initiatives combining technical innovation with careful policymaking and inclusive design practice enable the development of enhanced treatment systems that maintain medical standards and equality in care delivery.

## VI. FUTURE DIRECTIONS IN AI-POWERED SMART HEALTHCARE

Healthcare AI evolution advances through improved integrated systems to transform patient care through continuous personalized monitoring and intervention. The next generation of smart healthcare delivery systems will emerge from two promising technologies that merge IoT/wearable devices with autonomous monitoring capabilities for patients. Deep Q-Networks and reinforcement learning strategies will guide healthcare professionals to achieve predictive and preventive medicine by analysing dynamic data that comes from technological synergies between healthcare systems (Popolo n.d.,).

Technical barriers to linking IoT and AI systems have become progressively easier to overcome. Edge computing systems perform initial data processing tasks at wearable devices which protects battery life and reduces vital health notification delays. Federated learning frameworks let wearables use personal health data to support population health models within the devices thus resolving major privacy issues. Multiple wearable devices can share information through sophisticated algorithms which allow users to combine heart rate variability tracking from their smartwatch with measurements from a smart ring peripheral temperature sensor and blood flow sensors to recognize early cardiovascular event symptoms. Reinforcement learning demonstrates excellence within this setting since it optimizes interpretations of diverse signals through patient outcome analysis which enables the system to discover reliable combinations of wearable data for precise health event prediction among individual patients. Digital twin technology currently develops because patient wearable data feeds virtual simulation models which predict future health outcomes based on different treatment conditions (Sharma et al.,2024).

Development of smart healthcare focuses on turning AI-assisted systems into autonomous algorithms that can execute real-time clinical choices independently under diminished human supervision. Hospital-based AI technology now operates as a patient management system to handle basic healthcare tasks so clinical professionals only need to deal with advanced medical situations. Automated AI systems operating in intensive care units use simultaneous multiple-physiological parameter observation to spot delicate patient decline indicators that human medical professionals would possibly overlook in their busy cycles. The systems transform alerts into responsible actions by implementing preliminary treatment options such as ventilator parameter changes and changes to IV flow and medication dose limits within established boundaries. In these systems DQNs serve a fundamental purpose to learn ideal monitoring practices after analyzing numerous temporal clinical datasets for critical action indicators and suitable intervention predictions (McCall, 2022).

Next-generation remote patient monitoring platforms use autonomous monitoring to provide surveillance which extends outside traditional hospital facilities. Artificial intelligence systems observe patients with chronic diseases from home through the analysis of information gathered from wearable technology and smart house mechanisms as well as advanced computer vision systems which measure walking patterns and facial indications. Reinforcement learning-based monitoring systems adjust their examination protocols according to individual patient risk factors which direct advanced heart failure patients to receive greater observation intervals than patients who maintain stable diabetic health. The AI develops personalized models based on individual data patterns which helps it detect actual medical emergencies in advance by minimizing incorrect alerts. The autonomous systems activate emergency protocols by contacting essential contacts and providing essential first aid directions through smart speakers as well as dispatching emergency services depending on the situation (Taalat,2021).

The implementation of self-governing systems creates multiple technical as well as ethical issues that require thorough investigation. Security requirements must get embedded directly into AI systems for maintaining absolute safety during hazardous situations where the AI's learned insights appear advantageous. Human oversight systems should provide clinicians with suitable control while preventing the development of alert fatigue to ensure crucial warnings are interpreted. Protocols regarding legal responsibility need to define how autonomous systems will be held accountable for their clinical choices specifically when their decisions differ from standard procedures because their learning has occurred. The most fundamental concern about these systems requires complete validation through strict clinical trials to evaluate their accuracy and their impact on patient outcomes among different demographic groups (Xu et al.,2022).

Shifts in medical care will face their biggest breakthrough through intelligent systems which take IoT-generated continuous data to autonomously make real-time clinical diagnoses. Imagine a future where a patient's network of wearable devices detects early signs of atrial fibrillation, the autonomous AI system confirms the diagnosis through additional tests using smartphone-based sensors, initiates anticoagulation therapy through a smart medication dispenser, adjusts the treatment based on continuous monitoring of vital signs and potential side effects, and coordinates follow-up care with the patient's cardiologist—all with appropriate human oversight but minimal required intervention. The future of AI-enhanced healthcare which brings complete patient integration is progressively transitioning from fictional to actual clinical implementation (Job et al.,2024).

Continuous health monitoring together with adaptive treatments in healthcare requires reinforcement learning (RL) to execute its fundamental role since it enables optimum policy selection based on environmental feedback. In the future Deep

Q-Network-based systems will progress toward leadership roles over multiple specialized AI systems by guiding them to handle cardiovascular tasks and metabolic functions as the master RL system oversees the coordination process. A hierarchically structured system will establish a realistic approach to patient-specific care through agents that work together to optimize combined treatment approaches in true real time. Future technological breakthroughs—particularly in 5G networks and quantum computing—will further amplify these capabilities by providing the ultra-low latency and immense computational power required for large-scale, real-time health analytics. The rapid connection of 5G networks enables AI systems to analyze streaming data from hospital devices as well as wearables and implants in real time because quantum speedups with RTL appreciate difficult optimization solutions now arrive within seconds which takes regular computers days to finish this task. Modern healthcare AI advancements will bring autonomous healthcare AI systems to better accuracy and processing speed and enhanced scalability to establish a predictive medical practice that detects health threats prior to their critical phase. Advancement of healthcare AI systems depends on safety protocols with interpretability features and ethical governance to preserve trustworthiness. Medical technology development needs systems that demonstrate responsible autonomy to unite RL innovations with human medical expertise in practice (Liu, 2020).

Healthcare system enhancement requires solving technical integration problems with data unification testing as well as system connect ability and ethical assessments regarding autonomy together with privacy and equity standards. The highest value of future healthcare systems will emerge from disease prevention prior to symptom onset and delivering optimal care to patients at their most suitable biological times and locations. The book's concluding portion brings together relevant main concepts to present a synchronized perspective about the effects that reinforcement learning will have on healthcare evolution during the upcoming decade.

## CONCLUSION

The application of neural network learning technology in healthcare generates transformative power which enhances clinical decision-making processes through cost reductions by building patient-specific healthcare protocols based on sophisticated data analysis and variable treatment plan adjustments. The application of Healthcare AI systems analyzes sequential patient information for individualized treatment planning while minimizing healthcare expenses through better resource management and reducing treatment numbers and enabling early warning systems to stop complications before they occur. To implement DQNs effectively in patient-centered healthcare it is necessary to develop explainable AI systems and strict bias reduction procedures together with ethical protocols which will protect clinical oversight and safeguard patient privacy. Healthcare development requires building robust AI systems that unite DQNs pattern recognition features with clinical expertise so AI can team up with clinicians to handle standard healthcare tasks while doctors handle superior medical evaluations for delivering better healthcare results.

## REFERENCES


Abdellatif, A. A., Mhaisen, N., Chkirbene, Z., Mohamed, A., Erbad, A., & Guizani, M. (2021). Reinforcement learning for intelligent healthcare systems: A comprehensive survey. *arXiv preprint arXiv:2108.04087.*

Alabi, M. (2025). *Reinforcement Learning: Applications in Gaming*. Robotics, and Real-World Decision-Making.

Bandaru, V. K. R., Gondi, D. S., Gondi, K., & Indugu, V. V. R. (2021). Reinforcement Learning for Optimizing Personalized Treatment Plans in Oncology. *CIT. Journal of Computing and Information Technology*, *1*(1).

Banumathi, K., Venkatesan, L., Benjamin, L. S., Vijayalakshmi, K., Satchi, N. S., & Satchi, N. S.IV. (2025). Reinforcement Learning in Personalized Medicine: A Comprehensive Review of Treatment Optimization Strategies. *Cureus*, *17*(4).

Boppiniti, S. T. (2021). Evolution of Reinforcement Learning: From Q-Learning to Deep. *Available at SSRN* 5061696.

Carta, S., Ferreira, A., Podda, A. S., Recupero, D. R., & Sanna, A. (2021). Multi-DQN: An ensemble of Deep Q-learning agents for stock market forecasting. *Expert Systems with Applications*, *164*, 113820.

Deshmukh, R. (2024). Reinforcement learning in healthcare: Applications for personalized treatment planning and clinical decision support. *Shodh Sagar Journal of Artificial Intelligence and Machine Learning*, *1*(2), 19–24.

Ekundayo, F. (2024). Reinforcement learning in treatment pathway optimization: A case study in oncology. *International Journal of Science and Research Archive*, *13*(02), 2187–2205.

Faes, M., & Moens, D. (2020). Recent trends in the modeling and quantification of non-probabilistic uncertainty. *Archives of Computational Methods in Engineering*, *27*, 633–671.

Faiyazuddin, M., Rahman, S. J. Q., Anand, G., Siddiqui, R. K., Mehta, R., Khatib, M. N., & Sah, R. (2025). The Impact of Artificial Intelligence on Healthcare: A Comprehensive Review of Advancements in Diagnostics, Treatment, and Operational Efficiency. *Health Science Reports*, *8*(1), e70312.

Hider, M. A., Nasiruddin, M., & Al Mukaddim, A. (2024). Early Disease Detection through Advanced Machine Learning Techniques: A Comprehensive Analysis and Implementation in Healthcare Systems. *Revista de Inteligencia Artificial en Medicina, 15*(1), 1010–1042.

Job, S., Tao, X., Li, L., Xie, H., Cai, T., Yong, J., & Li, Q. (2024). Optimal treatment strategies for critical patients with deep reinforcement learning. *ACM Transactions on Intelligent Systems and Technology, 15*(2), 1–22.

Kalusivalingam, A. K., Sharma, A., Patel, N., & Singh, V. (2020). Optimizing Decision-Making with AI-Enhanced Support Systems: Leveraging Reinforcement Learning and Bayesian Networks. *International Journal of AI and ML, 1*(2).

Keerthika, K., Kannan, M., & Saravanan, T. (2024). Clinical Intelligence: Deep Reinforcement Learning for Healthcare and Biomedical Advancements. *Deep Reinforcement Learning and Its Industrial Use Cases: AI for Real-World Applications*, 137-150.

Laroche, R., Trichelair, P., & Des Combes, R. T. (2019, May). Safe policy improvement with baseline bootstrapping. In *International conference on machine learning* (pp. 3652-3661). PMLR.

Lin, Y., Zhang, Y., Wang, D., Yang, B., & Shen, Y. Q. (2022). Computer especially AI-assisted drug virtual screening and design in traditional Chinese medicine. *Phytomedicine, 107*, 154481.

Liu, S., See, K. C., Ngiam, K. Y., Celi, L. A., Sun, X., & Feng, M. (2020). Reinforcement learning for clinical decision support in critical care: Comprehensive review. *Journal of Medical Internet Research, 22*(7), e18477.

Lu, M., Shahn, Z., Sow, D., Doshi-Velez, F., & Lehman, L. W. H. (2021, January). Is deep reinforcement learning ready for practical applications in healthcare? A sensitivity analysis of duel-DDQN for hemodynamic management in sepsis patients. *AMIA ... Annual Symposium Proceedings - AMIA Symposium. AMIA Symposium, 2020*, 773.

McCall, A. (2022). *Reinforcement Learning: Applications in Gaming*. Robotics, and Real-World Decision-Making.

Mehmood, Y. (2025). Reinforcement learning in intelligent applications: Algorithms and case studies. *Journal of AI Spectrum, 2*(1), 12–22.

Nascimben, M. (2024). Machine learning approaches for personalized medicine.

Pandelu, A. P. (2024, December 28). *Day 62: Reinforcement Learning basics — agent, environment, rewards.* Medium. https://medium.com/@bhatadithya54764118/day-62-reinforcement-learning-basics-agent-environment-rewards-306b8e7e555c

Popolo, V., Trunfio, T. A., & Scala, A. A Literature Review on the Application of Reinforcement Learning in Healthcare Management.

Raghu, A., Komorowski, M., Ahmed, I., Celi, L., Szolovits, P., & Ghassemi, M. (2017). Deep reinforcement learning for sepsis treatment. *arXiv preprint arXiv:1711.09602.*

Rai, A. K., Sharma, M., Saravanan, V., Shalini, N., Kumar, M., & Singh, P. (2023, December). Personalized healthcare recommendations with Q-Learning reinforcement learning. In *2023 International Conference on Artificial Intelligence for Innovations in Healthcare Industries (ICAIIHI)* (Vol. 1, pp. 1-6). IEEE.

Rane, N., Choudhary, S., & Rane, J. (2024). Machine learning and deep learning: A comprehensive review on methods, techniques, applications, challenges, and future directions. *Techniques, Applications, Challenges, and Future Directions (May 31, 2024).*

Rosenbacke, R., Melhus, Å., McKee, M., & Stuckler, D. (2024). How Explainable Artificial Intelligence Can Increase or Decrease Clinicians' Trust in AI Applications in Health Care: Systematic Review. *JMIR AI*, *3*, e53207.

Roy, P. P., Teju, V., Kandula, S. R., Sowmya, K. V., Stan, A. I., & Stan, O. P. (2024). Secure healthcare model using multi-step deep q learning network in internet of things. *Electronics (Basel)*, *13*(3), 669.

Selvam, D. T., Vinothkumar, J., & Madhubala, S. (2024, November). Two-Phase Deep Q Learning Network for Secure Healthcare Model in the Internet of Things. In *2024 2nd International Conference on Advances in Computation, Communication and Information Technology (ICAICCIT)* (Vol. 1, pp. 365-370). IEEE.

Sharma, J., Kumar, D., & Gupta, T. (2024, July). Optimizing Pneumonia Detection: Integrating Quadratic Discriminant Analysis and Deep Q-Networks Through Reinforcement Learning. In *2024 2nd World Conference on Communication & Computing (WCONF)* (pp. 1-5). IEEE.

Singh, R., Arya, P., & Dubey, S. H. (2024). Artificial Intelligence in Pharmaceutics: Revolutionizing Drug Formulation and Optimization. *Journal of Drug Discovery and Health Sciences*, *1*(03), 138–145.

Sun, Y., Yan, J., Lu, L., Zhang, H., & Shang, Y. (2025). Semantic Fusion-Oriented Bi-Typed Multi-Relational Heterogeneous Graph Neural Network. *IEEE Access : Practical Innovations, Open Solutions.*

Talaat, F. M. (2022). Effective deep Q-networks (EDQN) strategy for resource allocation based on optimized reinforcement learning algorithm. *Multimedia Tools and Applications*, *81*(28), 39945–39961.

Tamrakar, P., Pathak, G. R., Lal, M., Goel, A., & Bhende, M. (2024, February). Personalized Healthcare Recommendations with Q-Learning Reinforcement Learning. In *International Conference on Machine Learning Algorithms* (pp. 182-193). Cham: Springer Nature Switzerland.

Xu, L., Zhu, S., & Wen, N. (2022). Deep reinforcement learning and its applications in medical imaging and radiation therapy: A survey. *Physics in Medicine and Biology*, *67*(22), 22TR02.

Yazdani, D., Omidvar, M. N., Yazdani, D., Branke, J., Nguyen, T. T., Gandomi, A. H., & Yao, X. (2023). Robust optimization over time: A critical review. *IEEE Transactions on Evolutionary Computation*.

Yazzourh, S. (2024). *Reinforcement learning and Bayesian outcome-weighted learning for precision medicine: integrating medical knowledge into decision-making algorithms* (Doctoral dissertation, Université de Toulouse).

# Chapter 13
# Learning to Heal:
## Deep Q-Networks as the Future of AI-Driven Healthcare

**Sapandeep Kaur Dhillon**
*Guru Nanak Dev University, Amritsar, India*

**Ikvinderpal Singh**
https://orcid.org/0000-0003-2154-9724
*Trai Shatabdi Guru Gobind Khalsa College, Amritsar, India*

**Parminder Kaur**
https://orcid.org/0000-0003-1954-3390
*Guru Nanak Dev University, Amritsar, India*

## ABSTRACT

*Deep Q-Networks (DQNs) in smart healthcare enable artificial intelligence to rapidly alter medical decisions and learn from mistakes. DQNs build smart healthcare agents by leveraging reinforcement learning rather than rules. Dynamic learning advances diagnosis, treatment, and hospital operations. DQNs enable artificial intelligence systems to assess activities by using rewards and punishments, thereby optimizing their strategies. They draw on deep learning and Q-learning. Robotic-assisted procedures and ICUs save lives through educated judgments. DQNs identify diseases, develop drugs and tailored therapies. AI bots use patient data to tailor treatment. Problems abound. Think about morality, openness in decision-making, and data security. Explainable artificial intelligence in human-AI decision systems increases dependability and utility. As wearable's and telemedicine interfaces offer smart, responsive healthcare, DQNs also do. Human knowledge remains enormous. The DQNs should help physicians. Beyond data analysis, systems help enhance patient care.*

DOI: 10.4018/979-8-3373-3311-3.ch013

## 1. INTRODUCTION: AI THAT LEARNS TO HEAL

Artificial intelligence (AI) is present-day reality altering access to, delivery of, and interpretation of healthcare, not a futuristic concept in medicine. Artificial intelligence has developed into a required tool in the modern clinical environment from helping diagnosis imaging and predictive analytics to streamlining back-office operations (AbdelAziz et al., 2025). Although artificial intelligence systems of today offer many benefits, their fixed aspect still primarily limits them. Most depend largely on pre-programmed rules or large historical datasets; once put into use, they cannot independently adapt to new data or changing situations. In the complex, erratic, always changing sector of healthcare, this rigidity is a big drawback.

The diversity of human physiology, the unpredictability of diseases, and the fast changing dynamics of healthcare systems demand a new kind of intelligence—one motivated not only by data but also by experience. Patients might not always follow recommended courses; medical crises strike at random and treatments that benefit one person could not benefit another. Even the most powerful static AI models have a hard time fitting this reality because they are not meant to learn and grow over time. Deep Q-Networks (DQNs) move to the front of the queue.

When it comes to artificial intelligence, DQNs are a big step forward. DQNs learn all the time by interacting with their surroundings, while standard models need to be retrained to adapt to new data. They use both deep learning and reinforcement learning together. Deep learning is great at handling unstructured data like medical photos or clinical notes. Reinforcement learning helps AI robots learn by doing—getting feedback, fixing mistakes, and planning the best actions for the future (Yu et al., 2021). This way of learning changes things in healthcare, where things are at stake and decisions need to be made quickly and correctly.

### 1.1 Moving from Static AI to Adaptive Intelligence

In healthcare, traditional AI is mostly made up of either uncontrolled or supervised machine learning. When trained on named datasets, these models are great at tasks like picture classification or finding strange things in pictures (Ma et al., 2023). Still, they can only do what their training data tells them to do. Once taught and used, they become tools that only do one thing. They can only react to new information after being retrained, which takes a lot of time and resources.

DQNs, on the other hand, work inside a loop with a lot of input. They decide what to do (like offering a therapy or assigning a resource), watch the results (like whether the patient gets better or worse), and change their methods based on what they see in the environment, such as the vital signs, test results, or treatment reactions.

Due to their ability to learn from both successes and failures in real time, DQNs are more like humans when it comes to making decisions than any other type of AI.

This level of adaptability changes not only the technology but also how we think about intelligence systems in healthcare. It clears the way for tools that do more than just serve as weapons in the care process.

## 1.2 How DQNs Work: Interactive Learning

DQNs are based on reinforcement learning (RL), which is done over and over again. In this model, an agent learns how to do its best in a certain setting by getting either positive feedback (rewards) or negative feedback (penalties). The agent's goal is to get the most total prize over time. To do this, it learns a policy, which is a set of rules that tells it what to do in every situation.

Q-learning is one of the most important RL methods. It works by guessing the expected future benefits (called Q-values) of doing a certain action in a certain state. DQNs improve Q-learning by using deep neural networks to get closer to these Q-values (Ma et al., 2023a). This lets the system handle very large and complicated state spaces, like those found in healthcare settings.

This approach enables DQNs to:

- Find trends in data too complex for conventional rule-based systems.
- Make sequential decisions in which the effects of choices are not immediately clear-cut.
- Learn rules that change with increasing data availability, therefore transforming over time.

In real life, this could mean that an AI system changes the settings of an ICU ventilator in real time based on physiological data or that a DQN adjusts the chemotherapy schedule based on how the patient is doing.

## 1.3 Transforming Possibilities in Medical Treatment

Deep learning combined with reinforcement learning opens numerous strong capabilities that could alter clinical practice (Lopez-Martinez et al., 2019):

### 1.3.1 Treatment and Customized Learning

Every patient is different; DQNs are designed to honor that difference. Real-time and longitudinal patient data combined allows DQNs to develop patient-specific models that change with the patient's state. Treatments can thus be constantly customized to increase safety and efficacy simultaneously.

### 1.3.2 Adaptive Resource Optimization

A lot of the time, healthcare systems are limited by things like a lack of staff, beds, or stable supply lines. DQNs can flexibly assign resources based on demand responses. In a pandemic, for example, a DQN might figure out the best way to set up ventilators across a network of hospitals based on how well treatments are working and how infections are spreading.

### 1.3.3 Real-Time Loops for Feedback

One of the best things about DQNs is that they can combine real-time data. This lets systems quickly change their course, which is very useful in places where time is of the essence, like operating rooms or emergency rooms.

### 1.3.4 Improved Clinical Intervention Support

With the most up-to-date information, DQNs can give doctors advice that is always changing. DQNs can give doctors probabilistic advice based on what they've seen or done in the past in tough or unclear situations where there isn't a lot of evidence or evidence that contradicts itself. This helps doctors be more confident as they face doubt.

## 1.4 Applications throughout the Medical Spectrum

DQNs have vast possible uses in many different spheres of healthcare (Jayaraman et al., 2024a):

- **Critical Care:** DQNs can support real-time monitoring and decision-making in intensive care units, including helping to decide when to wean a patient off mechanical ventilator.
- **Chronic Disease Management:** DQNs can customize drug regimens and lifestyle treatments depending on daily data from wearable devices for disorders including diabetes or hypertension.
- **Robotic-Assisted Surgery:** DQNs can tell robotic systems how to adapt to changes in the body's structure or unexpected medical problems, which makes the surgery more accurate and safer.

- **Hospital Administration:** DQNs may improve processes, cut down on wait times, and make patients happier, from planning operations to managing ER traffic.
- **Drug Discovery:** DQNs are also making progress in pharmaceutical research. Now, they can copy thousands of chemical interactions to find possible new medicines more quickly and accurately.

## 1.5 Adoption's Obstacles: Data, Trust, and Ethics

As powerful as DQNs are, they also have some problems and boundaries (Nguyen & Odigie, 2023). Before these methods can be widely used in healthcare, a number of important problems need to be fixed:

### 1.5.1 Data Requirements

Data-hungry models, DQNs need a lot of high-quality, labelled data to learn correctly. It is very hard to do this in healthcare because data is often separated, missing, or not dependable. Privacy concerns are another thing that makes sharing data annoying.

### 1.5.2 Computationally Costly

For computational intensity training DQNs, you need special tools and a lot of energy. For low- and middle-income countries, this can be hard, especially for institutions that aren't very good with technology.

### 1.5.3 Transparency and Confidence

It makes sense that clinicians don't want to rely on processes they don't understand. A "black box" quality of deep learning models, including DQNs, makes it hard to know who is responsible and how to understand them. If a DQN tells a doctor to do an operation that could be dangerous, the doctor needs to be ready to defend that advice to both the patient and the authorities.

### 1.5.4 Legal and Ethical Issues

AI applications in medicine raise serious ethical concerns. Should an artificial intelligence-driven therapy choice backfire, who bears liability? How can we make sure these systems lack prejudices that would negatively affect some patient groups?

How can we strike a mix between informed permission and patient autonomy against innovation?

These are social problems requiring multidisciplinary solutions involving ethicists, legislators, doctors, and technologists; they are not only technical ones.

## 1.6 Approaching a Medical New Paradigm

Integration of DQNs into healthcare aims to increase rather than replace human intellect (Ma et al., 2023a). These systems are intended to be smart partners that improve human judgement, lower mistakes, and increase access to first-rate treatment. DQNs can get even more skilled at negotiating the complexities of human health by always learning from every choice and its results.

This chapter aims to give a thorough introduction of this newly developing discipline. We start by building the theoretical basis of DQNs including their architectural, learning, and algorithmic aspects. We then look at practical uses and investigate how DQNs are now helping to enhance operations, diagnosis, and treatment. At last, we explore the obstacles that have to be removed to attain ethical, safe, and successful application of these technologies.

## 1.7 The Outlook: Gaining Healing Skills

Deep Q-Networks in smart healthcare have as their ultimate goal systems that learn to heal rather than only compute. Like great doctors, they see, adjust, and grow with time (Jayaraman et al., 2024a). By doing this, they assist to close the distance between medical knowledge and medical practice, between what is known and what is done.

Embedding learning into the fabric of healthcare systems opens fresh opportunities for:

- Precision medicine, whereby treatments are customised to the individual in real-time.
- Preventive care: patterns seen by artificial intelligence long before symptoms develop lead early therapies.
- Global health equity: with scalable, adaptable platforms, intelligent systems can provide sophisticated care to underdeveloped areas.

Guiding the evolution of DQNs with the same values that support the practice of medicine—empathy, responsibility, openness, and respect of human dignity—is essential as we explore this new frontiers. The objective is to create a wiser, more compassionate healthcare system as much as better machines.

## 2. DEEP Q-NETWORKS IN SMART HEALTHCARE

Artificial intelligence (AI) is changing healthcare by finding new ways to solve old problems, like making diagnosis better, easing processes, and tailoring treatment to each person. There are many types of artificial intelligence, but Deep Q-Networks (DQNs) are one of the most interesting because they can learn from their mistakes and keep changing to fit new, difficult healthcare situations. DQNs are different from standard AI systems because they don't just look at static datasets and follow predefined rules. Instead, they interact with clinical data streams, patient situations, and hospital operations to make the best decisions in real time. Because of this, DQNs are very helpful in healthcare, where decisions need to be made quickly and correctly even though situations are always changing (Jayaraman et al., 2024b).

DQNs combine reinforcement learning (RL), a model that lets computers learn by doing things and getting feedback, with deep learning (DL), a method that can understand very large and complicated medical data sets. By using all of these approaches together, DQNs help AI "learn to heal," which improves patient outcomes by taking actions based on data observed and choices made in the past. In this section, we look at the main ideas behind DQNs, how they have changed healthcare, and the detailed learning process that helps them get better in clinical settings.

### 2.1 Fundamental Ideas and DQN Functioning

DQNs are based fundamentally on three linked artificial intelligence ideas:

#### 2.1.1 Reinforcement Learning (RL)

Reinforcement learning is a model that comes from behavioural psychology. It involves an agent acting and dealing with its surroundings to figure out what actions get the best results. RL is about learning the best ways to do things by making mistakes (K et al., 2025). This is different from supervised learning, where a model learns from samples that have been marked.

In healthcare, the environment is the clinical context, and the agent is the AI system that makes choices about operations or therapy. The agent either gets rewards or punishments based on the outcomes of the choices it makes, like whether the patient heals or doesn't. The ultimate goal is to get the most long-term benefits, which will motivate the agent to choose tasks that improve health over time.

### 2.1.2 Deep learning (DL)

Deep learning is a subclass of machine learning whereby significant features from complicated and high-dimensional data are extracted by means of deep neural networks with several layers. Deep learning is especially suited for medical data since it frequently involves vast volumes of unstructured data including: medical images (MRI, CT scans, X-rays); electronic health records (EHRs); genomic data; continuous physiological data from monitors and wearable sensors (Stember & Shalu, 2020).

By allowing the AI to analyse these vast amounts of data and identify trends or anomalies difficult for humans or conventional methods to find, DL helps it to interpret.

### 2.1.3 Q-Learning

A model-free RL method, Q-learning teaches an agent to assess the quality (Q-value) of choosing a certain action in a given state. From then on, the Q-value shows the anticipated overall benefit from that activity. The agent creates a strategy based on highest Q-values, therefore guiding it towards best decision-making.

These Q-values are kept in a table in conventional Q-learning, which soon becomes unworkable as the number of states and actions increases—particularly in healthcare, where patient circumstances and treatment choices are wide and complex. DQNs solve this problem by approximating Q-values using deep neural networks, therefore allowing scalability in demanding settings (Nambiar et al., 2023).

## 2.2 Healthcare-Specific Components of DQNs

DQNs are implemented using a decision-making cycle especially fit for healthcare environments (Talaat, 2022). Three main components define this cycle:

### 2.2.1 Environment (Medical Facility)

In the real world, the AI system works in a complex clinical or medical setting, which is called the environment. It includes information about the patient's vital signs, lab results, imaging, and medication history. It also includes diagnostic tools and treatment recommendations.

- Workflows and health professionals.
- Outside factors including drug supplies, resource availability, and illness outbreaks.

The features of this area make it lively and hard to predict. Patients' conditions change quickly, treatments don't always work, and there are limits to what can be done, especially in critical care settings or during public health situations.

In an intensive care unit (ICU), for example, a DQN system constantly checks a patient's vital signs, the settings for their respirator, and the results of their tests. Based on this constantly changing stream of data, treatment plans are changed in real time.

### 2.2.2 Agent (AI Decision-Maker)

The fundamental DQN model that handles environmental inputs, chooses medical actions, and learns from results to guide next decisions is the agent—AI decision-maker. The agent wants two things:

- To maximise patient health outcomes—that is, lower death rates, hasten recovery, or raise quality of living.
- To maximise resource use—that is, the distribution of ICU beds or drugs.

In cancer, for instance, a DQN agent might examine tumour genetics, patient history, and past treatment responses to customise chemotherapy schedules that best maximise efficacy while minimising side effects.

### 2.2.3 Reward Mechanism

The reward system tells the agent whether or not its choices turned out as expected. This numerical signal motivates the artificial intelligence to learn which behaviours are good and which bad.

- Successful early diagnosis, stabilised vitals, or better patient survival rates could all bring positive advantages.
- Penalties result from treatment failures, negative events, or resource waste.

In emergency care, for example, a DQN system rewards correctly prioritizing patients who need treatment right away and punishes cases that is mis-triaged and cause problems.

## 2.3 The Medical Learning Cycle: Applications

Learning by an iterative five-step process, DQNs change constantly as fresh data comes in:

### 2.3.1 Notes and Data Gathering

The system starts with compiling thorough information from many sources, including Electronic Health Records (EHRs) including lab results, medical history, and demographics (Ma et al., 2023b).

- Wearable sensors' and monitors' real-time vital signs.
- Genetic data and medical imaging.
- Environmental factors such drug supply or personnel levels.

This large amount of data, which shows what is happening in the world, forms the state picture of the artificial intelligence.

For example, an ICU-focused DQN records blood pressure, oxygen saturation, ventilator settings, drug dosages, and lab values every hour. This gives a full picture of each patient's state.

### 2.3.2 Action Plan

The DQN chooses an action meant to improve patient outcomes considering the current situation. In the field of medicine, actions can be several and include: ordering diagnostic tests.

- Changing prescription dosages.
- Plan interventions or operations.
- Distribution of resources include nursing personnel or ICU beds.

The chosen action follows the learnt policy, which seeks to maximise projected future benefits.

In an emergency room triage system, the DQN might, depending on symptoms and vital signs, choose to fast-track a patient for surgery, admit to the hospital, or discharge.

### 2.3.3 Getting Advice

The DQN sees the patient's reaction and the clinical results following the selected action. Feedback is recorded as either a reward or a penalty.

- Positive changes in health bring rewards; negative or unfavourable events result in fines.
- The system cannot grasp the effect of its actions without this feedback loop.

For a diabetic patient, a DQN regulating insulin gets positive feedback if blood glucose levels stabilise and penalties if the patient has hypoglycemia.

### 2.3.4 Changing Q- Values

Based on the observed results, the system changes its internal Q-values, therefore enhancing its estimate of the efficiency of every activity in every state. This procedure sharpens the policy for next decisions.

For instance, a stroke detection DQN optimises its neural network weights depending on past successes and failures to increase recognition of ischaemic stroke patterns on MRI data.

### 2.3.5 Ongoing Education and Adjustment

The cycle repeated lets the DQN keep improving as it interacts with fresh patient data, adjusts to changing clinical guidelines, and handles new healthcare issues.

For instance, a DQN system changed treatment recommendations during the COVID-19 epidemic as knowledge of viral variations and successful treatments changed and learning to swiftly adapt to new clinical settings evolved.

## 2.4 Why DQNs Are Especially Fit for Healthcare

AI finds a particularly difficult environment in healthcare:

- Patient circumstances range greatly and change randomly.
- Data often is incomplete, noisy, and multi-modal.
- Decisions have to strike a mix between long-term results and current hazards.
- Ethical factors call for responsibility and openness.

DQNs solve these problems by means of adaptive learning that gradually improves decisions.

- Capacity to manage several sources of high-dimensional data.
- Optimisation of sequential decisions in which acts cause delayed consequences.
- Possibility to customise treatments by means of patient-specific patterns.

# 3. REAL-WORLD USES OF DEEP NETWORK SYSTEMS IN SMART HEALTHCARE

Deep Q-Networks (DQNs) are changing smart healthcare by letting artificial intelligence (AI) make decisions based on experience and adaptability. Traditional machine learning models depend on fixed, pre-collected datasets. DQNs, on the other hand, learn by interacting directly with their surroundings—they make choices, watch what happens, and adjust their strategy as needed. The idea behind this trial-and-error model comes from reinforcement learning. It helps DQNs do well in tough situations, like modern healthcare systems (Guan & Wang, 2024).

Because DQNs are flexible and can learn quickly, they are perfect for important tasks as healthcare moves towards more precise treatment and real-time improvement. These include early disease diagnosis, finding new medicines, hospital procedures, wearable health tracking, robotic-assisted surgery, and personalised therapy suggestions, such as managing the intensive care unit (ICU).

This section investigates in-depth these practical uses of DQNs, stressing how their predictive powers, higher accuracy, and adaptability change healthcare delivery.

## 3.1 Personalized Treatment Plan

### 3.1.1 Overview

Traditional medical methods often take a "one-size-fits-all" approach, but underlying medical problems, lifestyle choices, and genetic differences can all have a big impact on how patients respond to therapies. Customized therapy planning, or changing treatments based on how the patient acts, is the only way to get better results and fewer side effects.

### 3.1.2 Role of DQN

DQNs make personalised medicine possible by looking at different types of patient data, such as genetic information, imaging scans, electronic health records (EHRs), and long-term treatment results (Ma et al., 2023c). The DQN learns from this profile to suggest the best solutions; feedback systems help it keep making its suggestions better.

### 3.1.3 Example: AI in Oncology

Personalised medicine finds a convincing use in cancer treatment. Analysing tumour genetics, patient comorbidities, and past treatment responses, a DQN-based artificial intelligence system can suggest chemotherapy plans unique to the individual. It also affects the probability of adverse effects to prevent too harmful combinations.

### 3.1.4 Impact

Using DQNs, AI-assisted chemotherapy planning has shown in impact studies to lower treatment-related toxicity by 40% while raising patient survival. Through better drug choice, dose, and timing, the AI system improves clinical results and quality of life.

## 3.2 Optimization of ICU and ERGs

### 3.2.1 Overview

ERs and ICUs are high-stakes settings where quick choices are absolutely crucial. Key issues are controlling patient flow, forecasting degradation, and effective resource allocation.

### 3.2.2 Role of DQN

DQNs function as intelligent agents in ICU and ED environments, continually monitoring patient vitals (e.g., heart rate, oxygen saturation, respiration rate) together with contextual information like comorbidities and past interventions (Ma et al., 2023c). They advise preventative measures and project problems before they show up.

### 3.2.3 Example: Automated Ventilator Management

DQNs managing ventilator settings for patients with acute respiratory distress syndrome (ARD) is one effective deployment. Reducing the danger of ventilator-induced lung damage, the AI real-time monitors lung function and modulates oxygen flow, pressure, and volume.

### 3.2.4 Impact

ICU death rates have reportedly dropped up to 25% in hospitals implementing DQN-based ventilator control. AI-driven triage solutions in EDs can also effectively prioritise critical patients, lower crowding, and shorten wait times.

## 3.3 Medical Imaging and Diagnostics

### 3.3.1 Overview

Effective healthcare depends mostly on accurate and prompt diagnosis. Still, diagnostic mistakes are a major issue mostly caused by human tiredness or the excessive imaging data load.

### 3.3.2 Role of DQNs

Using convolutional neural network (CNN) architectures linked with reinforcement learning, DQNs process large-scale imaging datasets including X-rays, MRIs, and CT scans (Mall et al., 2023). By use of physician feedback, these algorithms learn to recognise tiny patterns linked with early-stage diseases, hence always improving.

### 3.3.3 Example: Radiology Decision Support

More consistently than conventional artificial intelligence, a DQN-based diagnostic tool applied in radiology can find brain tumours, lung nodules, and bone fractures (Xia et al., 2025). The DQN views a radiologist's disagreement with the AI's diagnosis as a feedback loop and adjusts its decision-making policy in line.

### 3.3.4 Impact

DQN-powered diagnostic tools, according to clinical studies, increase early diagnosis of diseases such lung cancer by up to 30%, therefore enabling doctors to intervene sooner and with more confidence.

## 3.4 Drug Discovery and Development

### 3.4.1 Overview

New drug development is famously sluggish, costly, and dangerous. Often with great failure rates, the conventional drug discovery process last over a decade and costs billions of dollars (Rehman et al., 2025).

### 3.4.2 Role of DQNs

DQNs help to speed drug discovery by negotiating large chemical and biological search areas. Simulating molecular interactions and leveraging previous data from both successful and failed medications helps them to find ideal routes across different environments (Fu & Chen, 2025).

### 3.4.3 Example: COVID-19 Therapeutics

Thousands of currently known compounds were screened for antiviral activity using DQN-based systems during the COVID-19 epidemic. These systems examined SARS-CoV-2 virus protein structures and projected which medications might prevent viral entry or replication.

### 3.4.4 Impact

This method, which was driven by AI, helped make vaccines and cut the time it took to find possible cures by a lot. In future pandemics, DQNs may be very helpful in figuring out the best ways to treat people before things get worse.

## 3.5 Hospital Resource Management

### 3.5.1 Overview

Tight resources define hospitals' operations. Maintaining patient safety and service quality depends critically on effective scheduling, bed allocation, and inventory control.

### 3.5.2 Role of DQNs'

DQNs change how hospitals work on the fly by guessing how many people will be admitted, how resources will be used, and how many staff members will be available (Wu et al., 2025). With outpatient care, elective surgeries, and emergency cases, they try to balance the needs of everyone.

### 3.5.3 Example: ER Triage and Staffing

A DQN-based triage system ranks arriving ED patients according to urgency and degree of severity. It simultaneously balances workloads to prevent burnout and maximises doctor and nurse schedules to guarantee coverage during peak hours.

### 3.5.4 Impact

Hospitals implementing such systems have noted lower ER wait times, more staff efficiency, and better patient satisfaction ratings.

## 3.6 Wearable Health Monitoring and Telemedicine

### 3.6.1 Overview

Wearable tech like glucose monitors, smartphones, and ECG patches have made it possible to keep an eye on patients when they're not in a hospital (Shajari et al., 2023). Still hard is getting real-time information from this data that can be used.

### 3.6.2 Role of DQNs'

DQNs look at the flowing data from wearables to find problems, predict health risks, and sound quick alarms. Their reinforcement learning core lets each person get their own health baselines, which makes the system more accurate over time.

### 3.6.3 Example: Diabetes Management Systems

A DQN-integrated insulin pump can learn from a patient's glucose readings, meal times, and how much they exercise and sleep. With this knowledge, the AI can change the insulin dose on its own and let the user or doctor know if help is needed.

### 3.6.4 Impact

These AI-powered solutions have been shown to cut emergency hospital visits for diabetes by 50%. This helps people better control their disease and lowers healthcare costs.

## 3.7 AI-Assisted Robotic Surgery

### 3.7.1 Overview

In difficult surgeries, robotic surgical devices improve control, dexterity, and accuracy. Including artificial intelligence into these systems brings intelligence and adaptation (Knudsen et al., 2024).

### 3.7.2 Role of DQNs'

Through constant evaluation of patient vitals and procedural data, DQNs regulate robotic motions during surgery. If unanticipated problems develop, the artificial intelligence changes surgical techniques in real time, therefore lessening reliance on preprogrammed guidelines.

### 3.7.3 Example: Adaptive Surgical Robots

DQNs track bleeding, tissue resistance, and patient stress signals in robotic-assisted orthopaedic or cardiac operations. Should the surgery stray from the intended course, the artificial intelligence adjusts the operation in real time to maintain effectiveness and safety.

### 3.7.4 Impact

Using DQN-augmented robotic systems, hospitals have seen a 40% drop in surgical problems and faster patient recovery periods, therefore rendering difficult operations safer and more accessible.

## 3.8 The Future of DQNs in Smart Healthcare

Deep Q-Networks have yet to be widely used in healthcare, but their promise is tremendous. DQNs will keep changing in their capacity to provide real-time, adaptive, patient-centered treatment as medical data gets more plentiful and linked (Fu & Chen, 2025a).

Future directions include:

- Self-learning hospitals, in which AI agents oversee all facets of operations—from patient care to logistics—whereby
- Global artificial intelligence-driven telemedicine, therefore increasing access to quality healthcare in underdeveloped areas away from each other.
- Wearable gadgets with autonomous health management systems with in-depth ability to predict and stop disease before it starts.
- Accelerated pharmaceutical research in which artificial intelligence independently creates, tests, and improves medicinal molecules on a mass production level.

Although technological issues including computing demand, data privacy, and explainability have to be solved, including DQNs into healthcare promises a paradigm change. These systems will enhance rather than replace medical experts, therefore allowing more exact, proactive, responsive treatment.

## 4. CHALLENGES IN IMPLEMENTING DEEP Q-NETWORKS (DQNS) IN HEALTHCARE

A reinforcement learning architecture, Deep Q-Networks (DQNs) have great potential to transform smart healthcare. Their capacity to dynamically learn from challenging, high-dimensional contexts sets them out as potent instruments for customising therapies, automating tests, streamlining hospital operations, and forward medical research. DQNs have transforming power, but their inclusion into practical healthcare environments presents difficult problems. These cover technical constraints, poor infrastructure, data privacy concerns, moral conundrums, and legal uncertainty. Every difficulty has to be methodically resolved to guarantee fair, safe, and efficient acceptance of this developed artificial intelligence technology.

### 4.1 Privacy and Security Issues

#### 4.1.1 The Challenge

One of the main problems with using DQNs in healthcare on a large scale is that they need to access huge amounts of patient data. The amount, type, and quality of data directly affect how well a DQN can be taught, which in turn affects how well decisions are made. Personal identities, medical histories, genetic information, and behavioural health records are all types of healthcare data that are naturally sensitive (Kathamuthu et al., 2022).

This brings up important issues:

- How patient data can be collected, kept, and used is controlled by laws like the Health Insurance Portability and Accountability Act (HIPAA) and the General Data Protection Regulation (GDPR). Other local privacy laws also apply.
- Patients' as well as healthcare providers' major concerns are cybersecurity issues including ransomware, phishing campaigns, and data breaches (Roy et al., 2024).
- Data abuse issues surface when companies or insurers access AI-driven insights—such as disease likelihood predictions—possibly resulting in discriminatory behaviour.

### 4.1.2 Real-world Example

In 2022, a cyberattack on a top hospital's AI-based imaging system let over 3 million patient data become public. Because of this, AI diagnosis services were temporarily shut down, and patients had to wait longer than expected to get important test results.

### 4.1.3 Potential Solutions

- Federated Learning lets DQNs learn from distributed patient data kept on local devices or hospital servers instead of sending sensitive data to central servers.
- Blockchain integration helps to provide tamper-proof, safe record-keeping, therefore facilitating open data sharing while preserving patient control.
- Advanced Access Controls & Encryption End-to--end encryption, role-based access controls, and frequent security audits help to reduce unwanted data access.

## 4.2 Lack of Explainability—the "Black Box" Problem

### 4.2.1 The Challenge

There is no way to understand the DQNs because they make decisions based on patterns they've learnt from reinforcement signals instead of rules that can be understood (Xu & Shuttleworth, 2024). This "black box" feature makes things less open and brings up big problems in hospital settings where trust and responsibility are very important (Marey et al., 2024).

Why if doctors don't know why AIs give advice, they might not want to accept it or follow it.

- Explainability becomes crucial for risk management in high-stakes settings such as intensive care or cancer.
- Patients might object to AI-based therapy if the justification for the choice is unknown or dubious.

### 4.2.2 Real World Example

An AI system taught with a DQN was able to find the best chemotherapy schedules for breast cancer patients. It once suggested a very aggressive treatment mix that doctors were surprised by. Clinicians didn't want to follow the advice because it wasn't clear what it meant, so the system's acceptance was put off.

### 4.2.3 Potential Solutions

- Artificial intelligence (XAI) that can be explained by using feature importance scores or attention maps to show which inputs the DQN thought were most important.
- Using DQNs with rule-based or decision-tree methods can make the results easier to understand and improve performance.
- Human-in-the-Loop (HITL) makes sure that doctors look over and agree with AI suggestions, which keeps responsibility.

## 4.3 High Computing Costs and Restraints on Infrastructure

### 4.3.1 The Challenge

Because deep neural networks and huge training data demand often high-end GPUs or even distributed computer clusters, the Challenge DQNs are computationally intense (Chan et al., 2023) (Su et al., 2024). Sadly, most hospitals and healthcare systems—especially in low-income environments—do not have the required infrastructure:

- Restricted access to cloud computing brought on by legal or bandwidth concerns.
- High expenses in obtaining and preserving local artificial intelligence gear.
- Challenges keeping real-time inference capacity for judgements requiring temporal sensitivity.

### 4.3.2 Real World Example

Insufficient GPU resources often caused an advanced DQN system intended to help with ICU ventilator adjustments at a regional hospital to lag at peak times, resulting in suboptimal decision support.

### 4.3.3 Potential Solutions

- Edge Computing: To cut latency and data transfer requirements, place light DQN models on local devices like wearables or bedside monitors.

- Use local processing combined with safe cloud backups to provide both performance and data security in hybrid artificial intelligence deployment models.
- Though still in early phases, quantum computing could potentially enable ultra-fast DQN training and decision-making.

## 4.4 Artificial Intelligence Decision-Making: Fairness and Bias

### 4.4.1 The Challenge

AI systems mirror the data they are fed. Should training datasets be lacking, uneven, or historically biased, the resulting DQN could support systematic inequalities in healthcare (Rajkomar et al., 2018). Typical causes of bias are:

- under-representation of minority groups in training data.
- Inaccurate labelling or antiquated therapy results distort reinforcement signals.
- Data imbalance wherein some demographic groups predominate among the training samples.

### 4.4.2 Real-world Example

A DQN model for dermatological diagnostics failed diagnosis in minority populations by greatly underperformance on darker skin tones while showing great accuracy on lighter skin tones (Obermeyer et al., 2019).

### 4.4.3 Potential Solutions

- Give inclusive data collecting across race, gender, age, and socioeconomic background top priority.
- Bias Audits: Review model performance often and independently among several patient groupings.
- Fairness-Aware Learning Algorithms: Use training approaches meant to discourage biased behaviour and advance just results.

## 4.5 Integration with Existing Healthcare Systems

### 4.5.1 The Challenge

Including DQNs into established medical procedures and legacy systems can be difficult (Topol, 2019):

- Many doctors depend on antiquated EHR systems not suitable for artificial intelligence.
- Easy data exchange is hampered by technical incompatibility and a dearth of APIs.
- Staff resistance results from unfamiliarity with artificial intelligence techniques or job displacement anxiety.

### 4.5.2 Real World Example

Staff resistance greeted a hospital's attempt to include a DQN-based artificial intelligence triage system. The new technology, according to nurses, upset established procedures and added complexity instead of relieving their workload.

### 4.5.3 Potential Solutions

- Phased Deployment: Assist users with low-risk jobs at first to build their confidence, then slowly add AI tools.
- Make tools that meet doctors' needs and include their feedback as the project is being built.
- Standardisation: HL7 FHIR (Fast Healthcare Interoperability Resources) and other formats that are suitable will make it easier to combine data (Jiang et al., 2017).

## 4.6 Ethical and Legal Implications

### 4.6.1 The Challenge

Pressing legal and ethical issues arise when DQNs make important medical decisions (Gerke et al., 2020):

- Who is responsible for an AI-related medical error—the developer, the institution, or the clinician?
- In life-and-death events, can artificial intelligence replace human judgement?

- Should patients agree especially for AI-guided treatments or be advised about them?

### 4.6.2 Real-World Example

A patient was sent home early after a DQN driven by artificial intelligence misclassified a cardiovascular ailment as low-risk. The condition got worse and legal action resulted. Under shared legal investigation were the hospital, AI vendor, and supervising physician.

### 4.6.3 Potential Solutions

- Clearly define responsibility lines separating consumers, hospitals, and developers.
- Create review boards to evaluate AI systems prior to implementation, ethical AI committees.
- Regulatory Frameworks: Governments have to pass thorough laws on artificial intelligence health guaranteeing openness, effectiveness, and safety (Mennella et al., 2024).

## 4.7 Real-Time Decision-Making and Unpredictability

### 4.7.1 The Challenge

DQNs shine at learning from past data, but real-time, erratic clinical scenarios offer a major constraint. In an emergency, where seconds count, the system must adjust without past knowledge of a like situation (Esteva et al., 2019).

- DQNs could “freeze,” or make bad decisions in unfamiliar circumstances.
- The latency in model updates suggests the artificial intelligence might be using obsolete learning.
- In important events, delayed response can be lethal.

### 4.7.2 Real World Example

A DQN trained on frequent trauma cases missed the symptoms of a rare but fatal allergic response in an emergency room, therefore postponing the delivery of epinephrine.

### 4.7.3 Potential Solutions

- Lifelong Learning Systems: AI that constantly learns from real-time data can over time adapt to new settings.
- Hybrid Systems: Combine edge case handling deterministic models with DQNs.
- Doctor-AI Cooperation: Make sure doctors are informed when the AI comes across unknown or doubtful circumstances.

## 4.8 The Future of DQN Implementation in Healthcare

Notwithstanding the difficulties, including DQNs into healthcare systems remains a quite exciting project. Dealing with present constraints calls for a multimodal strategy including technologists, doctors, legislators, and ethicists.

Future directions include:

- Differential privacy, federated learning, and homomorphic encryption adopted to protect patient data.
- Explainability by Design: Not as an afterthought, but rather from start, embed interpretability into DQN systems.
- Including artificial intelligence literacy into medical education can help medical practitioners to efficiently collaborate with intelligent technologies.
- Encouraging cross-sector alliances between hospitals, technology businesses, and academic institutions to test and scale DQN solutions would help to foster cooperative innovation.

Moreover, governments and regulatory agencies have to change concurrently to create rules guaranteeing patient safety and encouraging creativity. Public confidence will also be greatly influenced by open information regarding the use of artificial intelligence in care and strong ethical governance is therefore crucial.

# 5. THE FUTURE OF DEEP Q-NETWORKS IN AI-DRIVEN HEALTHCARE

By improving diagnostics, treatment personalising, hospital management, and medication discovery, Deep Q-Networks (DQNs) have started to change the scene of smart healthcare. Still, their full potential is hardly reached. More efficient, scalable, transparent models will characterize the next wave of healthcare innovation as artificial intelligence technologies develop. DQNs' future in healthcare is not just in small steps but also in a paradigm change whereby learning algorithms change in real-time, cooperate ethically with human specialists, and are easily available to healthcare systems all around.

This chapter investigates the transforming path of DQNs, stressing future developments, ongoing difficulties, and more general consequences for world healthcare.

## 5.1 Enhanced Model Efficiency and Scalability

### 5.1.1 Current Challenges

Widespread implementation of DQNs is greatly hampered by their great computing requirement. Training deep reinforcement learning models calls for advanced AI infrastructure, access to big-scale patient datasets, and substantial computing capability. Most healthcare facilities—especially in poor or rural areas—have difficulty fulfilling these criteria (Haripriya et al., 2025). Due to delays in training, network latency, and infrastructure incompatibility even in technologically advanced hospitals, DQNs for real-time decision assistance still presents challenges.

### 5.1.2 Emerging Solutions

Hardware innovation and algorithmic improvement will determine DQN scalability going forward. Several trends seem able to close the efficiency disparity:

- Quantum Computing for Reinforcement Learning: A route towards shockingly faster DQN training is provided by quantum processors, which can manage several computational states concurrently (Swayne, 2025). These systems will replicate difficult healthcare situations at hitherto unheard-of rates, allowing near-instant learning and real-time deployment in intensive care or emergency departments.
- Moving computation to local devices—such as wearable technology or hospital servers—edge artificial intelligence and federated learning lowers latency and enhances data privacy. Federated learning allows DQNs to train on distributed patient data across hospitals without revealing private information, hence increasing the scalability and privacy-consciousness of artificial intelligence.
- Next-generation artificial intelligence systems will lower memory use and computing costs by using approaches such model pruning, knowledge distillation, and sparse representations.

### 5.1.3 Long-Term Impact

Scalable DQNs will democratise AI-driven healthcare. Advanced diagnostic and decision-support systems will find their way to remote communities, field hospitals, and mobile health units in underdeveloped areas. In operating theatres, critical care, and emergency medicine, real-time decision-making will become reality and result in improved patient outcomes all around.

## 5.2 Explainable and Trustworthy AI in Medical Decision-Making

### 5.2.1 Current Barriers

The "black-box" character of DQNs raises one of the most urgent questions. Although these models can beat conventional systems in pattern recognition and decision-making, they hardly provide understanding of how judgements are taken (Noor et al., 2025). Where lives are on the line—in healthcare—trust, responsibility, and explainability are absolutely crucial.

DQN conclusions might not be recognised by doctors, patients, or legal institutions without clear logic or reasoning tracks. This opacity fosters mistrust and can prevent the acceptance of artificial intelligence even in cases of great performance.

### 5.2.2 Technological Advancements

Transparency will define the direction medical artificial intelligence takes. Several developments are under progress to provide DQNs more dependability and interpretability (Tanveer et al., 2022):

- Enhancements in explainable artificial intelligence (XAI) will show DQN decision-making routes. Saliency maps, idea attribution methods, and model distillation will let doctors identify which data points affected the suggestions of the AI.
- Integration of Decision-Support: Future DQNs will be smart assistants instead than replacements for doctors. DQNs will improve rather than replace human knowledge by offering second views, surface evidence, and alternate treatment approaches.
- Governments and healthcare accrediting authorities will mandate rules requiring AI systems to satisfy requirements for explainability, auditability, and safety. These rules will serve to foster public and professional confidence in DQNs.

### 5.2.3 Expected Outcomes

Clear DQN systems will help to increase patient comfort and doctor confidence. In oncology, for example, where treatment paths are convoluted and emotionally charged, AI-driven programs will have clear justifications. This will lower anxiety, improve treatment adherence, and help medical decisions to match patient values.

## 5.3 Personalized and Adaptive Healthcare AI Systems

### 5.3.1 Limitations Today

Conventional artificial intelligence algorithms can depend on fixed, historical data that misses the changing health profiles of individual individuals. This rigidity reduces the models' capacity to assist personalised medicine—a field aimed at customising treatment depending on a person's genetics, lifestyle, and current medical condition (Sagor et al., 2025).

### 5.3.2 The Next Frontier

Next generations of DQNs will be defined by adaptive learning and patient-centric intelligence(Rai et al., 2023):

- Self-Learning Models: Future DQNs will develop always. The model will dynamically adjust itself depending on real-time outcomes, lab findings, and physiological signals as patients receive treatment, therefore optimising treatment.
- Smartwatches, glucose monitors, and implanted biosensors will send health data to DQNs via wearable technology. These models will then independently fine-tune therapeutic schedules, detect abnormalities, or even alert emergency services.
- DQNs will create treatment programs customised to individual biology, not population-level averages by combining genomic data, lifestyle markers, and environmental variables.

### 5.3.3 Long-Term Benefits

Adaptive DQNs will rethink handling of chronic diseases. Diabetes patients, for instance, will get real-time medication changes depending on blood glucose patterns. Likewise, early therapies based on minor biomarker changes will help cardiac patients long before symptoms start. More exact, responsive, and preventative healthcare follows from this.

## 5.4 AI-Powered Drug Discovery and Clinical Trials

### 5.4.1 Current Inefficiencies

Often surpassing a decade and billions of dollars to create a single licensed medicine, the pharmaceutical sector deals with difficult budgets and deadlines (Fu & Chen, 2025b). Additionally sluggish are conventional clinical studies since participant recruitment, data collecting, and regulatory approvals cause significant delays.

### 5.4.2 AI-Driven Innovations

DQNs are especially suitable to simplify drug discovery and experimental design (Rehman et al., 2025):

- Reinforcement learning agents can replicate how thousands of therapeutic candidates interact with target proteins, therefore enabling molecular simulation and compound optimization. DQNs speed the identification of interesting molecules by learning ideal chemical arrangements.
- DQNs can replicate patient responses based on virtual avatars created from actual patient data. Before human testing, these models assist find perfect candidates, forecast side effects, and maximise trial design.
- Real-Time Monitoring: DQNs will constantly examine participant data in real-time to dynamically change protocols, identify side effects, and adjust dosages—so enhancing both safety and efficacy—during actual clinical trials.

### 5.4.3 Implications

These developments will lower the cost of development, allow quick reaction to public health emergencies (such as pandemics), and increase the feasibility of rare illness treatments. Faster access to life-saving medications will help patients; meanwhile, pharmaceutical businesses will face less R&D risk.

## 5.5 AI-Integrated Robotics for Autonomous Healthcare Services

### 5.5.1 Present-Day Constraints

Although automated rehabilitation tools and robotic surgery are available, most systems call for considerable human control. Robots find it difficult to respond to unanticipated surgical outcomes or offer context-specific care in dynamic settings like senior homes.

### 5.5.2 What's Coming

Future integration of DQNs with robotics will provide robots with adaptive, context-aware decision-making (Rogers, 2025):

- Because DQNs can re-calibrate in real time, robots will be able to handle shocks during surgery on their own, like tissue problems or bleeding problems.
- Rehabilitation Robotics: Machines will tailor therapy tasks to help people recover their motor skills after a stroke or injury based on real-time biometrics and their progress.
- Automated care for the elderly: smart companion robots with DQNs will keep an eye on vital signs, manage prescriptions, and provide mental support to older people, allowing them to live on their own longer.

### 5.5.3 Societal Impact

Robotics powered by AI will cut down on hospital readmissions, make caregiving easier, and make sure that patients get ongoing care. Robots with artificial intelligence that can move around and do easy surgeries or remote consultations in disaster or rural areas could make modern medicine more accessible (Soori et al., 2023).

## 5.6 Ethical and Regulatory Evolution in AI-Driven Healthcare

### 5.6.1 Persistent Dilemmas

DQN implementation in healthcare begs important issues (Mennella et al., 2024):

- When an artificial intelligence errors, who is responsible?
- Can artificial intelligence superseded advice from a doctor?
- How can we guarantee algorithms are not biased or discriminating?

### 5.6.2 Designed Frameworks

Ethics and regulation will change alongside technology advancement during the next ten years (Faheem et al., 2025):

- Harmonised AI healthcare regulations will develop, controlling transparency, liability, patient consent, and performance validation under international regulatory standards.
- Future artificial intelligence systems will incorporate built-in ethical reasoning layers, enabling them to identify morally difficult circumstances and defer to human judgement.
- DQNs will be trained on varied datasets using built-in fairness auditing tools that identify and remove algorithmic prejudice depending on race, gender, age, or socioeconomic level.

### 5.6.3 Broader Effects

These models will boost public trust in medicine driven by artificial intelligence. Not a goal, equitable treatment will become a reality; ethical failures will be methodically avoided. DQNs will be morally aligned allies rather than replacements for doctors.

## 5.7 The Road Ahead: A Fully AI-Integrated Healthcare System

Looking ahead, DQN development will signal a paradigm shift in healthcare delivery. Their inclusion into clinical practice, robotics, pharmaceutical R&D, and administrative management will profoundly change our perspective on medicine (Team, 2025).

Key Milestones

- 2025–2030: DQNs maximise treatments depending on real-time and genomic data, therefore artificial intelligence becomes a standard part of diagnostic and treatment planning.
- 2030–2040: Hospitals implement totally autonomous surgical and monitoring systems; artificial intelligence substantially shortens the time needed from disease detection to medication release.
- 2020 Onwards: Healthcare becomes a predictive, always changing, self-optimizing ecosystem. Treatments change dynamically, patients are watched in real-time, and human-AI cooperation is the standard.

## 6. CONCLUSION: THE TRANSFORMATIVE ROLE OF DEEP Q-NETWORKS IN AI-DRIVEN HEALTHCARE

A class of reinforcement learning models, deep Q-Networks (DQNs), has become a transforming agent in artificial intelligence-driven healthcare. They reflect a change in the concept and approach of patient care, not only a technical improvement. Learning effective decision-making strategies via trial and error helps DQNs provide dynamic adaptation to the always changing complexity of clinical settings. DQNs offer tools that can change every part of healthcare service in a field where speed, customization, and accuracy are very important.

This chapter looked at how DQNs are used now, how they work technically, where they might go in the future, and some of the problems that come with them in medical settings. After putting these talks together, it's clear that DQNs are not just supporting technologies; they are key parts of how future medicine will be designed.

### 6.1 Important Notes: Our Learnings

#### 6.1.1 DQNs Support AI-Driven Real-Time, Decision-Making in Healthcare

Unlike traditional rule-based AI models, DQNs learn and improve their behaviour by interacting with their surroundings all the time. This makes them very useful in settings with a lot of change and data, like healthcare, where patients' conditions can change quickly and decisions need to take that into account.

- DQNs allow chemotherapy dosage to be tailored depending on patient response.
- Track patient vitals and advise real-time interventions.
- Forecasting patient demands helps you to maximise hospital resources—including ICU bed allocation.
- Dynamically change programs depending on progress data to help in rehabilitation.

DQNs help us to approach proactive rather than reactive healthcare systems by combining learning, flexibility, and autonomy.

### 6.1.2 Real-World Applications Are Rapidly Expanding

DQNs are moving from theory to practice right from research labs to hospital hallways. Particularly in radiology and oncology, they are now under trial or use in systems for cancer diagnosis and treatment advice.

- Emergency room triage automation uses artificial intelligence to classify patients according to degree of severity.
- Hospital logistics—where DQNs simplify patient flow, supply chain management, and scheduling.

Furthermore, DQN-based systems are starting to be used by pharmaceutical firms to replicate molecular interactions and maximise compound screening in medication development. DQNs in wearable technology examine sensor data in real-time to direct patient behavior—such as diabetic insulin dose adjustments.

### 6.1.3 Issues Needed Resolved for Scalable Application

Though promising, the road to wide-scale DQN acceptance is paved with difficulties that need to be addressed if we are to guarantee efficacy, fairness, and safety.

a. Explainability

DQNs serve as black boxes, much as most deep learning models. Models must provide openness if healthcare professionals are to trust and implement these solutions. Making AI decisions interpretable and justified in healthcare settings depends on explainable artificial intelligence (XAI) methods include surrogate models or attention processes.

b. Legal and ethical constraints

Who is responsible when a decision made by artificial intelligence hurts a patient? This question shows how important it is to create strong legal and moral systems. Also, AI systems that are trained on biassed data could accidentally make healthcare disparities worse if they are not designed with fairness in mind.

c. Accessibility and infrastructure

A lot of medical sites, especially in poor rural areas, don't have the computers they need to train and use DQNs. Increasing access to these technologies for everyone will depend on things like edge AI, shared learning, and cloud infrastructure.

d. Security and privacy of data

A lot of patient data is needed for DQNs to learn effectively. It still takes a lot of careful balancing to keep this info safe and help a lot of people learn. Differential privacy and safe multiparty computation are two methods that need more work, even though they offer some interesting possibilities.

### 6.1.4 DQNs' Future Is Especially Very Bright

Looking forward, DQNs are supposed to transform various aspects of healthcare:

- Autonomous surgical robots directed by DQNs will dynamically adjust in real-time to problems, anatomical variance, and patient-specific nuances.
- Using behavioural and physiological data to suggest lifestyle changes or preventive therapies, artificial intelligence systems will predict health issues before they start.
- Future DQNs will not only learn once but also constantly adjust to each patient's changing health profile, therefore guaranteeing treatment that change with the individual.

DQNs will integrate into daily healthcare faster as they grow more transparent, ethically aligned, and data-efficient.

## 6.2 The DQN Future Roadmap for Healthcare

To make sure that DQNs are effectively integrated and spread in healthcare, a detailed and collaborative road map is necessary. This plan calls for a planned change, changes in regulations, and growth in technology.

### 6.2.1 Funding Scalable AI Implementation Infrastructure

Modern healthcare architecture has to change to meet the computing needs of DQN training and inference. Edge artificial intelligence technologies should be used by hospitals to support speedy, localised decision-making.

- Enable cooperative training using federated learning models without sacrificing data privacy.
- For high-intensity computation—especially in underfunded environments—use cloud computing.

Driving this change will depend on government financing, public-private alliances, and policy incentives with an eye towards artificial intelligence.

### 6.2.2 Improvement of Model Transparency and Interpretability

Adoption of artificial intelligence in healthcare will depend mostly on explainable artificial intelligence. Thus, DQNs have to be integrated with visualisation tools and explanation modules that enable users grasp artificial intelligence reasoning.

- Doctors have to participate in the design and assessment of DQN systems so that their observations show in model outputs.
- Not only prediction accuracy, but also evaluations of trust, usability, and intelligibility should be included of clinical trials of artificial intelligence systems.

Open artificial intelligence is not only a moral need but also a pragmatic one for user adoption.

### 6.2.3 Regulatory Reform and Ethical Leadership

The evolution of worldwide guidelines for medical artificial intelligence will determine the direction DQNs in healthcare take:

- Standardised paths for AI approval, auditing, and post-market surveillance must be established by regulatory bodies such the FDA, EMA, and WHO.
- Ethical frameworks must make sure DQNs are meant to enhance rather than replace human carers.
- Responsability Systems should be in place to allocate accountability for results driven by artificial intelligence and stop abuse.

Legal clarity, ethical foresight, and institutional control taken together will preserve the integrity of AI-powered healthcare systems.

### 6.2.4 Promoting Multidisciplinary Cooperation

Since healthcare is by nature interdisciplinary, DQN implementation must mirror this reality. Good teamwork should involve: data scientists creating and honing models.

- Medical professionals and clinicians will guarantee clinical validity and offer topic knowledge.
- Policymakers and ethicists to steer growth towards social responsibility.
- Consumers and the public will help to define expectations, provide comments, and guarantee that artificial intelligence meets actual human needs.

The foundation of sustainable innovation will be cooperative research projects, cross-sector consortia, co-designed artificial intelligence systems.

## 6.3 Final Thoughts: The AI-Powered Healthcare Revolution

We live on the brink of a medical revolution. Like the discovery of antibiotics or the development of medical imaging, the emergence of artificial intelligence—and especially Deep Q-Networks—will revolutionise what medicine means in the twenty-century. These systems will become really essential for healthcare, not only help it.

For Patients, Healthcare will becoming extremely personal. Every therapeutic route will be optimised in real-time for each patient's genetic profile, lifestyle, environment, and medical history, so no two individuals will get same treatment. DQNs will allow safer, more humane, more effective treatments.

### 6.3.1 Regarding Clinicians

Doctors will have brilliant, relentless helpers. These systems will offer second views, identify odd trends, handle administrative chores, and increase a physician's ability to precisely diagnose and treat. DQNs will strengthen the medical professionals rather than replace them.

Hospitals will grow to be sophisticated ecosystems for healthcare institutions. Automatically optimal patient flow will be achieved. Forecasts of disease epidemics made by predictive models Robotic systems will manage everyday maintenance. DQNs will enable universities to grow more responsive, financially sustainable, and efficient.

Globally, artificial intelligence will enable low-income and high-income areas close their healthcare disparity. Rural clinics can get the same decision-making help as elite hospitals thanks to scalable DQN-powered systems housed on mobile devices or edge servers. AI will enable world health equity to reach a realistic target rather than only a dream.

Finally, a future defined by cooperation between artificial and human intelligence.

Deep Q-Networks into healthcare symbolises a new era of cooperation rather than the displacement of doctors by machines. One in which patients gain from the synergy; doctors learn from machines, and machines learn from data. DQNs promise not in the algorithms themselves but in our careful, forward-looking, human application of them.

DQNs are not a far-off dream; as this chapter has demonstrated, they are presently here saving lives and enhancing treatment. Still, their greatest potential is only ahead. Overcoming technical, ethical, and social obstacles will help us to create a future in which healthcare is intelligent, fair, and sensitive to all.

The revolution is starting here. The instruments are on hand. The issue now is not whether DQNs will revolutionise healthcare but rather how swiftly, fairly, and sensibly we will let them to do so.

## REFERENCES


AbdelAziz, N. M., Fouad, G. A., Al-Saeed, S., & Fawzy, A. M. (2025). Deep Q-Network (DQN) Model for Disease Prediction Using Electronic Health Records (EHRs). *Sci*, *7*(1), 1. Advance online publication. DOI: 10.3390/sci7010014

Chan, K. Y., Abu-Salih, B., Qaddoura, R., Al-Zoubi, A. M., Palade, V., Pham, D.-S., Ser, J. D., & Muhammad, K. (2023). Deep neural networks in the cloud: Review, applications, challenges and research directions. *Neurocomputing*, *545*, 126327. DOI: 10.1016/j.neucom.2023.126327

Esteva, A., Robicquet, A., Ramsundar, B., Kuleshov, V., DePristo, M., Chou, K., Cui, C., Corrado, G., Thrun, S., & Dean, J. (2019). A guide to deep learning in healthcare. *Nature Medicine*, *25*(1), 24–29. DOI: 10.1038/s41591-018-0316-z

Faheem, F., Haq, M., Derhab, M., Saeed, R., Ahmad, U., & Kalia, J. S. (2025). Integrating Ethical Principles Into the Regulation of AI-Driven Medical Software. *Cureus*, *17*(2), e79506. DOI: 10.7759/cureus.79506

Fu, C., & Chen, Q. (2025a). The future of pharmaceuticals: Artificial intelligence in drug discovery and development. *Journal of Pharmaceutical Analysis*, *101248*. Advance online publication. DOI: 10.1016/j.jpha.2025.101248

Fu, C., & Chen, Q. (2025b). The future of pharmaceuticals: Artificial intelligence in drug discovery and development. *Journal of Pharmaceutical Analysis*, *101248*. Advance online publication. DOI: 10.1016/j.jpha.2025.101248

Gerke, S., Minssen, T., & Cohen, G. (2020). Ethical and legal challenges of artificial intelligence-driven healthcare. *Artificial Intelligence in Health*, *295*. Advance online publication. DOI: 10.1016/B978-0-12-818438-7.00012-5

Guan, S., & Wang, G. (2024). Drug discovery and development in the era of artificial intelligence: From machine learning to large language models. *Artificial Intelligence Chemistry.*, *2*(1), 100070. DOI: 10.1016/j.aichem.2024.100070

Haripriya, R., Khare, N., & Pandey, M. (2025). Privacy-preserving federated learning for collaborative medical data mining in multi-institutional settings. *Scientific Reports*, *15*(1), 12482. DOI: 10.1038/s41598-025-97565-4

Jayaraman, P., Desman, J., Sabounchi, M., Nadkarni, G. N., & Sakhuja, A. (2024a). A Primer on Reinforcement Learning in Medicine for Clinicians. *NPJ Digital Medicine*, *7*(1), 1–10. DOI: 10.1038/s41746-024-01316-0

Jayaraman, P., Desman, J., Sabounchi, M., Nadkarni, G. N., & Sakhuja, A. (2024b). A Primer on Reinforcement Learning in Medicine for Clinicians. *NPJ Digital Medicine*, *7*(1), 1–10. DOI: 10.1038/s41746-024-01316-0

Jiang, F., Jiang, Y., Zhi, H., Dong, Y., Li, H., Ma, S., Wang, Y., Dong, Q., Shen, H., & Wang, Y. (2017). Artificial intelligence in healthcare: Past, present and future. *Stroke and Vascular Neurology*, *2*(4). Advance online publication. DOI: 10.1136/svn-2017-000101

Kathamuthu, N. D., Chinnamuthu, A., Iruthayanathan, N., Ramachandran, M., & Gandomi, A. H. (2022). Deep Q-Learning-Based Neural Network with Privacy Preservation Method for Secure Data Transmission in Internet of Things (IoT) Healthcare Application. *Electronics (Basel)*, *11*(1), 1. Advance online publication. DOI: 10.3390/electronics11010157

Knudsen, J. E., Ghaffar, U., Ma, R., & Hung, A. J. (2024). Clinical applications of artificial intelligence in robotic surgery. *Journal of Robotic Surgery*, *18*(1), 102. DOI: 10.1007/s11701-024-01867-0

Lopez-Martinez, D., Eschenfeldt, P., Ostvar, S., Ingram, M., Hur, C., & Picard, R. (2019). *Deep Reinforcement Learning for Optimal Critical Care Pain Management with Morphine using Dueling Double-Deep Q Networks* (No. arXiv:1904.11115). arXiv. https://doi.org//arXiv.1904.11115DOI: 10.48550

Ma, S., Lee, J., Serban, N., & Yang, S. (2023a). *Deep Attention Q-Network for Personalized Treatment Recommendation* (No. arXiv:2307.01519). arXiv. https://doi.org//arXiv.2307.01519DOI: 10.48550

Ma, S., Lee, J., Serban, N., & Yang, S. (2023b). *Deep Attention Q-Network for Personalized Treatment Recommendation* (No. arXiv:2307.01519). arXiv. https://doi.org//arXiv.2307.01519DOI: 10.48550

Ma, S., Lee, J., Serban, N., & Yang, S. (2023c). *Deep Attention Q-Network for Personalized Treatment Recommendation* (No. arXiv:2307.01519). arXiv. https://doi.org//arXiv.2307.01519DOI: 10.48550

Mall, P. K., Singh, P. K., Srivastav, S., Narayan, V., Paprzycki, M., Jaworska, T., & Ganzha, M. (2023). A comprehensive review of deep neural networks for medical image processing: Recent developments and future opportunities. *Healthcare Analytics*, *4*, 100216. DOI: 10.1016/j.health.2023.100216

Marey, A., Arjmand, P., Alerab, A. D. S., Eslami, M. J., Saad, A. M., Sanchez, N., & Umair, M. (2024). Explainability, transparency and black box challenges of AI in radiology: Impact on patient care in cardiovascular radiology. *The Egyptian Journal of Radiology and Nuclear Medicine*, *55*(1), 183. DOI: 10.1186/s43055-024-01356-2

Mennella, C., Maniscalco, U., De Pietro, G., & Esposito, M. (2024). Ethical and regulatory challenges of AI technologies in healthcare: A narrative review. *Heliyon*, *10*(4), e26297. DOI: 10.1016/j.heliyon.2024.e26297

Nambiar, M., Ghosh, S., Ong, P., Chan, Y. E., Bee, Y. M., & Krishnaswamy, P. (2023). *Deep Offline Reinforcement Learning for Real-world Treatment Optimization Applications* (No. arXiv:2302.07549). arXiv. https://doi.org//arXiv.2302.07549DOI: 10.48550

Nguyen, D. S. W., & Odigie, R. (2023). Toward Artificial General Intelligence: Deep Reinforcement Learning Method to AI in Medicine. *Journal of Computer and Communications*, *11*(9), 9. Advance online publication. DOI: 10.4236/jcc.2023.119006

Noor, A. A., Manzoor, A., Mazhar Qureshi, M. D., Qureshi, M. A., & Rashwan, W. (2025). Unveiling Explainable AI in Healthcare: Current Trends, Challenges, and Future Directions. *Wiley Interdisciplinary Reviews. Data Mining and Knowledge Discovery*, *15*(2), e70018. DOI: 10.1002/widm.70018

Obermeyer, Z., Powers, B., Vogeli, C., & Mullainathan, S. (2019). Dissecting racial bias in an algorithm used to manage the health of populations. *Science*, *366*(6464), 447–453. DOI: 10.1126/science.aax2342

Rai, A. K., Sharma, M., Saravanan, V., Shalini, N., Kumar, M., & Singh, P. (2023). *Personalized Healthcare Recommendations with Q-Learning Reinforcement Learning*. 1–6. https://doi.org/DOI: 10.1109/ICAIIHI57871.2023.10489223

Rajkomar, A., Hardt, M., Howell, M. D., Corrado, G., & Chin, M. H. (2018). Ensuring Fairness in Machine Learning to Advance Health Equity. *Annals of Internal Medicine*, *169*(12), 866–872. DOI: 10.7326/M18-1990

Rehman, A. U., Li, M., Wu, B., Ali, Y., Rasheed, S., Shaheen, S., Liu, X., Luo, R., & Zhang, J. (2025). Role of artificial intelligence in revolutionizing drug discovery. *Fundamental Research (Beijing)*, *5*(3), 1273–1287. DOI: 10.1016/j.fmre.2024.04.021

Rogers, T. N. (2025, May 27). Robots take on some of the 'busy work' at US hospitals. *Financial Times*. https://www.ft.com/content/aabb7d4b-1e2d-47b9-97f4-c3fc96448aa7

Roy, P. P., Teju, V., Kandula, S. R., Sowmya, K. V., Stan, A. I., & Stan, O. P. (2024). Secure Healthcare Model Using Multi-Step Deep Q Learning Network in Internet of Things. *Electronics (Basel)*, *13*(3), 3. Advance online publication. DOI: 10.3390/electronics13030669

Sagor, D. H., Chowdhory, U. G., Dey, A., & Sagor, D. H. (2025). *AI and Machine Learning in Healthcare: Advancing Diagnostics, Personalized Treatment, and Predictive Modeling* (No. 2025040007). *Preprints*. https://doi.org/DOI: 10.20944/preprints202504.0007.v1

Shajari, S., Kuruvinashetti, K., Komeili, A., & Sundararaj, U. (2023). The Emergence of AI-Based Wearable Sensors for Digital Health Technology: A Review. *Sensors (Basel)*, *23*(23), 9498. DOI: 10.3390/s23239498

Soori, M., Arezoo, B., & Dastres, R. (2023). Artificial intelligence, machine learning and deep learning in advanced robotics, a review. *Cognitive Robotics*, *3*, 54–70. DOI: 10.1016/j.cogr.2023.04.001

Stember, J., & Shalu, H. (2020). *Deep reinforcement learning to detect brain lesions on MRI: A proof-of-concept application of reinforcement learning to medical images* (No. arXiv:2008.02708). arXiv. https://doi.org//arXiv.2008.02708DOI: 10.48550

Su, X., Fang, X., Cheng, Z., Gong, Z., & Choi, C. (2024). Deep reinforcement learning based latency-energy minimization in smart healthcare network. *Digital Communications and Networks*. Advance online publication. DOI: 10.1016/j.dcan.2024.06.008

Swayne, M. (2025, March 26). National Quantum Computing Centre's Paper Explores Quantum Computing's Transformative Potential in Healthcare And Pharmaceuticals. *The Quantum Insider*. https://thequantuminsider.com/2025/03/26/national-quantum-computing-centres-paper-explores-quantum-computings-transformative-potential-in-healthcare-and-pharmaceuticals/

Talaat, F. M. (2022). Effective deep Q-networks (EDQN) strategy for resource allocation based on optimized reinforcement learning algorithm. *Multimedia Tools and Applications*, *81*(28), 39945–39961. DOI: 10.1007/s11042-022-13000-0

Tanveer, H., Faheem, M., & Khan, A. H. (2022). Explainable AI in Medical Decision-Making: Challenges and Opportunities. *Iconic Research and Engineering Journals*, *5*(12), 423–435.

Team, D. R. L. (2025, January 14). *The State of Reinforcement Learning in 2025*. DataRoot Labs. https://datarootlabs.com/blog/state-of-reinforcement-learning-2025

Topol, E. J. (2019). High-performance medicine: The convergence of human and artificial intelligence. *Nature Medicine*, *25*(1), 44–56. DOI: 10.1038/s41591-018-0300-7

Wu, Q., Han, J., Yan, Y., Kuo, Y.-H., & Shen, Z.-J. M. (2025). Reinforcement learning for healthcare operations management: Methodological framework, recent developments, and future research directions. *Health Care Management Science*. Advance online publication. DOI: 10.1007/s10729-025-09699-6

Xia, Q., Zheng, H., Zou, H., Luo, D., Tang, H., Li, L., & Jiang, B. (2025). A comprehensive review of deep learning for medical image segmentation. *Neurocomputing*, *613*, 128740. DOI: 10.1016/j.neucom.2024.128740

Xu, H., & Shuttleworth, K. M. J. (2024). Medical artificial intelligence and the black box problem: A view based on the ethical principle of "do no harm.". *Intelligent Medicine*, *4*(1), 52–57. DOI: 10.1016/j.imed.2023.08.001

Yu, C., Liu, J., Nemati, S., & Yin, G. (2021). Reinforcement Learning in Healthcare: A Survey. *ACM Comput. Surv.*, *55*(1), 5:1-5:36. https://doi.org/DOI: 10.1145/3477600

Chapter 14
# Drug Discovery and Optimization With AI

**Dipesh Uike**
https://orcid.org/0000-0001-5322-7813
*Dr. Ambedkar Institute of Management, Studies, and Research, India*

**Neha Dhule**
https://orcid.org/0009-0001-4410-4085
*Datta Meghe Institute of Management Studies, India*

**S. Sugapriya**
*Velammal Engineering College, India*

**P. Selvakumar**
https://orcid.org/0000-0002-3650-4548
*Department of Science and Humanities, Nehru Institute of Technology, Coimbatore, India*

**Manpreet Kaur**
https://orcid.org/0009-0005-6038-723X
*Chandigarh Group of Colleges, Jhanjeri, India*

**Manjunath T. C.**
https://orcid.org/0000-0003-2545-9160
*Rajarajeswari College of Engineering, India*

**Amruta Mahalle**
https://orcid.org/0009-0001-4246-4060
*Datta Meghe Institution of Management Studies, India*

## ABSTRACT

*Across many scientific disciplines, and application is in modern development long, costly over a can cost billions of dollars. predictive analytics, are now playing pivotal roles in revolutionizing this process by making. The drug discovery process typically includes generating hypotheses about drug interactions. Using vast datasets derived from genomics, proteomics, chemical libraries, and biomedical literature, AI algorithms can process and analyze complex biological information in a fraction of the time it would take using conventional methods. response to emerging diseases, where speed is critical—as demonstrated during the COVID-19 pandemic.omics data to reveal previously unknown associations between biological markers and diseases.*

DOI: 10.4018/979-8-3373-3311-3.ch014

*interpret thousands of scientific articles, extracting valuable insights about genes, proteins, and potential disease mechanisms. By integrating this information with experimental data, error experimentation. predictive ability helps researchers filter out unsuitable compounds early, reducing the risk of late-stage failures.*

## THE ROLE OF AI IN MODERN DRUG DISCOVERY

Across many scientific disciplines, and application is in modern development long, costly over a can cost billions of dollars. predictive analytics, are now playing pivotal roles in revolutionizing this process by making. The drug discovery process typically includes generating hypotheses about drug interactions. Using vast datasets derived from genomics, proteomics, chemical libraries, and biomedical literature, AI algorithms can process and analyze complex biological information in a fraction of the time it would take using conventional methods. response to emerging diseases, where speed is critical—as demonstrated during the COVID-19 pandemic.omics data to reveal previously unknown associations between biological markers and diseases. interpret thousands of scientific articles, extracting valuable insights about genes, proteins, and potential disease mechanisms. By integrating this information with experimental data, error experimentation. predictive ability helps researchers filter out unsuitable compounds early, reducing the risk of late-stage failures.AI can also aid in structure-based drug design proteins (as demonstrated by DeepMind's AlphaFold) and simulate how candidate molecules bind to these structures. This leads to more precise drug design and optimization, especially for targets that were previously considered "undruggable."Virtual screening is another critical area where AI shows exceptional promise. Instead of physically testing millions of compounds in the lab—a process that is time-consuming and expensive—AI-powered virtual screening allows researchers to computationally evaluate vast libraries of molecules against a biological target.Machine learning models trained on binding affinity data can score and rank compounds based on their likelihood of success (Abbas et al., 2022). Some AI systems can even suggest modifications to improve binding efficacy or selectivity, enhancing hit-to-lead development.because repurposed drugs have already passed safety trials, allowing them to move faster into clinical development. In the realm of makeup, lifestyle, and health records. By identifying biomarkers and ensures that the right s.By integrating data from prior trials, patient registries, and real-world evidence, AI can forecast potential risks and suggest design modifications to enhance trial efficacy. Furthermore, AI-powered tools can monitor ongoing trials, identifying early signs of efficacy or adverse reactions, thus facilitating adaptive trial designs and timely decision-making.Pharmaceutical giants and biotech startups alike are increasingly investing in common, with examples such as the partnership between GSK and Exscientia or Sanofi's collaboration with Atomwise.(Agamah et al., 2020) These alliances leverage from molecule generation to clinical decision support.AI is also being used by regulatory agencies to evaluate submissions more efficiently.

## CHALLENGES IN TRADITIONAL DRUG DISCOVERY

However, it is also widely recognized as one of the most complex, time-consuming, and expensive scientific endeavors. Despite decades of innovation, the traditional approach to discovering and developing new drugs continues to face numerous challenges that hinder efficiency and success. These challenges span scientific, logistical, financial, and regulatory domains, making drug discovery a high-risk venture with uncertain outcomes. the rigorous preclinical and clinical testing required. This figure includes costs for research and development (R&D), regulatory compliance. A significant portion of these costs arises from the trial-and-error nature of the traditional discovery process. Many compounds fail at various stages—especially during clinical trials—causing companies to absorb losses after substantial investment. Moreover, as scientific understanding of diseases grows more complex, the resources needed to develop targeted therapies, biologics, and personalized treatments continue to escalate.(Bajwa et al., 2021)Pharmaceutical companies often pass these costs onto healthcare systems and consumers, contributing to rising drug prices globally. This has sparked public and political debate, emphasizing the need for more affordable and efficient drug discovery models.Each stage requires rigorous validation, often involving years of laboratory work, animal studies, and human testing. Delays are common, whether due to unexpected toxicity in animal models, inadequate efficacy in clinical trials, or regulatory hurdles. The lengthy timelines not only delay access to potentially life-saving therapies but also increase the financial risk for pharmaceutical developers The traditional pipeline suffers from a notoriously high failure rate. For every 10,000 compounds initially screened in the laboratory, only one typically reaches the market. The attrition rate is particularly steep in the later stages—especially during clinical trials, where over 90% of candidates fail. Reasons for failure are varied and include poor pharmacokinetics, unexpected toxicity, lack of efficacy, and adverse side effects. Sometimes, promising drugs that succeed in animal models fail in humans due to differences in physiology. These setbacks are costly and can demoralize research teams, while also delaying potential treatments for patients in need.Traditional drug discovery relies heavily on in vitro experiments and animal models to assess safety and efficacy before human trials. However, these models often fall short in accurately predicting human outcomes. For instance, many drugs that show promise in rodents or primates fail in human trials due to differences in metabolism, immune responses, or disease pathology. (Capecchi et al., 2020)This lack of translatability contributes significantly to high failure rates in later stages. Moreover, ethical concerns around animal testing have led to increased demand for alternative models, further complicating the development pipeline(Ball & Dal Pan, 2022). The scientific community is increasingly calling for more predictive, human-relevant systems such as organ-on-chip platforms and computational modeling, though these are still in early stages of validation. far more complex than previously thought. This complexity poses significant challenges for target identification and validation. signaling pathways, genetic heterogeneity, and environmental interactions involved in disease mechanisms. Identifying the right target, understanding its role in the disease, and developing a molecule that can modulate it effectively is a daunting task. In many cases, a lack of reliable biomarkers further complicates efforts to track disease progression or therapeutic response. Even with advances in genomics and proteomics, identifying a target that is both druggable and clinically relevant remains challenging. Many putative targets lack adequate validation, and investments in developing drugs against poorly understood targets can result in costly failures.

Additionally, target-based drug discovery often leads to a reductionist approach that may overlook the broader network of biological interactions. A drug might successfully modulate a target but still fail in clinical trials due to unintended effects on other pathways or compensatory biological mechanisms.While necessary to protect public health, these regulations often result in long review timelines, extensive documentation, and repeated rounds of evaluation.Meeting compliance standards requires a dedicated regulatory affairs team and significant investment in clinical trial management, pharmacovigilance, and post-marketing studies. These requirements can slow down development and increase operational complexity, particularly for smaller biotech companies and academic institutions with limited resources. is frequently siloed, with limited sharing or integration. This fragmentation limits the potential for collaborative insight and can lead to redundancy in research efforts. Moreover, a lack of standardized data formats, inconsistent reporting, and varying quality of research make it difficult to build comprehensive datasets that could be used to inform future studies. The absence of interoperability between databases and platforms further hinders the ability to perform large-scale meta-analyses or apply data-driven approaches to discovery.

## HOW AI IS REVOLUTIONIZING DRUG DISCOVERY

R&D costs, long development timelines, and high attrition rates, AI is offering new ways to innovate and accelerate every stage of the drug discovery pipeline. By harnessing powerful algorithms—particularly those rooted predict outcomes, and personalize treatments. The result is a paradigm shift in how medicines are developed and deliveredsuch as a protein or gene associated with a disease. (Cardozo et al., 2022)Traditionally, this has involved years of experimental research, genetic studies, and painstaking biological validation. AI, particularly ML algorithms, is dramatically expediting this process.data, to uncover hidden patterns and associations between biological markers and diseases. Natural Language Processing (NLP) tools can mine scientific literature, clinical reports, and databases to identify candidate targets that may not have been previously considered. This allows researchers to generate more hypotheses in less time, prioritize the most promising targets, and reduce early-stage failures. and clinical trial data—AI systems can also validate targets with real-world evidence. This cross-verification improves the likelihood of downstream success and ensures that selected targets are both druggable and clinically relevant.Designing a novel drug molecule that can effectively interact with a biological target is an intricate process. and reinforcement learning (RL). kinase inhibitors and then propose entirely new molecules with similar or improved binding affinity, solubility, or stability.AI also enables in silico optimization—where virtual compounds are rapidly modified and tested computationally to improve their drug-like characteristics. This not only reduces reliance on costly laboratory synthesis and screening but also shortens the lead optimization phase. In this way, AI turns the creative task of drug design into a precise, predictive, and scalable process.Machine learning models, particularly support vector machines, random forests, and deep neural networks, can be trained to predict the binding affinity of compounds to specific targets.(Dara et al., 2022) These models can rapidly score and rank millions of compounds in silico synthesis and experimental testing.

Additionally, AI can incorporate 3D structural information of proteins and ligands—such as those generated by AlphaFold—to perform structure-based drug screening. This combination of accurate protein folding predictions and ML-based docking simulations leads to more effective and selective hit identification, significantly increasing the efficiency of early drug discovery.Deep learning models trained on historical ADMET data can assess how a molecule will behave in the body, flagging potential issues such as liver toxicity, poor solubility, or blood-brain barrier penetration. Some AI systems can even simulate metabolic pathways and predict which enzymes will interact with a compound, offering insights that would typically require weeks of lab work.By screening out unsuitable compounds earlier, AI helps developers focus resources on the most viable drug candidates, saving both time and money while increasing the likelihood of clinical success.g interaction networks—AI can identify new therapeutic uses for approved or shelved drugs.Machine learning algorithms can detect similarities in molecular structure, gene expression, or clinical response between different diseases and suggest how an existing drug might be effective in a new context. This approach significantly reduces development timelines and costs because repurposed drugs have already undergone safety testing. AI can suggest combinations that enhance efficacy, reduce resistance, or mitigate side effects—insights that are nearly impossible to achieve manually.This level of personalization improves patient outcomes and reduces the trial-and-error approach to prescribing drugs. AI-driven platforms are now being used to identify biomarkers that predict therapeutic response, monitor disease progression, and even adapt treatment protocols in real-time.based on the specific mutations present. Similarly, in neurology, AI can help differentiate between similar diseases (e.g., types of dementia) and suggest optimal treatment strategies. helping to optimize trial design, recruitment, and management. By analyzing EHRs, population health data, and prior trial results, AI can identify ideal patient populations, predict enrollment challenges, and recommend sites with higher recruitment potential.Machine learning models can simulate trial outcomes based on different protocols, helping sponsors select the most effective and efficient designs. AI also supports real-time monitoring of ongoing trials, detecting early signs of efficacy, adverse effects, or protocol deviations.Furthermore, AI enables adaptive trial designs—where the parameters of the trial can be modified based on interim results—thereby improving speed and flexibility without compromising scientific integritytware allow users to perform complex tasks—such as molecular docking.

## TARGET IDENTIFICATION WITH AI: UNLOCKING THE MOLECULAR KEYS TO DISEASE

Traditionally, this process has relied on laborious experimental approaches, such as gene knockouts, protein assays, and phenotype screening(Dash et al., 2019). However, these methods are time-consuming, limited in scale, and prone to human bias and error combination with bioinformatics and genomics, target identification has been transformed into a highly efficient, data-driven discipline capable of revealing novel insights at unprecedented speed and scale.Historically, target identification was driven by hypothesis-based research, often focusing on well-known biological pathways or previously studied proteins. While effective in some cases, this approach is inherently limited by existing knowledge and may overlook novel or less-understood targets. AI disrupts this model by enabling hypothesis-free, data-centric exploration. By processing vast amounts of biological, of big data, where biomedical information is generated at a rate that far exceeds human capacity for analysis., transcriptomics, proteomics, metabolomics, and epigenomics. This integration allows researchers to form a holistic view of disease mechanisms and identify key regulatory nodes that may serve as potential drug targets.Genomics provides a blueprint of the DNA sequence, revealing mutations and genetic variants associated with diseases. Transcriptomics captures gene expression changes, showing which genes are up- or down-regulated in disease states. Proteomics and metabolomics further refine this picture by revealing how proteins and metabolites interact within cells. identify correlations, causal relationships, and critical points of intervention.Bioinformatics has long served as the computational backbone of genomics and molecular biology. It provides the tools to align sequences, identify variants, and interpret gene function.(Fisher & Rosella, 2022) However, traditional bioinformatics approaches often require predefined hypotheses and cannot scale efficiently to massive datasets. AI, when integrated with bioinformatics, augments this process by automating data interpretation and uncovering hidden patterns. gene-disease associations. Meanwhile, unsupervised learning methods can cluster gene expression profiles from patient samples to detect novel subtypes of diseases and reveal targetable molecular signatures.In genome-wide CRISPR or RNAi screens, AI can analyze the phenotypic consequences of gene knockouts across various cell types or disease models. By correlating genetic perturbations with cellular outcomes, AI helps identify genes essential for survival or proliferation in disease-specific contexts—especially in cancer, where synthetic lethality is a key therapeutic strategy. Deep learning models can further process scRNA-seq data to identify cell-specific gene expression patterns and regulatory networks, providing insights into tissue-specific targets and the heterogeneity of disease mechanisms. Not all potential targets are equally viable for drug development. Factors such as druggability, safety, tissue specificity, and biological redundancy must be considered. AI can assist in prioritizing targets by evaluating these criteria simultaneously.For instance, models can predict the "druggability" of a protein by analyzing its structural features, cellular location, and existing small molecule binding data. Other algorithms assess off-target effects and potential toxicity by simulating the downstream impact of modulating a given target. (Fogel, 2018)This prioritization process allows researchers to focus resources on targets with the highest therapeutic potential and the lowest risk of adverse effects.I also plays a role in experimental validation by designing optimal in vitro and in vivo studies, identifying relevant disease models, and even controlling automated laboratory equipment in high-throughput assays. Some platforms combine AI with robotics to carry out autonomous experimentation cycles, rapidly confirming AI-generated hypotheses. Platforms such as BenevolentAI, Recursion, Insitro, and Deep Genomics have built entire discovery engines based on AI-driven genomics and bioinformatics. These platforms ingest proprietary and public data to identify novel targets in oncology, neurology, rare diseases, and beyond.BenevolentAI, for example, uses NLP and knowledge graph-based AI models to mine AI to understand how genetic mutations disrupt RNA splicing and protein translation, identifying targets for genetic diseases with no current treatments.Academic institutions are also integrating AI tools into their drug discovery programs, often through partnerships with tech companies or the use of open-source platforms. These collaborations accelerate theof basic research into clinical candidates by enabling data-rich exploration of disease biology.

## COMPOUND SCREENING WITH AI: REVOLUTIONIZING DRUG DISCOVERY

Traditionally, this has been accomplished through compound screening methods, such as high-throughput screening (HTS), where libraries of thousands to millions of compounds are tested for their ability to bind to a target of interest. However, while HTS has proven to be effective, it is also resource-intensive, costly, and time-consuming. With the explosion of biological data and advancements in artificial intelligence (AI), compound screening has entered a new era. AI is rapidly transforming the screening process, enabling more efficient, faster, and cost-effective identification of drug candidates. of AI models that can predict compound behavior, reducing the reliance on experimental screening methods.Compound screening has traditionally been divided into two main categories: high-throughput screening (HTS) and virtual screening. HTS involves and requires sophisticated robotics to automate the screening process.(Fogel, 2018) While HTS is powerful, it is resource-heavy, requiring significant infrastructure, time, and human effort, as well as the synthesis of compounds that might not be relevant to the disease. of the computational models and the structural information available for the target. those trained on large datasets of molecular structures, biological activity, and known compound-target interactions. AI models can be used in tw ways: (1) predicting the activity of a compound against a target and (2) optimizing compound properties for better efficacy, bioavailability, and safety. Machine learning algorithms,patterns in compound efficacy and predict how new, untested compounds will behave.reduces the need for costly physical screening.can provide a more comprehensive understanding of how compounds interact with biological targets across different disease states and patient populations. Incorporating genomic and transcriptomic data allows AI models to better predict how compounds will interact with targets that are expressed differently in various tissues or under different disease conditions. For instance, in cancer research, gene expression profiles can inform more personalized screening of particular patient populations. test vast numbers of compounds, HTS has several limitations, including high costs, time consumption.

AI is playing an increasingly prominent role in optimizing HTS by improving both its efficiency and the accuracy of its results. streamlining the screening process and increasing the hit rate.architecture, are used to analyze molecular images and protein structures. By analyzing these images, CNNs can identify key features that contribute to a compound's ability to bind to a target. These models can understand the sequential nature of chemical structures, providing deeper insights into how compounds interact with biological targets. they interact in more biologically relevant conditions. and autoimmune disorders. AI is uniquely positioned to address this challenge by enabling the design of multi-target compounds through multi-objective optimization models.These AI models can simultaneously evaluate the binding affinity of a compound to several targets, optimizing its structure to achieve desired biological outcomes. Machine learning algorithms can also predict off-target effects and potential toxicity, ensuring that the multi-target compounds developed are not only effective but also safe. This approach holds significant promise in areas like cancer therapy, where targeting multiple signaling pathways or mutations may improve treatment efficacy and reduce resistance. with known clinical histories and matching them to disease-specific data, AI can identify novel uses for drugs that are already approved or in clinical trials.For example, AI-driven systems can cross-reference databases like DrugBank or ChEMBL with genetic for new indications3D structures of proteins and predicts how small molecules will interact with them, leading to the identification of promising drug candidates for diseases like Ebola and multiple sclerosis.Furthermore, AI-powered screening platforms are now available as cloud-based services, democratizing access to high-quality screening tools for academic institutions, small biotech companies, and research organizations. These platforms allow users to access AI-driven virtual screening, HTS optimization, and multi-target design capabilities, even without in highly regulated industries like pharmaceuticals, where transparency and validation are critical for regulatory approval.help enhance the to uncover novel therapeutic possibilities that would be impossible through traditional methods.

## DE NOVO DRUG DESIGN WITH AI: PIONEERING THE FUTURE OF DRUG DISCOVERY

Which start with known compounds and iteratively optimize them for better efficacy and safety, space of drug candidates and address the unmet medical needs for diseases that are difficult to treat with existing therapies. The traditional de novo drug design process has long been a challenging and resource-intensive endeavor, often requiring deep knowledge of medicinal chemistry and molecular biology, as well as extensive trial-and-error experimentation. efficient, and more accurate creation of drug-like molecules with specific therapeutic targets.AI- their bioactivity, and the optimization of their properties—all in a much shorter time structures based on learned patterns from vast databases of known molecules. drug-like (Garralda et al., 2017)molecules that could potentially interact with biological targets of interest, such as proteins, receptors, or enzymestraction in the field of drug discovery due to their ability to create novel, bioactive molecules that exhibit properties conducive to drug development. VAEs can be trained on large chemical databases to learn the essential features of molecules that contribute to their biological activity. Once trained, VAEs can generate novel molecules by sampling from the learned latent space and decoding it into valid chemical structures. The generated molecules are often diverse and can have desirable drug-like properties. VAEs are particularly effective in ensuring that the generated molecules are chemically valid and adhere to the rules of medicinal chemistry.(Gawriljuk et al., 2021). AI-driven molecular generation is powered by generative models like VAEs, GANs, and other deep learning techniques, which learn the key features of successful drug candidates and then generate molecules that incorporate these features.AI-based molecular generation involves the optimization of several properties to make the generated compounds suitable for drug development:Binding on protein-ligand docking simulations can predict how well a new molecule will bind to a target based on its structure.(Haleem et al., 2022a)Drug-Like Properties: Beyond potency, generated molecules must exhibit favorable pharmacokinetic properties (e.g., good absorption, distribution, metabolism, and excretion, or ADME). AI models can be trained to optimize drug-like properties by evaluating generated molecules against known drug characteristics. (Liang et al., 2022) For example, a compound with poor solubility may be adjusted by modifying its chemical structure to improve its solubility and bioavailability.

*Figure 1. The Impact of Generative AI in Drug Discovery*

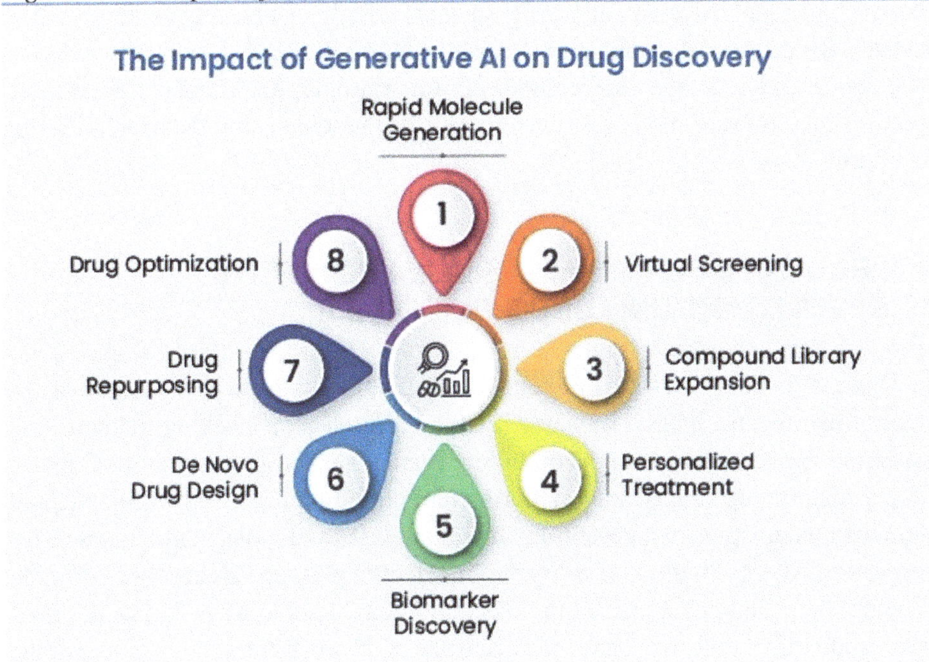


**Toxicity Prediction**: One of the major challenges in drug design is ensuring that generated compounds do not exhibit toxic By incorporating toxicity predictions into the generation process, AI can guide the creation of safer drug candidates.. AI-driven generative models can account for synthetic constraints by predicting how easily a molecule can be synthesized in the laboratory. By incorporating synthetic pathways into the generative process, AI models can propose drug-like molecules that are not only effective but also practical for production. part of known drug classes, enabling researchers to explore previously unexplored areas of chemical space. Traditional drug discovery methods, on the other hand, often rely on known molecular motifs or frameworks that have been historically successful in producing bioactive compounds. a combination of known drugs and disease-specific data, AI can propose new molecular variants that could serve as potential treatments for diseases beyond the original indication.AI's ability to generate novel molecules with diverse structures and properties also facilitates the discovery of new combinations of drugs. For example, AI can generate molecular combinations that may work synergistically to treat complex diseases like cancer or HIV, providing new avenues for polypharmacology.such as the presence of multiple targets, patient-specific variability, and environmental factors.Moreover, AI-generated molecules must be experimentally validated in the lab, and the process of moving from in silico predictions to in vivo testing still requires significant resources and time. . (Mak et al., 2021)As AI models become more sophisticated and trained on increasingly diverse and comprehensive datasets, the process of designing novel molecules will become more accurate and efficient. The use of quantum computing, for example, could enable even more precise simulations of molecular interactions, further enhancing the capabilities of AI in drug discovery.

## MOLECULAR DOCKING AND SIMULATION WITH AI: REVOLUTIONIZING DRUG DISCOVERY

This interaction, known as protein-ligand binding, is critical for the development of therapeutic agents. However, traditional molecular docking methods and molecular dynamics simulations often face challenges these computational methods are undergoing significant transformation, providing faster, more reliable, and more detailed insights into protein-ligand interactions and molecular dynamics. By integrating AI with traditional computational techniques, researchers are now able to model the dynamic nature of biomolecular interactions in ways that were previously impossible. AI can enhance the accuracy of docking predictions, improve the efficiency of simulations, and even predict the behavior of molecules under various conditions, paving the way for more effective drug discovery. of drug discovery, this helps identify potential lead compounds by evaluating the strength and stability of the binding interaction.(Haleem et al., 2022b)However, molecular docking is not without its limitations. It is primarily based on static models, assuming that both the ligand and the protein do not undergo significant conformational changes upon binding. In reality, proteins and ligands are dynamic, and their interactions often involve flexibility. This is where molecular dynamics simulations come into play. Molecular dynamics (MD) simulations provide a more accurate picture by modeling the physical movements of atoms in a system over time. MD simulations offer insights into how proteins and ligands move and interact, accounting for flexibility and the changes in conformation that occur during binding.Both docking and simulation are computationally demanding, (Madgule et al., 2023)often requiring high-performance computing resources. While these methods have been used successfully for decades,(Javaid et al., 2022) they have not been fully optimized in terms of computational speed and predictive accuracy—this is where AI becomes a game-changer.Traditional molecular docking relies on rigid docking, where the protein is treated as a fixed structure, and the ligand is flexed to find the best binding pose. However, this approach ignores the flexibility of both the protein and the ligand, which can lead to inaccurate binding predictions. AI, specifically machine learning and deep learning, is now being employed to address these limitations.AI algorithms can be used to predict the binding affinity of a ligand to a target protein more accurately by considering both the flexibility of the ligand and the protein. This allows AI to generate more accurate and reliable docking scores, which can guide researchers in selecting the best drug candidates. notoriously difficult to model using traditional docking methods, but AI can help identify key interactions and optimize docking predictions, even in these(Nag et al., 2022) challenging cases. While molecular docking provides a snapshot of the interaction between a protein and a ligand, molecular dynamics simulations offer a more dynamic and realistic representation. MD simulations expensive, often requiring long simulation times and extensive resources to model the interactions accurately.of protein-ligand dynamics. Machine learning models can be trained on experimental and high-level computational data to refine force fields, enabling more accurate simulations with reduced computational costs.

AI-driven methods such as reinforcement learning are also being explored to improve MD simulations. parameters dynamically to focus on regions of interest, like active sites of proteins. (Sugumaran et al., 2024)This approach has the potential to accelerate simulations, reduce resource consumption, and provide more detailed insights into the molecular behavior of the system being studied. calculating binding free energy is computationally expensive and time-consuming, as it requires running extensive simulations. AI algorithms can predict binding free energy more efficiently by learning from a large set of simulation data and applying this knowledge to new systems. This could drastically reduce the time required for energy calculations and enhance the accuracy of drug discovery predictions However, AI can enhance these processes by identifying binding patterns, recognizing key interaction features, and predicting how small changes in a molecule might impact its binding affinity. which residues in a protein's active site are most likely to interact with a ligand, or which molecular features of the ligand will optimize binding. AI can also assist in predicting allosteric sites—regions on a protein that are not part of the active site but can still influence ligand binding. This opens up new avenues for drug discovery, particularly in targeting proteins that were previously considered "undruggable."

## AI-POWERED PHARMACOKINETICS AND PHARMACODYNAMICS: TRANSFORMING DRUG DEVELOPMENT

Pharmacokinetics (PK) and pharmacodynamics (PD) are two essential components in the study of drug action and behavior within theoptimizing drug development, ensuring that new drugs are both effective and safe for patients.Traditionally, the assessment of PK and PD properties of drug design, reduce costs, and facilitate the development of more personalized therapies.Pharmacokinetics is primarily concerned with how a drug is absorbed into the bloodstream, distributed throughout the body, metabolized by the liver, and eventually excreted, primarily through the kidneys. (Sreenivasulu et al., 2022) Understanding these processes is critical for determining the optimal dosing regimen of a drug, predicting potential drug-drug interactions, and assessing the overall safety and efficacy of a new therapeutic agent.AI models rely on chemical structure, molecular descriptors, and biological activity data to learn patterns in how molecules are absorbed, distributed, metabolized, and excreted.Absorption solubility, permeability, and stability in the gastrointestinal tract. AI models can predict a compound's oral bioavailability, which is a key measure of absorption efficiency, by analyzing its chemical structure and using large datasets of known compounds. for identifying potential drug-drug interactions, as certain drugs can inhibit or induce these enzymes, leading to adverse effects or altered drug efficacy. Machine learning models can predict which enzymes a compound is most likely to interact with, allowing researchers in a way that alters their pharmacokinetic properties, potentially leading to reduced efficacy or increased toxicity. AI can be trained on vast datasets containing information about known DDIs and the molecular features of compounds involved in those interactions. AI can help researchers design safer drug regimens, minimize adverse interactions, and optimize therapeutic outcomes for patients. By identifying the molecular targets of drugs and understanding how they interact with cellular pathways, AI can predict how well a drug will perform in human patients. For example, AI models can predict how a drug will modulate signaling pathways in cancer cells, enabling researchers to design more effective cancer therapies.Toxicity is a critical concern in pharmacodynamics, as many drug candidates fail in the clinical stages due to adverse effects. (Teles et al., 2022)Traditional methods of predicting toxicity often rely on animal models, which can be time-consuming and not always predictive or other adverse effects, allowing researchers to discard toxic candidates early in the development process.

Another aspect of pharmacodynamics that AI is enhancing is selectivity—the ability of a drug to target a specific biological molecule or pathway without affecting others. This is particularly important for minimizing side effects and improving therapeutic outcomes. AI models can predict the selectivity of a drug by analyzing its molecular structure and comparing it to known binding sites in different proteins. By identifying the most relevant targets for a drug and predicting how it will interact with them, AI can help design drugs that are more specific and effective while reducing the risk of off-target effects.view of the molecular landscape, offering insights into gene expression, protein activity, and metabolic changes that influence drug behavior in the body(Thakkar et al., 2021). Looking ahead, the role of AI in pharmacokinetics and pharmacodynamics will only continue to grow. As more high-quality datasets become available and AI algorithms become more advanced, the ability to predict ADME properties and drug effects will improve dramatically. providing deeper insights into drug dynamics and improving predictions of both PK and PD propertiesAI-powered pharmacokinetics and pharmacodynamics ageneration of drug discovery, ensuring that new therapies reach patients faster and with greater precision.

## CASE STUDIES OF SUCCESSFUL AI-DRIVEN DRUG DISCOVERY: LESSONS LEARNED AND BEST PRACTICES

AI-driven drug discovery, offering valuable insights into how these technologies can be effectively applied in pharmaceutical development. In this section, we analyze these successful case studies, discuss lessons learned, and identify best practices that can guide future AI-driven initiatives in drug discovery—an unprecedented timeline compared to traditional drug discovery methods, which typically take years.Approach: Insilico Medicine used its AI-based platform, which integrates molecules that could potentially inhibit the viral protein.Outcome: The AI-driven platform successfully identified INS018_055, a small molecule that demonstrated activity against the virus in preclinical studies. Insilico Medicine collaborated with other biotech firms to advance the compound through further testing, including in vitro assays. Though the drug is still undergoing clinical trials, the speed and success of the initial stages were groundbreaking. The case illustrated the potential of AI to rapidly identify drug candidates in response to urgent public health needs. screening and predicting protein-ligand interactions, AI enables researchers to sift through vast libraries of compounds in a fraction of the time it would take through traditional methods. biological data, such as protein structures, genetic data, and chemical libraries, to generate more accurate predictions and enhance discovery AI specialists, biotechnologists, and pharmaceutical experts. Working together across disciplines ensures that AI platforms are being used effectively and that the results are actionable.

*Figure 2. Benefits of Generative AI in Drug Discovery*

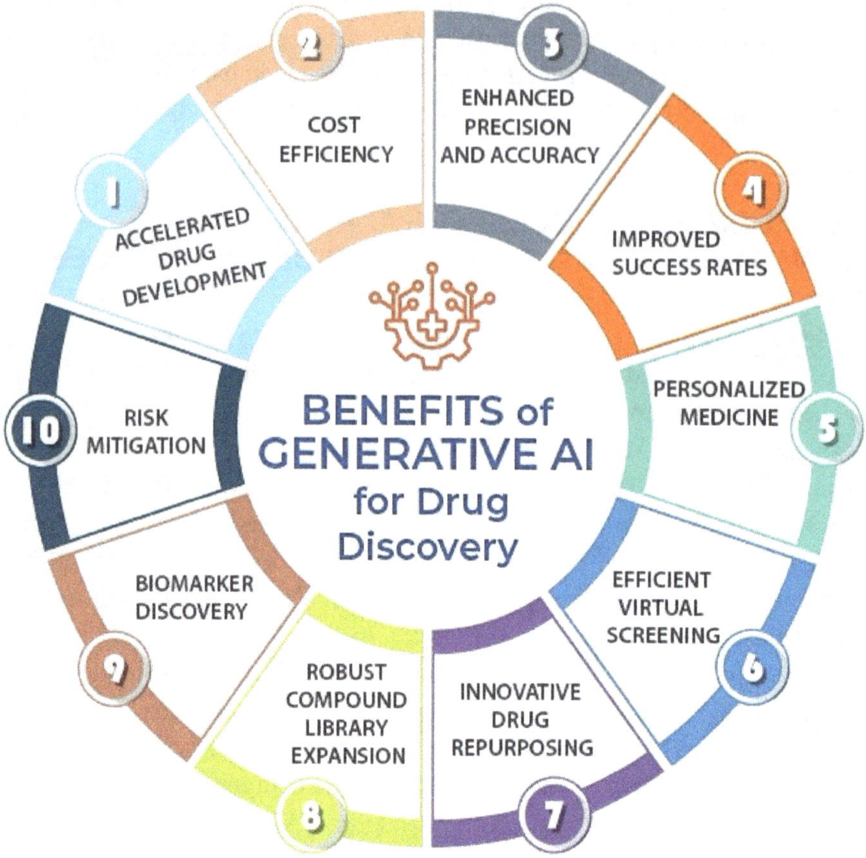


Iterative Development: AI models should be continuously refined and improved based on experimental results and real-world data. This iterative approach ensures that the models remain relevant and accurate throughout the drug development process. or the treatment of rheumatoid arthritis, was found by BenevolentAI to potentially target key inflammatory pathways involved in COVID-19, offering a novel approach to managing the disease. The platform focuses on identifying promising drug candidates by predicting how existing drugs might interact with new disease targets. For COVID-19, Benevolent AI integrated data from thousands of research papers and clinical studies, identifying potential connections between the immune system's response to SARS-CoV-2 and the signaling pathways modulated by Baricitinib.The AI model flagged Baricitinib as a candidate for treating COVID-19 due to its ability to block certain immune system pathways that exacerbate lung inflammation in COVID-19 patients.Outcome: After AI identified Baricitinib as a potential treatment, clinical trials were quickly launched. The drug was subsequently granted emergency use authorization by the U.S. FDA for COVID-19 patients requiring supplemental oxygen. The rapid identification of Baricitinib as a viable treatment underscored the power of AI in drug repurposing, especially during urgent public health crises.

## AI IN RARE DISEASE DRUG DISCOVERY: EMPOWERING ORPHAN DRUG DEVELOPMENT AND PRECISION MEDICINE

Organization (WHO), there are over 7,000 known rare diseases, with approximately 400 million people globally affected. While individually rare, these diseases share common Historically, the development of treatments for rare diseases has been slow, costly, and fraught with challenge (Sarker, 2021)s. However,of Artificial Intelligence AI plays a critical role in orphan drug development and precision medicine, helping to overcome many of the limitations inherent in rare disease research. This discussion explores how AI is reshaping the landscape of rare disease drug discovery, with a focus on orphan drug development, precision medicine, and the lessons learned from successful AI applications in this field (Varadi et al., 2022). the sheer number of such diseases means that millions of individuals worldwide suffer from conditions that lack effective treatments. Several key challenges hinder the development of drugs for rare diseases:Limited Patient Populations: One of the most significant hurdles in rare disease research isthe small number of patients, which makes it difficult to recruit participants for clinical trials. This limited patient pool often results in insufficient data, making it challenging to develop statistically significant findings or assess the safety and efficacy of a drug.Lack of Disease Understanding: Many rare diseases are poorly understood at the molecular and lead to disease and identifying potential intervention points requires deep biological and molecular insight.High Development Costs: The costs associated with drug development for rare diseases are often prohibitively high, given the small market size and the difficulty in enrolling patients in clinical trials. Pharmaceutical companies are often unwilling to invest in these areas due to limited financial incentives.

Furthermore, AI models can be used to predict how genetic mutations lead to functional disruptions, such as the misfolding of proteins, which could inform the development of drugs that target these molecular defects.known mechanisms of action, AI can uncover potential matches between existing drugs and rare disease targets.For instance, in 2020, BenevolentAI, an AI-driven drug discovery company, used its (Vaz & Balaji, 2021)AI platform to repurpose an existing drug, Baricitinib, for the treatment of COVID-19. Similarly, AI has been used to identify potential repurposing candidates for rare diseases like Cystic Fibrosis and Amyotrophic Lateral Sclerosis (ALS). Drug repurposing is particularly valuable for rare diseases, as it can significantly reduce the time and cost of development, since the safety profiles of these drugs are already well-established.ical trials for rare diseases are often small and difficult to design due to the limited number of patients. AI can help optimize clinical trial design by predicting patient responses based likelihood of success in clinical trials and reducing the time required to demonstrate efficacy.

## AI-POWERED PERSONALIZED MEDICINE: TAILORED TREATMENT STRATEGIES AND PATIENT STRATIFICATION

Across several domains, including patient stratification, biomarker identification, tailored treatment strategies, and predictive modeling for drug efficacy and adverse reactions. This and increase the overall efficiency of medical interventions.Traditional medicine often adopts a generalized approach where patients with the same disease receive the same treatment, regardless of individual differences. While this method works for . This leads to several challenges:Variable Treatment Responses: Patients with the same disease may respond differently to the same treatment. For example, chemotherapy may work for some cancer patients but have little or no effect on others, or it may cause severe side effects in some patients.Inefficient Resource Allocation:(Vijayakumar et al., 2024) The traditional model may lead to the overuse of healthcare resources on treatments that are ineffective for certain patient subgroups, delaying the identification of the most effective therapeutic approach.

Lack of Early Diagnosis: In many diseases, particularly rare or complex ones, early diagnosis is challenging, leading to the progression of the disease before appropriate interventions can be madePatient stratification refers to the process of dividing patients into subgroups based on specific characteristics, such as genetic(Ramakrishnan et al., 2022) variations, biomarkers, disease stage, or lifestyle factors. AI can be particularly effective in this regard by analyzing large datasets to identify meaningful patterns that may be too complex for human clinicians to detect. Match patients with specific treatment regimens that have been shown to work best for their subtype of the disease.Reduce treatment failures by avoiding ineffective or harmful therapies for certain subgroups.For instance, in oncology, AI has been used to identify distinct subtypes of cancers based on molecular markers, allowing doctors to target therapies that are more likely to be effective for a particular molecular profile. I helps bridge this gap by analyzing large-scale genomic datasets, identifying genetic mutations, and determining how these mutations may impact disease progression and drug response. By applying machine learning algorithms to vast genomic databases, AI can uncover previously hidden relationships between genetic variants and disease characteristics.For example, AI has been instrumental in identifying novel cancer biomarkers, which are c targeted therapies, such as

HER2-targeted treatmentscystic fibrosis, where AI has helped identify new genetic mutations linked to the disease, providing insights into potential therapeutic targets. experience adverse drug reactions (ADRs). Traditional methods of drug development and treatment often fail to predict individual responses, leading to inefficient treatment plans and adverse outcomes. genetic profile, medical history, and lifestyle. This approach can predict drug efficacy, optimal dosages, and potential side effects more accurately than traditional methods. By analyzing factors like genetic mutations and existing comorbidities, AI models can optimize treatment protocols, ensuring the best possible therapeutic outcomes with minimal side effects.(Rácz et al., 2021) Additionally, AI can help predict and monitor drug interactions, an important consideration in elderly patients or those with multiple chronic conditions. Predictive models can assess the risk of adverse reactions and suggest alternative therapies, improving patient safety.AI-powered technologies enable real-time monitoring of patient health, which is a crucial component of personalized medicine. With the advent of wearables, implantable devices, and mobile health apps, patient data can be continuously collected and analyzed. AI algorithms process this real-time data to provide ongoing insights into the patient's health status, treatment adherence, and response to therapy.

## OPPORTUNITIES FOR AI IN DRUG DISCOVERY: IMPROVED EFFICIENCY, REDUCED COSTS, AND MORE

In this analysis, we will explore the numerous opportunities that AI presents in drug discovery, including the potential to streamline the process, reduce failure rates, and develop more personalized and effective treatments for patients.scientific literature, databases, and biological knowledge, with much of the work relying on the expertise of scientists to hypothesize possible targets based on observed disease mechanisms.learning models, can analyze these vast datasets to identify patterns and relationships between biological targets and diseases that are difficult for humans to discern. For example, by combining information from genetic studies, biological pathways, and drug-target interactions, AI can pinpoint the most promising targets with a higher degree of confidence and speed.Furthermore, AI can assist in target validation by using advanced algorithms to simulate the biological effects of modulating a given target in a disease model, reducing the need for expensive and time-consuming wet lab experiments. By predicting how changes in target activity might influence disease progression, AI can guide experimental research more efficiently, thus shortening the discovery timeline.AI enables researchers to analyze biological, chemical, and clinical data to uncover hidden connections between existing drugs and diseases that were not previously considered. By analyzing historical clinical trial data, AI models can predict which approved drugs might be effective for conditions they were not originally designed to treat, significantly reducing the time required(Zhang et al., 2022a) for developing new treatments.Additionally, AI facilitates compound screening by improving the virtual screening process, which involves testing large libraries of compounds against biological targets. Traditional high- and their targets, enhancing the likelihood of identifying novel compounds with drug-like properties.Once potential drug candidates are identified, the next step is to optimize their efficacy, safety, and pharmacokinetic properties. Traditionally, lead optimization involves synthesizing and testing hundreds or thousands of compounds to find the most promising candidates for clinical trials.(Weissler et al., 2021) This process can be resource-intensive and slow.AI-driven structure-activity relationship (SAR) analysis is transforming lead optimization by enabling rapid analysis of the relationship between a compound's structure and its biological activity. Using machine learning algorithms trained on large datasets of chemical compounds and their biological effects, AI can predict how structural modifications will affect a compound's efficacy, toxicity, and other pharmacological properties. This allows researchers to make data-driven decisions and refine compounds more efficiently, potentially reducing the number of iterations needed before reaching an optimal drug candidate.Additionally, AI technologies can assist in molecular design by generating novel compounds with desired properties using generative models. These models use existing chemical libraries to design new molecules that fit specific criteria, such as potency, stability, and bioavailability. By employing reinforcement learning, AI can optimize the design of drug molecules to improve their chances of success in clinical trials.(Yang et al., 2022)AI-driven molecular design also offers the advantage of reducing attrition rates in clinical trials by identifying compounds with a higher likelihood of success early in the development process. This helps avoid the significant financial and time losses associated with pursuing ineffective drug candidatesOne of the primary causes of drug failure in clinical trials is toxicity, which often becomes apparent only in later stages of development. Predicting the toxicity of a drug candidate early in the discovery process can save significant time and resources. AI is well-suited to this task by analyzing preclinical data, historical drug toxicity profiles, and patient data to predict the potential adverse effects of a drug before it enters clinical trials.

## FUTURE DIRECTIONS FOR AI IN DRUG DISCOVERY: EMERGING TRENDS, TECHNOLOGIES, AND THE PATH FORWARD

Characterized by emerging trends and cutting-edge technologies that promise to streamline development, enhance predictive accuracy, and unlock novel therapeutic possibilities. This section explores the future directions of AI in drug discovery, highlighting key innovations, trends, and challenges that will shape the industry in the coming years.variations and biomarkers that predict responses to specific drugs.(Patel et al., 2020)By incorporating this information, AI can help design personalized treatment regimens, ensuring higher efficacy and fewer side effects.n metabolism, genetic predisposition, and comorbid conditions. Additionally, AI can enable the development of combination therapies that are optimized for individual patients, targeting multiple pathways or disease mechanisms simultaneously. targeted and more efficient therapeutic interventions. Over time, the integration of real-time patient data, such as information from wearable devices, could allow AI systems to continuously update and adjust treatment recommendations based on evolving patient profiles. (e.g., graph neural networks, attention-based models, and transformers) will allow for even more accurate and efficient predictions of molecular interactions, drug efficacy,Pan et al., 2022) and safety profiles.properties—such as higher binding affinity, better bioavailability, and reduced toxicity—faster and more efficiently than ever before. drug discovery pipelines. The combination of generative AI and molecular docking simulations will enable the rapid generation and testing of novel drug candidates, accelerating the pace of drug development. understanding of disease mechanisms. By merging genomic data with clinical data, imaging, and environmental factors, AI can build more accurate models of disease biology, providing new targets for drug discovery and identifying potential biomarkers for patient stratification.This multi-omics approach will likely lead to the development of more accurate disease etiologies, such as cancer, neurodegenerative disorders, and autoimmune diseases, where the interplay between genetics, the environment, and lifestyle is still not fully understood.algorithms continuously integrate new data from various sources, such as clinical trials, patient monitoring devices, and even social determinants of health, to update disease models and personalize treatment options(Namanja et al., 2019). This dynamic, data-driven approach will ensure that drug discovery efforts are based on the most current and holistic understanding of disease.

## CONCLUSION

The application of AI, from early-stage target identification to late-stage clinical trials, is fundamentally altering the way drugs are discovered, developed, and brought to market. This speed is not only valuable in terms of cost reduction but also in enhancing the potential for innovation. —AI can uncover relationships between disease mechanisms and potential treatments that might have otherwise been overlooked.Additionally,. AI aids in the predictive modeling of how certain evelopment, ensuring resources are focused on the most viable candidates.AI's ability to identify and validate therapeutic targets is another cornerstone of its impact on drug discovery. Traditionally, identifying the correct molecular targets for diseases has been s with higher precision and accuracy. capable of identifying druggable targets, which can be particularly useful in diseases with complex genetic underpinnings, such as cancer or neurodegenerative disorders. The precision with which AI identifies targets allows for the development of more specific and less toxic drugs, reducing the side effects that are often associated with broad-spectrum treatmentsMoreover, AI plays a pivotal role in target validation, helping researchers confirm whether a potential target is truly involved in disease processes and whether modulating it will lead to a therapeutic effect. Through techniques such as gene editing and CRISPR, AI can guide experimental approaches to validate targets and evaluate their effectiveness in cellular models, ultimately improving the chances of success in clinical trials.Furthermore, lead optimization, which involves refining lead compounds to enhance their efficacy, selectivity, and safety, is greatly improved by AI. Structure-activity relationship (SAR) analysis, traditionally a labor-intensive process, is now made more efficient through AI algorithms that can analyze molecular structures and predict As a result, AI is reducing the time and cost required to develop lead compounds into viable drugs.Moreover, AI's ability to predict pharmacokinetics and pharmacodynamics of compounds provides researchers with early insights into how drugs will behave in the human body. This predictive capability allows for the optimization of drugs to ensure they are not only effective but also safe for human use, reducing the likelihood of late-stage clinical trial failuresPatient recruitment and stratification are among the most critical aspects of clinical trial design, given treatment, improving the precision of clinical trials and minimizing the risk of failure due to patient heterogeneity. This dynamic approach can improve patient safety and accelerate the identification of successful treatments.Furthermore, AI can aid in clinical trial simulations, predicting the outcomes of trials based on previous data and helping to optimize trial designs before they are implemented in the real world. This can significantly reduce the number of patients needed in trials, lowering costs and improving trial success rates.

# REFERENCES


Abbas, A. A., Hansen, B. A., Koesmahargyo, V. A. X., Yadav, V. A., Rosenfield, P. A., Patil, O. A., Dockendorf, M. A., Moyer, M. A., Shipley, L. A., Perez-Rodriguez, M. A., & Galatzer-Levy, I. A. X. (2022). Facial and vocal markers of schizophrenia measured using remote smartphone assessments: Observational study. *JMIR Formative Research*, *6*(1), e26276. Advance online publication. DOI: 10.2196/26276 PMID: 35060906

Agamah, F. E., Mazandu, G. K., Hassan, R., Bope, C. D., Thomford, N. E., Ghansah, A., & Chimusa, E. R. (2020). Computational/in silico methods in drug target and lead prediction. *Briefings in Bioinformatics*, *21*(5), 1663–1675. DOI: 10.1093/bib/bbz103 PMID: 31711157

Bajwa, J., Munir, U., Nori, A., & Williams, B. (2021). Artificial intelligence in healthcare: Transforming the practice of medicine. *Future Healthcare Journal*, *8*(2), e188–e194. DOI: 10.7861/fhj.2021-0095 PMID: 34286183

Ball, R. A., & Dal Pan, G. (2022). "Artificial intelligence" for pharmacovigilance: Ready for prime time? *Drug Safety*, *45*(5), 429–438. DOI: 10.1007/s40264-022-01157-4 PMID: 35579808

Capecchi, A., Probst, D., & Reymond, J.-L. (2020). One molecular fingerprint to rule them all: Drugs, biomolecules, and the metabolome. *Journal of Cheminformatics*, *12*(1), 43. Advance online publication. DOI: 10.1186/s13321-020-00445-4 PMID: 33431010

Cardozo, G. A., Tirloni, S. A., Pereira Moro, A. A., & Marques, J. A. (2022). Use of artificial intelligence in the search for new information through routine laboratory tests: Systematic review. *JMIR Bioinformatics and Biotechnology*, *3*(1), e40473. Advance online publication. DOI: 10.2196/40473 PMID: 36644762

Dara, S. A., Dhamercherla, S., Jadav, S. S., Babu, C. M., & Ahsan, M. J. (2022). Machine learning in drug discovery: A review. *Artificial Intelligence Review*, *55*(3), 1947–1999. DOI: 10.1007/s10462-021-10058-4 PMID: 34393317

Dash, S., Shakyawar, S. K., Sharma, M., & Kaushik, S. (2019). Big data in healthcare: Management, analysis and future prospects. *Journal of Big Data*, *6*(1), 54. Advance online publication. DOI: 10.1186/s40537-019-0217-0

Fisher, S., & Rosella, L. C. (2022). Priorities for successful use of artificial intelligence by public health organizations: A literature review. *BMC Public Health*, *22*(1), 2146. Advance online publication. DOI: 10.1186/s12889-022-14422-z PMID: 36419010

Fogel, D. B. (2018). Factors associated with clinical trials that fail and opportunities for improving the likelihood of success: A review. *Contemporary Clinical Trials Communications, 11*, 156–164. DOI: 10.1016/j.conctc.2018.08.001 PMID: 30112460

Garralda, E., Dienstmann, R., & Tabernero, J. (2017). Pharmacokinetic/pharmacodynamic modeling for drug development in oncology. *American Society of Clinical Oncology Educational Book, 37*, 210–215. DOI: 10.1200/EDBK_180460 PMID: 28561730

Gawriljuk, V. O., Foil, D. H., Puhl, A. A., Zorn, K. M., Lane, T. R., Riabova, O., Makarov, V., Godoy, A. S., Oliva, G., & Ekins, S. A. (2021). Development of machine learning models and the discovery of a new antiviral compound against yellow fever virus. *Journal of Chemical Information and Modeling, 61*(8), 3804–3813. DOI: 10.1021/acs.jcim.1c00460 PMID: 34286575

Haleem, A., Javaid, M., Qadri, M. A., Singh, R. P., & Suman, R. (2022a). Artificial intelligence (AI) applications for marketing: A literature-based study. *International Journal of Intelligent Networks, 3*, 119–132. DOI: 10.1016/j.ijin.2022.08.005

Haleem, A., Javaid, M., Singh, R. P., & Suman, R. (2022b). Medical 4.0 technologies for healthcare: Features, capabilities, and applications. *Internet of Things and Cyber Physical Systems, 2*, 12–30. DOI: 10.1016/j.iotcps.2022.04.001

Javaid, M., Haleem, A., Singh, R. P., Suman, R., & Rab, S. (2022). Significance of machine learning in healthcare: Features, pillars and applications. *International Journal of Intelligent Networks, 3*, 58–73. DOI: 10.1016/j.ijin.2022.05.002

Jiang, M., Wang, S., Zhang, S., Zhou, W., Zhang, Y., & Li, Z. (2022). Sequence-based drug-target affinity prediction using weighted graph neural networks. *BMC Genomics, 23*(1), 449. Advance online publication. DOI: 10.1186/s12864-022-0868-9 PMID: 35715739

Liang, L., Hu, J., Sun, G., Hong, N., Wu, G., He, Y., Li, Y., Hao, T., Liu, L., & Gong, M. (2022). Artificial intelligence-based pharmacovigilance in the setting of limited resources. *Drug Safety, 45*(5), 511–519. DOI: 10.1007/s40264-022-01170-7 PMID: 35579814

Madgule, M., Vinayaka, N., Sonkhaskar, Y. M., Patel, D. R., Karthikeyan, R., & Selvakumar, P. (2023). Mechanical properties and microstructure of activated TIG welded similar joints of Inconel alloys by desirability approaches. *Materials Today: Proceedings, 77*, 528–533. DOI: 10.1016/j.matpr.2022.11.251

Nag, S., Baidya, A. T. K., Mandal, A., Mathew, A. T., Das, B., Devi, B., & Kumar, R. A. (2022). Deep learning tools for advancing drug discovery and development. *3 Biotech, 12*(5), Article 110. https://doi.org/DOI: 10.1007/s13205-022-03165-8

Namanja, A. T., Xu, J., Wu, H., Sun, Q., Upadhyay, A. K., Sun, C., Van Doren, S. R., & Petros, A. A. X. (2019). NMR-based fragment screening and lead discovery accelerated by principal component analysis. *Journal of Biomolecular NMR, 73*(12), 675–685. DOI: 10.1007/s10858-019-00279-9 PMID: 31541395

Patel, L., Shukla, T., Huang, X., Ussery, D. A., & Wang, S. A. (2020). Machine learning methods in drug discovery. *Molecules (Basel, Switzerland), 25*(22), 5277. Advance online publication. DOI: 10.3390/molecules25225277 PMID: 33198233

Rácz, A., Bajusz, D., Miranda-Quintana, R. A., & Héberger, K. (2021). Machine learning models for classification tasks related to drug safety. *Molecular Diversity, 25*(3), 1409–1424. DOI: 10.1007/s11030-021-10239-x PMID: 34110577

Ramakrishnan, T., Gift, M. D. M., Chitradevi, S., Jegan, R., & Jose, P. S. H. (2022). Nagaraja, Sharma, H. N., Selvakumar, P., & Hailegiorgis, S. M. (2022). Study of numerous resins used in polymer matrix composite materials. *Advances in Materials Science and Engineering*, •••, 1088926. Advance online publication. DOI: 10.1155/2022/1088926

Sarker, I. A. (2021). Deep learning: A comprehensive overview on techniques, taxonomy, applications and research directions. *SN Computer Science, 2*(6), 420. Advance online publication. DOI: 10.1007/s42979-021-00815-1 PMID: 34426802

Sreenivasulu, A., Manimozhi, T., Satheesh Kumar, P., Selvakumar, P., & Singh, P. (2022). The model of smart sensing device for sensitive nanoclusters modification in sensing properties. In *2022 2nd International Conference on Advance Computing and Innovative Technologies in Engineering (ICACITE)* (pp. 1043–1047). IEEE. https://doi.org/DOI: 10.1109/ICACITE53722.2022.9823846

Sugumaran, K. M. D., Pandiyarajan, V., Sonkhaskar, Y. B., Selvakumar, P., & M. S. (2024). Analysis of electromyography signals for control of mechanical prosthesis using machine learning techniques. In *2024 2nd International Conference on Intelligent Data Communication Technologies and Internet of Things (IDCIoT)* (pp. 1059–1067). IEEE. https://doi.org/DOI: 10.1109/IDCIoT59759.2024.10467707

Teles, H. R., Ferreira, L. A., Valli, M. A. X., Coelho, F., & Andricopulo, A. A. X. (2022). Hierarchical clustering and target-independent QSAR for antileishmanial oxazole and oxadiazole derivatives. *International Journal of Molecular Sciences, 23*(16), 8898. Advance online publication. DOI: 10.3390/ijms23168898 PMID: 36012163

Thakkar, A., Johansson, S., Jorner, K., Buttar, D., Reymond, J.-L., & Engkvist, O. (2021). Artificial intelligence and automation in computer aided synthesis planning. *Reaction Chemistry & Engineering*, *6*(1), 27–51. DOI: 10.1039/D0RE00340A

Varadi, M., Anyango, S., Deshpande, M., Nair, S., Natassia, C., Yordanova, G., Yuan, D., Stroe, O., Wood, G., Laydon, A., Žídek, A., Green, T., Tunyasuvunakool, K., Petersen, S., Jumper, J., Clancy, E., Green, R., Vora, A., Lutfi, M., & Velankar, S. (2022). AlphaFold protein structure database: Massively expanding the structural coverage of protein-sequence space with high-accuracy models. *Nucleic Acids Research*, *50*(D1), D439–D444. DOI: 10.1093/nar/gkab1061 PMID: 34791371

Vaz, J. M., & Balaji, S. (2021). Convolutional neural networks (CNNs): Concepts and applications in pharmacogenomics. *Molecular Diversity*, *25*(3), 1569–1584. DOI: 10.1007/s11030-021-10225-3 PMID: 34031788

Vijayakumar, G., Rajkumar, M., Chandar, N. R., Selvakumar, P., & Duraisamy, R. (2024). Environmentally friendly TDS removal from wastewater by electrochemical ion exchange batch-type recirculation (EIR) technique. *Environmental Science. Water Research & Technology*, *10*(3), 826–835. DOI: 10.1039/D3EW00793F

Weissler, E. H., Naumann, T., Andersson, T., Ranganath, R., Elemento, O., Luo, Y., Freitag, D. F., Benoit, J., Hughes, M. C., Khan, F., Slater, P., Shameer, K., Roe, M., Hutchison, E., Kollins, S. H., Broedl, U., Meng, Z., Wong, J. L., Curtis, L., & Ghassemi, M. (2021). The role of machine learning in clinical research: Transforming the future of evidence generation. *Trials*, *22*(1), 537. Advance online publication. DOI: 10.1186/s13063-021-05489-x PMID: 34399832

Yang, Z., Shi, Y., Li, P., Pan, K., Li, G., Li, X., Yao, S., & Zhang, D. (2022). Application of principal component analysis (PCA) to the evaluation and screening of multiactivity fungi. *Journal of Ocean University of China*, *21*(3), 763–772. DOI: 10.1007/s11802-022-5096-x PMID: 35582545

Zhang, C., Lu, Y., & Zang, T. A. (2022). CNN-DDI: A learning-based method for predicting drug-drug interactions using convolution neural networks. *BMC Bioinformatics*, *23*(Suppl 3), 88. Advance online publication. DOI: 10.1186/s12859-022-04612-2 PMID: 35255808

Chapter 15
# Future Trends in AI and Smart Healthcare

**Amandeep Kaur**
*Chandigarh Group of Colleges Jhanjeri, Mohali, India*

**Ramandeep Sandhu**
https://orcid.org/0000-0003-2595-4030
*Lovely Professional University, Phagwara, India*

**Gaganpreet Kaur**
https://orcid.org/0009-0006-2957-5352
*Chandigarh Group of Colleges Jhanjeri, Mohali, India*

**Deepika Ghai**
https://orcid.org/0000-0002-1113-822X
*Lovely Professional University, Phagwara, India*

## ABSTRACT

*The healthcare industry will experience revolutionary medical practices through Artificial Intelligence (AI) integration up to 2030. This chapter analyzes future tendencies in AI coupled with smart healthcare through a discussion about advanced technologies helping medical staff with prediction capabilities, tailored treatment solutions, and immediate clinical choices. Through Systematic Literature Review (SLR) methodology, this chapter sets out major investigation paths that highlight federated learning as a data protection and Explainable AI (XAI) method for decision processes and digital twin modeling for precise healthcare delivery. This chapter identifies AI-powered diagnostic technologies, along with robotic surgery systems and wearable health monitoring. Remote patient care services can be improved through the combination of Internet of Medical Things (IoMT) technology with*

DOI: 10.4018/979-8-3373-3311-3.ch015

*5G-enabled smart healthcare infrastructure. The chapter also presents the essential framework needed to deploy AI in healthcare and achieve ethical standards and security requirements for healthcare data.*

# 1. INTRODUCTION

## 1.1 Background of AI in Healthcare

### 1.1.1 Definition of Artificial Intelligence

The definition is 'representing human thinking with computers which is called Artificial Intelligence (AI).' An important part of AI involves understanding (learning), using rules (reasoning), and being able to make improvements (self-correction) (Russell & Norvig, 2016). AI in medicine is often defined as technologies including robotics, machine learning, and natural language processing and their role is to analyze medical data, assist with diagnostics, and improve care for patients.

### 1.1.2 Historical Context of AI in Medicine

From what we understand, AI in medicine began in the 1970s when systems such as MYCIN (Shortliffe, 1974), meant for detecting infection and supplying antibiotic suggestions, were introduced. Using ML, access to data, machine power, and algorithm complexity have all progressed steadily over the years. Imaging, genomics, and personalized medicine have adopted AI applications more than any other industries because of the recent rise of big data and machine learning (Topol, 2019). Table 1 shows the timeline of AI development in healthcare.

*Table 1. Timeline of AI Development in Healthcare*

| Year | Milestone |
|---|---|
| 1970s | Development of MYCIN |
| 1990s | Introduction of neural networks in diagnostics |
| 2010s | Rise of deep learning and big data analytics |
| 2020s | Widespread adoption of AI in clinical settings |

## 1.2 Significance of AI Integration by 2030

### 1.2.1 Potential Impact on Healthcare Delivery

AIs's ability to take care of healthcare delivery and make treatment plans more personalized. (Singhal & Carlton, 2019) said that using AI in healthcare may help the U.S. economy by saving up to $100 billion a year by 2025 with higher production and lower costs. With AI helping integration, there can be instant decisions, successful patient results, and competent use of resources.

### 1.2.2 Importance of Research and Development

Even after big improvements, its full potential cannot be achieved unless more is done in research and development with a special focus on healthcare AI. The National Institutes of Health also pointed out that working across different fields is necessary to make AI technology that can help with challenging molecules and health issues (Allen Jr, 2019). In addition, research on AI is necessary to guarantee that AI systems work well, are fair and help address health disparities between groups. Table 2 projects the benefits of AI integration in healthcare.

*Table 2. Projected Benefits of AI Integration in Healthcare*

| Benefits | Description | Estimated Impact |
|---|---|---|
| Improved Diagnostics | Enhanced accuracy in disease detection | 20% reduction in misdiagnoses |
| Personalized Treatment | Tailored therapies based on individual data | 30% increase in treatment efficacy |
| Operational Efficiency | Streamlined workflows and reduced administrative burden | 25% cost savings |

## 1.3 Objectives of the Chapter

### 1.3.1 Explore Future Trends

In this chapter, we intend to find out about future AI and smart healthcare technology trends that could affect how medicine is practiced. The chapter will examine the way healthcare works, especially through advances in predictive analytics, personalized medicine, and remote patient care.

### 1.3.2 Identify Key Technologies and Innovations

Also, the chapter will highlight and explain significant technologies and innovations set to disrupt routine healthcare practices. AI-based medical tools, robotic surgeries, and devices for health tracking are prepared to improve healthcare and make health outcomes better.

## 2. SYSTEMATIC LITERATURE REVIEW (SLR)

To study AI in healthcare, researchers use SLR as a structured way to identify, study, and combine studies on the topic. The authors of the 2006 book Common Sense, Petticrew and Roberts, describe the SLR as asking research questions, specifying what should be included and excluded from the study, searching widely through literature, and combining the results (Petticrew & Roberts, 2008).

### 2.1 Criteria for Literature Selection

The literature chosen for this chapter consists of articles, conference papers, and reports that were published in the last decade of research. AI will be explored as the main topic related to applications that run personalized diagnosis and treatment. Questions about relevance, research methods, and importance to the field are formed when scoring the studies. Figure 1 shows the flowchart of the SLR process.

## 3. CURRENT LANDSCAPE OF AI IN HEALTHCARE

### 3.1 Machine Learning and Deep Learning

Let's highlight and study important components of AI and how they operate in a specific case. There is a good deal of information about this topic available online. They are going to let us discuss ML initially, which is a major branch of AI. It consists of various sets of algorithms like supervised learning, unsupervised learning, and Reinforcement learning. Essential in medicine to healthcare are predictive analytics, risk categorization, and personalized suggestions on how to treat patients (Jordan & Mitchell, 2015), as in the field of machine learning.

a) Supervised Learning:- When we use labeled data and feed the model correct answers, that is called supervised learning. It is a typical way of doing things in healthcare, like when classifying diseases and calculating risks. Specialists can collect and review historical patient data to train algorithms to estimate the risk of diabetes and heart disease (Kourou et al., 2015).

b) Unsupervised Learning:- There is also unsupervised learning which explores the patterns in unlabeled data. The point of using it is to discover any patterns that may exist within the data. Health care can also use unsupervised learning to group patients with similar features and find new kinds of health problems. To illustrate, if you use these algorithms together, they can sort patients whose responses to different treatments vary (Hastie, 2009).

*Figure 1. Flowchart of the SLR Process*

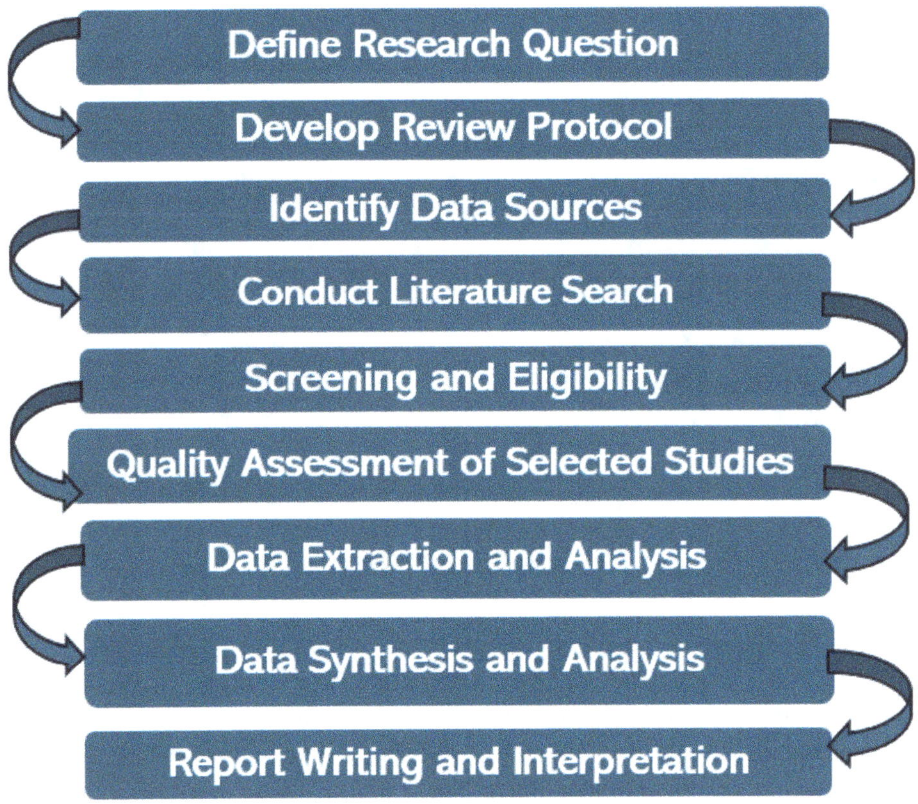


c) Reinforcement Learning:- An agent learning to act in an environment to get a reward is known as reinforcement learning in Machine Learning. Healthcare can use reinforcement learning to enhance the way treatments are managed as time goes by. For example, adaptive programs can be made based on the patient's response which improves the outcome (Sutton & Barto, 1998).

Deep learning is when neural networks with several layers (meaning deep) are applied in machine learning. The main reason artificial intelligence became important in healthcare is that it can work with large amounts of unorganized data like pictures from a medical scan or genetic material. In similar ways, CNNs have been used in radiology to find abnormalities in images with accuracy much like that of a radiologist (Esteva et al., 2017). Figure 2 shows the overview of machine learning and deep learning in healthcare.

*Figure 2. Overview of Machine Learning and Deep Learning in Healthcare*

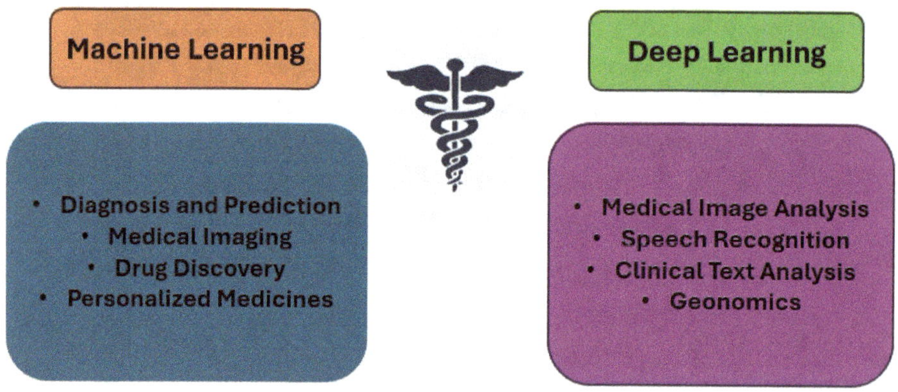


## 3.2 Natural Language Processing (NLP)

Natural Language Processing (NLP) is another important type of AI technology concerned with communication between computers and humans. NLP is used in healthcare settings to study doctors' notes, draw meaning from unorganized health information, and allow patients to understand and share details with their doctors. NLP is used in many fields which include:

a) Clinical Documentation:- NLP can also assist with transcribing doctor-patient interactions and pulling out essential details from electronic records. With automation, healthcare providers are relieved from dealing with a lot of paperwork and can focus on patient treatment. An example of an NLP algorithm is turning free text notes into organized data for analysis of patient information and monitoring health progress (Iroju et al., 2015).

b) Sentiment Analysis:- NLP is commonly used to analyze patient feedback and reviews to see what patients think about the care they have received. Healthcare organizations may be able to enhance customer service by looking into how patients feel. One example is using sentiment analysis to find out if positive feedback occurs a lot to help quality improvement (Keramatfar et al., 2019).
c) Clinical Decision Support:- Using real-time suggestions from NLP, clinical decision support systems can improve services by processing patient files and medical reports. By analyzing clinical notes and various research articles, NLP algorithms can give guidance to healthcare providers in deciding the right course of treatment and diagnosis (Iroju et al., 2015). Because of NLP, the way patients move through services can become simpler, and clinical records can be made more precise. Table 3 shows the applications of NLP in healthcare.

*Table 3. Applications of NLP in Healthcare*

| Application | Description | Benefits |
|---|---|---|
| Clinical Documentation | Automating transcription and data extraction | Reduces administrative burden and errors |
| Sentiment Analysis | Analyzing patient feedback | Enhances patient satisfaction and care |
| Clinical Decision Support | Real-time recommendations based on data | Improves diagnostic accuracy and treatment |

## 4. CURRENT APPLICATIONS IN MEDICAL PRACTICE

### 4.1 Diagnostics and Imaging

In radiology, pathology, and dermatology, diagnostics, and imaging have advanced because of progress in AI. AI algorithms can review medical images pick out tumors, give information about fractures, and recognize several unusual conditions with a high rate of accuracy. (Rajpurkar et al., 2017) carried out a study where a deep learning algorithm outperformed radiologists in finding pneumonia in chest X-rays, demonstrating the point.

a) Radiology:- Radiology makes use of AI systems to help with analyzing imaging investigations. Using wearable devices, radiologists may discover potential issues sooner and analyze medical images more quickly. The system looks for parts of X-rays or MRIs that might hint at a disease which radiologists inspect further.

It not only helps doctors give a more accurate diagnosis, but it also speeds up operations in the radiology department (Lakhani, 2017).

b) Pathology:- AI is making changes to pathology, in the same way, it affects all other industries: by replacing how we interpret tissue samples that are often misdiagnosed. These types of systems with AI are able to process images of whole slides and look for cancerous and unusual cells. Health professionals can process and examine thousands of images, giving pathologists quick information for making fast diagnoses. Research shows that AI can lead to better outcomes in diagnostic accuracy and thus it can raise the standard of care (Cruz-Roa et al., 2014).

c) Dermatology:- Developing AI in dermatology is directed at having it assist with the diagnosis of various skin conditions. If a large database of skin images that distinguish benign moles from melanomas is given to deep learning models, the models can accurately find melanomas and benign moles. Identifying skin cancer early is very important for the patient's recovery and that's what the increased capability allows. In another research, AI was proven to perform as well as or even better than dermatologists in determining skin cancer from images (Esteva et al., 2017). Figure 3 shows AI applications in medical imaging.

*Figure 3. AI Applications in Medical Imaging*

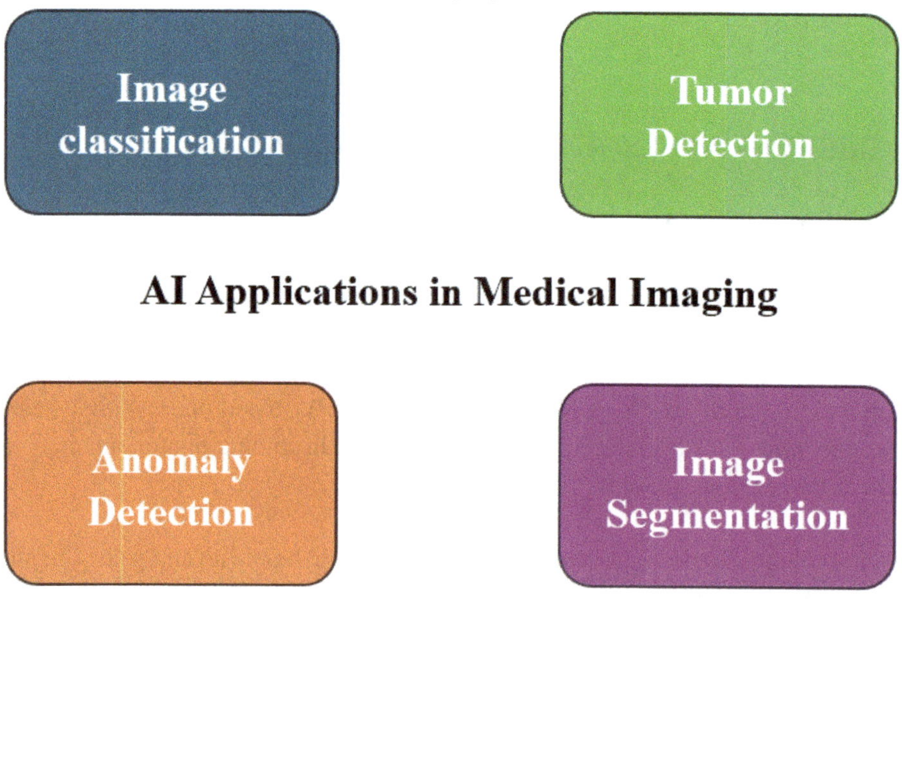

## 4.2 Treatment Planning and Management

AI helps to design and carry out personalized treatment plans for patients using their information. Machine learning is used to look at past patient information which helps find the best-suited way to treat certain conditions. For example, artificial intelligence makes it possible for oncologists to find targeted therapy suited to each patient based on their DNA and cancer characteristics (Kourou et al., 2015 ; Faiz et. al., 2023).

a) Personalized Medicine:- AI is used in medicine to create a personalized treatment for each person. AI can examine a patient's genetic, environmental, and lifestyle factors to discover which therapies will be most effective for them. Confirming the effectiveness of medicines not only makes treatments better but also cuts down on side effects from ineffective medicines (Collins & Varmus, 2015).
b) Decision Support Systems:- Providers can count on AI-driven decision support systems to help them build a treatment plan that includes patients' preferences and accounts for other conditions the patient has as well as the likelihood of drug interactions. As a result, the systems gather significant clinical information and make evidence-supported recommendations to support the treatment choice. In some cases, AI will help doctors notice drug interactions among medications and advise selecting alternate treatments based on the patient's history (Bates et al., 2001). Table 4 shows AI applications in treatment planning.

*Table 4. AI Applications in Treatment Planning*

| Application | Description | Benefits |
|---|---|---|
| Personalized Treatment | Tailored therapies based on patient data | Increases treatment efficacy and patient satisfaction |
| Decision Support Systems | Optimizing treatment plans | Reduces errors and improves outcomes |

# 5. CHALLENGES AND LIMITATIONS

## 5.1 Data Privacy and Security Concerns

Even though AI can enhance healthcare, the main issue is safeguarding patient data. Since AI models use confidential patient data during training, there is a chance data could be stolen or accessed by someone unauthorized. Healthcare organizations in the U.S. must comply with strict data protection rules set by regulations like HIPAA (Edemekong et al., 2018).

a) Ethical Considerations: AI creates an ethical requirement in healthcare as well. Dealing with informed consent, who owns our data and algorithmic discrimination is necessary before using AI. A situation can arise if the AI systems receive biased inputs, causing them to create biased outcomes; this leads to unfair results for some patient populations (Obermeyer et al., 2019).
b) Standardization and Interoperability: There is a strong ethical reason to use AI in healthcare as well. AI should not be used without paying attention to issues of consent, who owns the data, and algorithmic bias. If the data used to train AI is biased, the outcomes will be biased as well which can negatively affect some patients (Obermeyer et al., 2019).

## 5.2 Integration with Existing Systems

A further issue is getting existing healthcare systems to work with the current AI technologies. There are a lot of legacy systems used by healthcare organizations and some of these cannot work well with new AI solutions. It often results in obstacles for moving data, disrupts the way things are done, and raises the expense of system upgrades (Bates et al., 2001).

a) Resistance to Change: The healthcare provider, the IT team, and the regulatory body must be involved for AI to succeed. AI is not always seen as completely positive support by healthcare experts who do not know enough about its benefits at the beginning. Because staff will be working with AI, they need to receive training and education. Bringing healthcare professionals into the development and execution of the process can spread positive changes in an organization.
b) Cost Implications: Adopting artificial intelligence costs money and it is even more costly for small healthcare practices. Getting an AI system involves financial costs, staff training, and making sure the infrastructure is ready. Though the costs upfront can be heavy, the advantages of AI make it worth spending, as it leads to improved efficiency, less error, and improved patient outcomes (Bates et al., 2001). Figure 4 shows the challenges in AI integration in healthcare.

*Figure 4. Challenges in AI Integration in Healthcare*

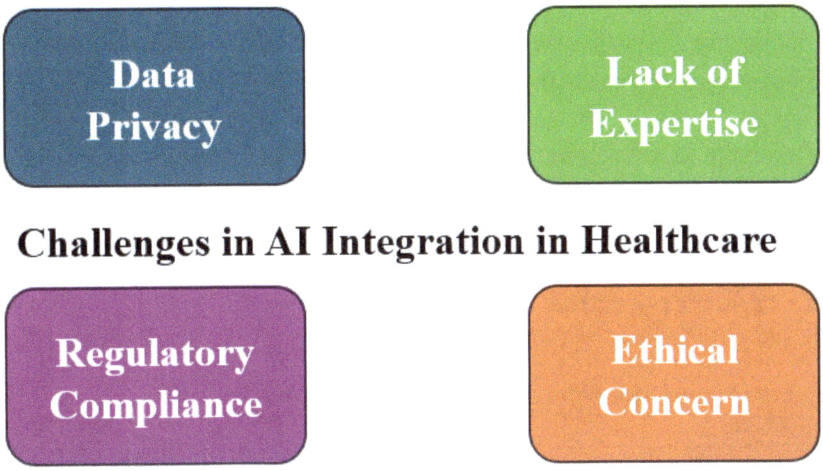


## 6. FUTURE TRENDS IN AI AND SMART HEALTHCARE

### 6.1 Advanced Technologies Shaping Healthcare

#### 6.1.1 Predictive Analytics

Gathering previous experience and applying statistical algorithms and machine learning helps predict future results; this is called 'Predictive Analytics'. Using predictive analytics, many risks for patients can be spotted and it becomes easier to detect disease outbreaks in advance and track the success of treatments.

a) Definition and Applications:- Information from electronic health records (EHRs), wearable devices, and other sources is used to analyze the data and forecast the patient's health outcome. In this example, a model would predict the chance of readmission after discharge by health professionals, so that special interventions could be put in place to avoid interruptions in patient care (Churpek et al., 2016). In population health management, predictive analytics are used to anticipate disease trends so that proper interventions can be created by public health officials.
b) Case Studies:- Healthcare has noted diabetes management through predictive analytics to be one of its leading examples. Dr. Harper and her team at the University of California, San Francisco built a model that can estimate wheth-

er someone is likely to get type 2 diabetes based on patient information, their habits, and clinical records. According to the model's accuracy of more than 80%, healthcare professionals can use preventive care for patients who are at high risk (Kahn et al., 2014).

An example is using predictive analytics to identify sepsis in patients. The researchers at JAMA discovered that using machine learning in an early warning system helped doctors predict sepsis in patients up to 12 hours ahead with very positive results and very low mortality (Henry et al., 2015). Figure 5 shows the predictive analytics workflow in healthcare.

*Figure 5. Predictive Analytics Workflow in Healthcare*

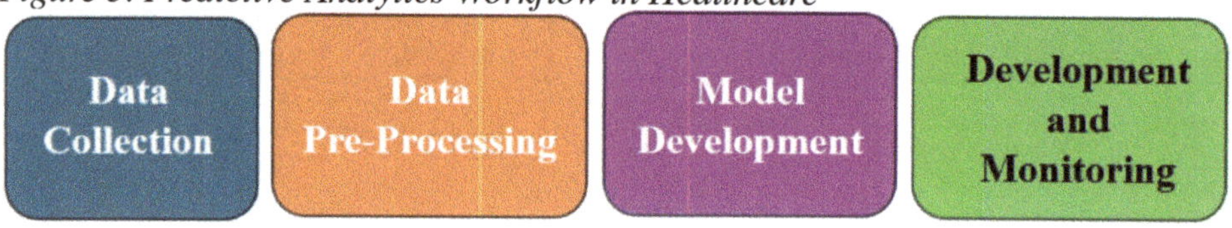


## 6.2 Personalized Medicine

Personalized (or precision) medicine focuses on delivering the right medical care at the right time for each patient. It encompasses various factors, including genes, environment, and lifestyle, to enhance the effectiveness of treatment and minimize negative effects.

a) Tailored Treatment Solutions:- Since personalized medicine is based on someone's genetic makeup, doctors can select treatments according to a patient's genes. As another example, for oncology, studying the genes from tumor cells can reveal mutations that feed into tumor progression. This enables doctors to use medicines targeting the needed mutations which may increase the chances of effective treatment. According to a historic trial, people with non-small cell lung cancer who used targeted therapy because of their genetic makeup lived longer than those treated with regular chemotherapy (Mok et al., 2009).
b) Role of Genomics:- With genomics, personalized medicine tries to identify the genetic factors in diseases. Due to Next Generation Sequencing (NGS), analyzing someone's genome is much easier and less expensive than before. Evidence from this information forms the foundation of treatments and ways to prevent infectious diseases. An example is that if women have the BRCA1 and BRCA2

gene mutation, they are identified for special screenings and measures to handle breast and ovarian cancer (King et al., 2003). Table 5 shows the applications of personalized medicine.

*Table 5. Applications of Personalized Medicine*

| Applications | Description | Benefits |
|---|---|---|
| Oncology | Targeted therapies based on tumor genetics | Improved treatment efficacy and reduced side effects |
| Cardiovascular Disease | Genetic risk assessment for heart disease | Tailored prevention strategies and interventions |
| Pharmacogenomics | Drug response prediction based on genetic factors | Enhanced drug efficacy and reduced adverse reactions |

## 6.3 AI-Powered Diagnostic Technologies

### 6.3.1 Machine Learning Algorithms

Progress in diagnosis is brought about by new machine learning developments. Using them, healthcare services can view and manage complicated medical information to reach a proper diagnosis (Ghai et al., 2022).

a) Deep Learning in Diagnostics:- Still, using deep learning in medical imaging has enjoyed a lot of success. CNN is normally used for image analysis, in short, for detecting tumors, fractures, and other anomalies. For example, a deep learning model matches the way dermatologists are able to identify skin lesions (Esteva et al., 2017).
b) Natural Language Processing for Diagnostics:- Also, some new diagnostic approaches involve using natural language processing (NLP). Unstructured clinical notes can be processed with NLP to help doctors make decisions for diagnosis. A good example is using NLP, which helps discover the main symptoms and prior health issues of patients from their records, allowing clinicians to make an accurate diagnosis (Iroju et al., 2015). Figure 6 shows AI-powered diagnostic technologies.

*Figure 6. AI-Powered Diagnostic Technologies*

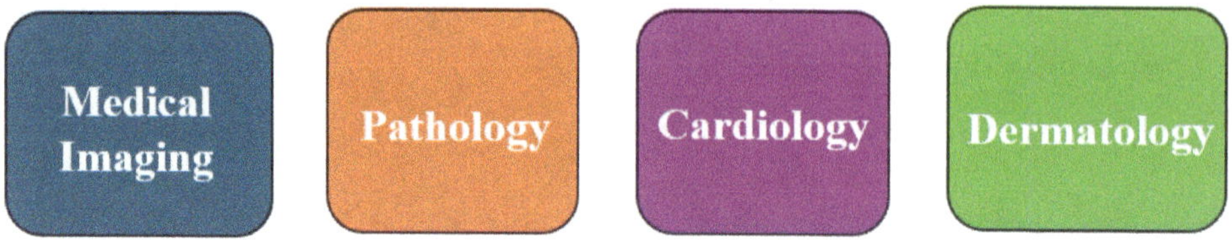


## 6.4 Innovations in Imaging and Diagnostic Tools

Imaging and diagnostic tools are being revolutionized by how accurately and efficiently the machine can find out about other things. Some of these developments come from using automated picture review and real-time diagnostic tools powered by AI algorithms.

a) Automated Image Analysis: AI helps make it possible for images to be analyzed quickly by machines, which supports faster and easier diagnosis. This information helps the radiologist notice the most important findings by spotting tumors or lesions. Mammogram analysis for breast cancer is carried out by some AI tools, and their accuracy matches that of seasoned radiologists (Yala et al., 2019).
b) Real-Time Diagnostic Support Systems: Getting information in real-time is now possible for doctors because of AI-powered diagnostic support systems. With patient data, these systems can offer up potential diagnoses and therapy choices according to recent clinical guidelines and scientific findings (Sandhu et al., 2025). Some clinical decision support systems, powered by AI, inform physicians about the chances of drugs interacting and advise on tests to be conducted due to a patient's symptoms (Bates et al., 2001). Table 6 shows innovations in imaging and diagnostic tools.

*Table 6. Innovations in Imaging and Diagnostic Tools*

| Innovation | Description | Benefits |
|---|---|---|
| Automated Image Analysis | AI tools for processing medical images | Reduces diagnosis time and improves accuracy |
| Real-Time Diagnostic Support | Immediate feedback for clinicians | Enhances decision-making and patient safety |

## 6.5 Robotic Surgery Systems

### 6.5.1 Current Developments in Robotics

Due to their cutting-edge design, medical robots now help during surgery with more precision and accurate control. The use of systems allows surgeons to do surgeries more accurately and this leads to better care for patients after their treatments. The da Vinci Surgical System is commonly used by doctors to perform prostate and uterus surgeries and other minimally invasive procedures, as it has shown superior results to traditional methods (Tomulescu, 2009).

a) Enhanced Precision and Control:- Surgical robots make it simple for medical staff to look at the surgical site from any direction while managing surgical tools with accuracy. Because mistakes in neurosurgery or cardiac surgery can be dangerous, using robotic systems gives doctors the greatest opportunity for precise handling. According to a report by (Autorino et al., 2013), robotic systems result in better medical outcomes and a decline in problems during surgery.

### 6.5.2 Future Prospects and Enhancements

Due to its ambition for improved robotic surgery, it ended up devoted to improving AI and machine learning. Advancements may be made through:

a) AI-Enhanced Surgical Assistance:- The information may be applied to direct robots during surgeries, with AI algorithms doing the job normally handled by people. Artificial intelligence can give immediate advice to surgeons during surgery and alert them to possible hazards thanks to past information (Huang et al., 2020).
b) Teleoperated Surgery: A new trend in surgery is using robotics to allow doctors to operate from afar, which means surgical services can reach communities that are hard to reach with healthcare (Soewu et al., 2025). Using this technology, doctors could manage patients outside their own country in places with better healthcare and better results (Haidegger et al., 2011). Figure 7 shows future trends in robotic surgery.

*Figure 7. Future Trends in Robotic Surgery*

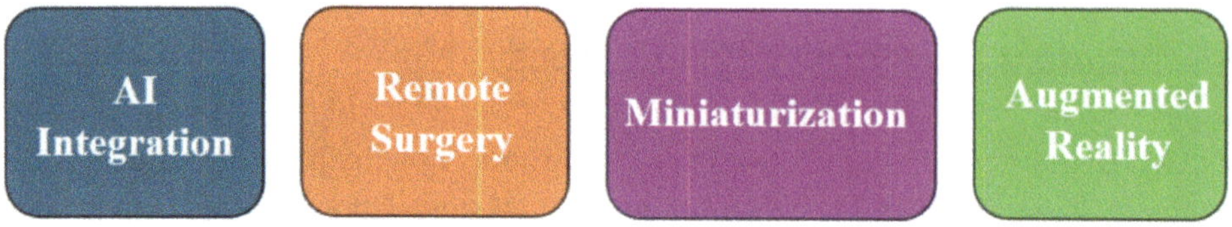


# 7. KEY DISRUPTIVE INNOVATIONS

## 7.1 Wearable Health Monitoring Devices

### 7.1.1 Types of Wearables

Today, many individuals are using wearable health monitors that help them see several health statistics as they happen. Such equipment can be sorted into different categories.

a) Smartwatches:- Apple Watch, Fitbit, and similar smartwatches have sensors that can observe your heart rate, hours of exercise, and sleep. Usually, these devices include features such as ECG (electrocardiogram) monitoring, as well as blood oxygen level monitoring, so users can learn about their heart health. As an example, the Apple Watch Series 4 lets users do an electrocardiogram on their wrist and provides useful information about atrial fibrillation (Bartschke et al, 2021).
b) Biosensors:- Specialized equipment for this is called a biosensor which can sense biological changes and provide real-time health feedback. They may be put on top of the skin or inserted into the body to keep track of health indicators. Continuous glucose monitors are biosensors used in diabetes management to always check blood glucose levels. There is evidence from prior studies that continuous glucose monitoring can help people with diabetes better control their blood sugar and have fewer low blood sugar episodes (Bergenstal et al., 2010).
c) Fitness Trackers:- Their main purpose is to follow physical activity and exercise, so fitness trackers focus on that. Most wearables register how many steps are taken, how many calories are burned, and how far the wearer moves. Devices like the Fitbit Charge and Garmin Vivo smart bands are highly valued by fitness enthusiasts because they help them learn how active they are every day. Table 7 shows the types of wearable health monitoring devices.

*Table 7. Types of Wearable Health Monitoring Devices*

| Device Type | Description | Key Features |
|---|---|---|
| Smartwatches | Multifunctional devices with health monitoring | Heart rate monitoring, ECG, sleep tracking |
| Biosensors | Devices that detect biological signals | Continuous glucose monitoring, hydration levels |
| Fitness Trackers | Devices focused on physical activity tracking | Step counting, calorie tracking, distance |

### 7.1.2 Impact on Patient Engagement and Monitoring

With self-powered and comfortable health monitors, patients can now closely monitor their health. With these, users receive instant information about their health which supports good hygiene habits.

a) Enhanced Patient Engagement:- Being able to wear a device promotes user involvement in health care and gives people chances to define what they want to achieve for their health. Nicely, an individual can create a daily step goal and receive reminders when getting close to that goal. Those who have wearable tech are more apt to keep up with a fitness routine and better health practices (Cadmus-Bertram et al., 2015).
b) Remote Monitoring and Data Collection:- Due to remote patient monitoring with wearables, clinicians gain useful information that helps guide their actions. With wearables, those with chronic diseases are able to keep providers informed about their vital signs and symptoms, so the provider may recommend actions early if required. It is especially valuable in taking care of people with hypertension, diabetes, and heart disease (Bashshur et al., 2014). Figure 8 shows various impacts of wearable devices on patient engagement.

*Figure 8. Impact of Wearable Devices on Patient Engagement*

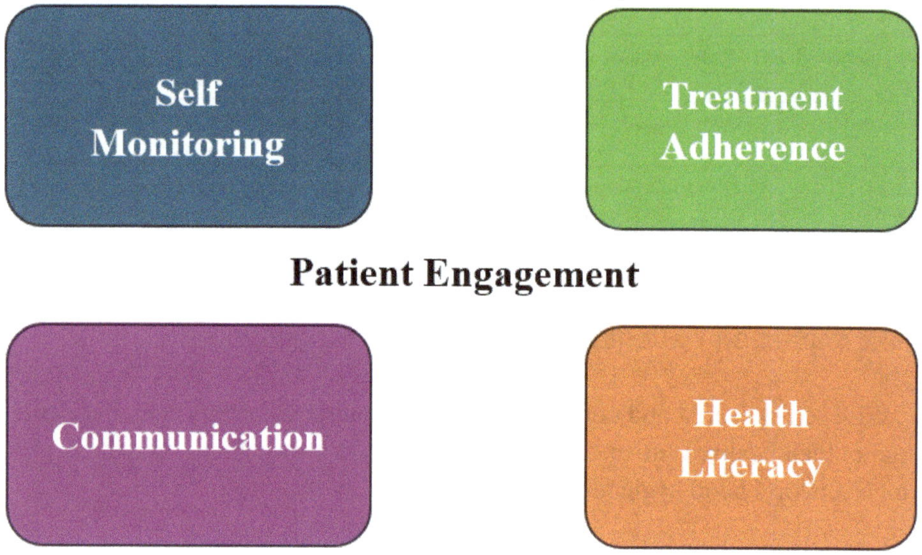


## 7.2 Internet of Medical Things (IoMT)

### 7.2.1 Definition and Key Components

IoMT includes all medical devices that are linked with each other using the internet for sharing healthcare information. Quality care is possible by using medical devices, smart equipment, remote systems for monitoring, and wearables.

a) Key Components:- The key components of IoMT include:
    - Using Sensors:- Several medical devices that can collect health data and share it with others in the system.
    - Data Analytics Platforms:- Software used to look at data from connected devices and make decisions based on insights.
    - Cloud Computing:- For instance, using the Cloud for securely managing and accessing your data remotely from any location.

### 7.2.2 Integration with 5G Technology

The healthcare industry is set for a revolution because IoMT connects with 5G, a fast and real-time data transfer technology.

a) Benefits of High-Speed Connectivity:- 5G is much faster for data transfer and takes less time per round-trip than any other wireless technology has before. Internet connectivity that is fast is necessary for the IoMT to pass data from connected devices to healthcare providers as quickly as needed. Consequently, the vital signs of patients can be watched in real-time, right away, so doctors can act promptly (Devi et al., 2023).
b) Real-Time Data Transmission:- In remote patient monitoring and telemedicine, real-time data transmission proves very effective. When used with 5G, medical professionals will instantly receive updates on patients and prompt action is possible when things change. Having this skill in emergencies can be particularly helpful since immediate information benefits patient care. To illustrate, surgeons performing remote surgeries can achieve low delay and operations can be carried out from anywhere with confidence and a high level of skill (Devi et al., 2023).

## 7.3 Remote Patient Care Services

### 7.3.1 Advancements in Telemedicine

When COVID-19 appeared, virtual healthcare started being used more in the medical field. Telemedicine consists of video consultations, remote monitoring, and mobile applications and also includes working with doctors in other countries using virtual platforms, amongst similar services.

a) Video Consultations:- With video information, patients have the chance to talk to healthcare providers at home. According to this strategy, access to care is improved, especially in places where it is limited and patients and caregivers are equally protected from contracting infections. It has been found through studies that telemedicine is just as effective for psychiatric and chronic disease treatment as face-to-face visits (Koonin et al., 2020).
b) Remote Monitoring:- Health technology allows healthcare providers to check patients' health data in locations other than the doctor's office. Patient health can be checked continuously using devices that include blood pressure monitors and pulse oximeters which send the data to the healthcare providers. Following this approach will make it possible to quickly see and manage any health concerns before they become serious (Bashshur et al., 2014).

### 7.3.2 Benefits and Challenges of Remote Care

Despite all the good points, remote patient care services are still not without their problems.

a) Benefits
- Reaching Patients at a Distance:- Obviously, remote services help patients who are far from traditional healthcare services to get treatment.
- Cost-Effectiveness:- Telemedicine often leads to lower healthcare bills because patients need fewer hospital visits or face-to-face appointments.
- Improved Patient Satisfaction:- Convenient and flexible remote consultations lead to more happiness and satisfaction on the part of patients (Bashshur et al., 2014).

b) Challenges
- Technology Barriers:- Even so, a lack of money or internet access means that some patients cannot use telemedicine services.
- Regulatory and Reimbursement Issues:- Not having the same healthcare regulations and reimbursement policies for people receiving telemedicine is unfortunately rather common.
- Data Security Concerns:- Data security and privacy issues may occur when health information is shared over the Internet (Koonin et al., 2020). Table 8 shows the benefits and challenges of remote patient care services.

*Table 8. Benefits and Challenges of Remote Patient Care Services*

| **Benefits** | **Description** |
|---|---|
| Increased Access to Care | Bridges gaps for patients in remote areas |
| Cost-Effectiveness | Reduces the need for in-person visits |
| Improved Patient Satisfaction | Enhances convenience and flexibility |
| Challenge | Description |
| Technology Barriers | Limited access to technology for some patients |
| Regulatory Issues | Variability in telemedicine regulations |
| Data Security Concerns | Risks associated with transmitting sensitive data |

# 8. DATA PROTECTION AND ETHICAL CONSIDERATIONS

## 8.1 Federated Learning as a Data Protection Method

### 8.1.1 Concept and Mechanism

Federated learning is a recent method in machine learning that allows various organizations to collaboratively prepare one model by jointly learning and everyone keeps their information securely private. Federated learning works by sending patient data to a server instead of the gradients which are made by each institution training on its own dataset. An advantage is keeping the raw data at the institution which helps maintain data privacy and security (McMahan et al., 2017). Figure 9 shows the process of federated learning process.

*Figure 9. Federated Learning Process*

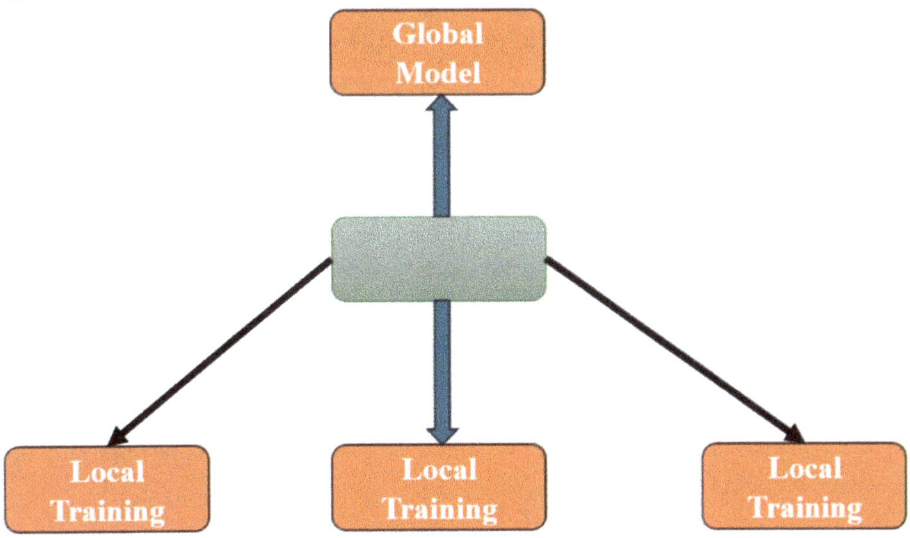


## 8.2 Explainable AI (XAI)

### 8.2.1 Importance of Transparency in AI Decision-Making

Techniques and methods to help people understand the outputs from AI systems (famously referred to as XAI or explainable AI). It is very important for healthcare to be transparent since the impact of some decisions can be significant for patients.

When making healthcare decisions, professionals need to rely on AI systems and should know the explanation for the recommendations (Lipton, 2018).

a) Building Trust:- AI decision-making makes healthcare providers and patients more trustful. Having this information expressed in human language helps clinicians recognize the reasoning behind an AI recommendation and accept and apply it more confidently. It is necessary to do this to bring AI into clinical use effectively (Miller, 2019).
    b. Regulatory Compliance:- Because of this, regulatory groups are now insisting more strongly that AI systems be open and understandable. According to proposed EU regulations, AI-driven decisions should not be made without clear prerequisites and a clear explanation; this is especially important in essential areas such as healthcare (Act, 2021).

### 8.2.2 Techniques for Implementing XAI

Various measures can be used to make AI explainable in healthcare situations.

a) Model-Agnostic Methods:- LIME and SHAP are example algorithms that explain how any machine learning algorithm made its decision. With these techniques, healthcare providers can examine the effect that every feature has on the result to understand which aspects matter in the decision-making process (Ribeiro et al., 2016; Lundberg & Lee, 2017).
b) Interpretable Models:- Explainability can be improved by turning to methods such as decision trees or linear regression, which are naturally interpretable. The upside is that these models provide a clear view of the way features help in the prediction, which benefits clinicians in better grasping how decisions are made (Doshi-Velez & Kim, 2017). Table 9 shows techniques for implementing explainable AI.

*Table 9. Techniques for Implementing Explainable AI*

| Techniques | Description | Benefits |
|---|---|---|
| LIME | Local Interpretable Model-agnostic Explanations | Provides insights into individual predictions |
| SHAP | Shapley Additive Explanations | Quantifies feature contributions to predictions |
| Interpretable Models | Decision trees, linear regression | Offers straightforward insights into decision-making |

## 8.3 Ethical Standards and Security Requirements

### 8.3.1 Framework for Responsible AI Deployment

A healthcare AI system should maintain ethical standards and have secure features while it is deployed. That's why this framework must include these major components.

a) Ethical Guidelines:- Regulations are needed for both making and rolling out AI systems, so they are used responsibly. These guidelines must always put patient well-being, informed agreement, and equity in getting AI-related healthcare treatments first. Patients, healthcare providers, and ethicists are among those who should take part in developing detailed ethical guidelines, so it's important for organizations to use AI to do so (Jobin et al., 2019).
b) Risk Assessment:- By the very nature of AI, it is essential to do a thorough risk analysis to identify possible ethical and security risks. Because of these reasons, this process needs to address AI's impact on patient safety, data privacy, and possible biases in AI decisions. Even so, companies can take steps to prevent risks that AI systems may cause and protect the trust in their applications (Binns, 2018).
c) Continuous Monitoring and Evaluation:- A way to regularly observe and evaluate AI systems is required to check if they follow ethical rules and security measures. Evaluating AI applications, collecting user feedback, and making improvements to maintain transparency are very important (Garcia-Gonzalez et al., 2022). Figure 10 shows the framework for responsible AI deployment.

*Figure 10. Framework for Responsible AI Deployment*

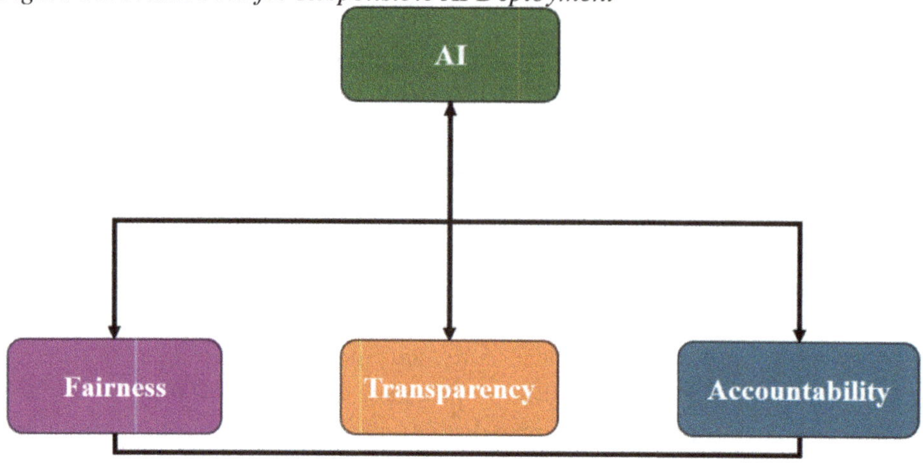


## 9. DIGITAL TWIN MODELING IN HEALTHCARE

### 9.1 Overview of Digital Twin Technology

A digital twin is what happens when a real-world item, system, or process gets represented by a virtual version. Real-time information about the physical building is fed into the digital version, so it can be looked at, studied, and tried out in various scenarios. Originally, this approach started in manufacturing and engineering, and only recently has it been picked up by healthcare to benefit patients and reduce running expenses (Grieves, 2014).

The healthcare system, patients, and medical devices can all be represented by a digital twin. Digital twins gather information from several sources including medical records, devices on the body, and medical scans to assess the patient's condition and see what different treatment plans might achieve (Patel & Misra, 2020).

### 9.2 Applications of Digital Twin in Healthcare

Digital twin technology has a wide range of applications in healthcare, including:

a) Patient Monitoring and Management:- Through digital twins, patient models can be set up to monitor the health of a patient. As an example, digital twins for chronic heart patients could mix patients' wearable gadget information, lab findings, and medical history to understand the patient's condition. Because of this, records are actively managed, and troublesome situations can be dealt with on time to avoid complications (Hassani et al., 2022).

b) Surgical Planning and Simulation:- Surgeons can conduct surgery exercises in the digital twin tool before performing in the operating room on a patient. Surgeons gain practice through practicing digital replicas of patients' anatomies based on medical images and this experience improves their surgical method. This application is especially helpful in complicated surgeries, since being precise matters a lot (Ding et al., 2024).

c) Drug Development and Testing:- Developing drugs could use digital twins since they could be tested with different patients' biological systems. To judge how a drug may work and its safety, researchers can use digital twin technology in three dimensions which helps speed up the development of new drugs (Patel & Misra, 2020). Table 10 shows the applications of digital twin technology in healthcare.

*Table 10. Applications of Digital Twin Technology in Healthcare*

| Application | Description | Benefits |
|---|---|---|
| Patient Monitoring | Real-time health monitoring through digital twins | Proactive management and timely interventions |
| Surgical Planning | Simulation of surgical procedures | Improved precision and outcomes |
| Drug Development | Modeling drug interactions within a digital twin | Accelerated drug development and testing |

## 9.3 Personalized Healthcare Delivery

### 9.3.1 Role in Treatment Planning

When providers have a detailed picture of a patient's health, digital twins allow them to plan treatment that best fits the patient's needs. Their clinical worth is derived from their ability to use data from various places and aid physicians in selecting the appropriate care for each patient since each patient requires a different treatment (Sandhu et al., 2024).

a) Tailored Treatment Strategies: In oncology, a digital twin might hold the cancer patient's genomic information, details on their tumor, and the kinds of treatment they have received and simulate responses to each therapy. This means that treatment can be developed specifically for a patient by an oncologist (Patel & Misra, 2020).

b) Predictive Analytics for Treatment Outcomes:- More than likely, digital twins use past data and current information to expect the outcome of treatment in advance. An analysis of others' health outcomes from a particular treatment can guidance when choosing the best way to proceed with a patient (Hassani et al., 2022).

## 10. CONCLUSION

### 10.1 Summary of Key Findings

Healthcare can be changed by AI through better patient treatment, improved ways of working, and increased chances of good results. The exploration produced the following key discoveries:

a) Diagnosis:- AI helps enhance methods for diagnosis, making treatment plans, and organizing patient information with machine learning, text analysis, and simulators of digital twins. Technology allows medical experts to rely on lots of data to determine an accurate diagnosis and design a suitable treatment plan (Patel & Misra, 2020).
b) Digital Twin Modeling:- In healthcare, a digital twin is made to track patient health and give each person improved personalized care. It assists in managing chronic illnesses ahead of time and planning successful surgeries with simulation (Hassani et al. 2022).
c) Data Protection and Ethical Considerations:- Many are concerned about using AI in healthcare because it raises issues of privacy, data accuracy, security, and ethics. Patient trust can be restored by using responsible AI technologies such as explainable AI and federated learning (Jobin et al., 2019).
d) Infrastructure and Interoperability:- The infrastructure for AI in healthcare must be safe, have enough computing power, store data securely and connect different healthcare platforms to successfully handle requests and give results. So, having these parts is important to allow the smooth sharing of data and the use of AI tools within clinical tasks (Devi et al., 2023).

### 10.2 Implications for Healthcare Operators and Policymakers

Healthcare operators and policymakers can learn a lot from what was uncovered in this study.

a) Investment in Technology:- Therefore, the benefits of technology and infrastructure in healthcare organizations are now more crucial, simply because the healthcare sector cannot change much with the market but is vital for all people. Advanced systems for handling data, system resources, and networks that are safe for AI applications are part of big data integration (Patel & Misra, 2020).
b) Training and Education:- They must always upgrade their skills and knowledge through training and education to apply AI in healthcare correctly. Healthcare workforce policymakers should have opportunities for education and learning in AI (Bates et al., 2001).
c) Regulatory Frameworks:- Regulations should be developed by Residential authorities for AI projects that touch on important aspects like data privacy, security, and ethics. Taking care of the usage of AI, and requiring it to follow existing laws, boosts the trust of the public in AI (Jobin et al., 2019).
d) Equity in Healthcare:- Ensuring AI technologies help every group of patients, particularly those who are unrepresented, must be one of the biggest goals in using them. To this day, policymakers should support using AI to reduce unequal health care and make it more accessible (Garcia-Gonzalez et al., 2022). Table 11 shows the implications for healthcare operators and policymakers

*Table 11. Implications for Healthcare Operators and Policymakers*

| Implication | Description | Action Required |
|---|---|---|
| Investment in Technology | Prioritize investments in AI technologies | Allocate resources for infrastructure and tools |
| Training and Education | Continuous education for healthcare professionals | Support AI literacy initiatives |
| Regulatory Frameworks | Establish clear guidelines for AI deployment | Develop policies addressing data privacy and ethics |
| Equity in Healthcare | Ensure accessibility of AI technologies | Promote initiatives to address health disparities |

By including AI in healthcare, it is possible to improve patient care, organize healthcare operations, and address gaps in health care. Still, healthcare operators and policymakers can use AI by investing in new technologies, employee education, and reforming regulations. Additional study and research will be necessary to guide AI technology to bring better outcomes to healthcare.

## REFERENCES


Autorino, R., Kaouk, J. H., Stolzenburg, J. U., Gill, I. S., Mottrie, A., Tewari, A., & Cadeddu, J. A. (2013). Current status and future directions of robotic single-site surgery: A systematic review. *European Urology*, *63*(2), 266–280.

Bartschke, A., Börner, Y., & Thun, S. (2021). Accessing the ECG data of the apple watch and accomplishing interoperability through FHIR. In German Medical Data Sciences: Bringing Data to Life (pp. 245-250). IOS Press.

Bashshur, R. L., Shannon, G. W., Smith, B. R., Alverson, D. C., Antoniotti, N., Barsan, W. G., & Yellowlees, P. (2014). The empirical foundations of telemedicine interventions for chronic disease management. *Telemedicine Journal and e-Health*, *20*(9), 769–800.

Bates, D. W., Cohen, M., Leape, L. L., Overhage, J. M., Shabot, M. M., & Sheridan, T. (2001). Reducing the frequency of errors in medicine using information technology. *Journal of the American Medical Informatics Association : JAMIA*, *8*(4), 299–308.

Bergenstal, R. M., Tamborlane, W. V., Ahmann, A., Buse, J. B., Dailey, G., Davis, S. N., & Wood, M. A. (2010). Effectiveness of sensor-augmented insulin-pump therapy in type 1 diabetes. *The New England Journal of Medicine*, *363*(4), 311–320.

Binns, R. (2018, January). Fairness in machine learning: Lessons from political philosophy. In *Conference on Fairness, Accountability and Transparency* (pp. 149-159). PMLR.

Cadmus-Bertram, L. A., Marcus, B. H., Patterson, R. E., Parker, B. A., & Morey, B. L. (2015). Randomized trial of a Fitbit-based physical activity intervention for women. *American Journal of Preventive Medicine*, *49*(3), 414–418.

Churpek, M. M., Adhikari, R., & Edelson, D. P. (2016). The value of vital sign trends for detecting clinical deterioration on the wards. *Resuscitation*, *102*, 1–5.

Collins, F. S., & Varmus, H. (2015). A new initiative on precision medicine. *The New England Journal of Medicine*, *372*(9), 793–795.

Cruz-Roa, A., Basavanhally, A., González, F., Gilmore, H., Feldman, M., Ganesan, S., & Madabhushi, A. (2014, March). Automatic detection of invasive ductal carcinoma in whole slide images with convolutional neural networks. In *Medical Imaging 2014: Digital pathology* (Vol. 9041, p. 904103). SPIE.

Devi, D. H., Duraisamy, K., Armghan, A., Alsharari, M., Aliqab, K., Sorathiya, V., & Rashid, N. (2023). 5G technology in healthcare and wearable devices: A review. *Sensors (Basel)*, *23*(5), 2519.

Devi, R. D. H., Naresh, R., & Kumar, C. V. (2023). Advanced 5G Technology in Healthcare Field. *Resource Management in Advanced Wireless Networks*, *227*, 227.

Ding, H., Seenivasan, L., Killeen, B. D., Cho, S. M., & Unberath, M. (2024). Digital twins as a unifying framework for surgical data science: The enabling role of geometric scene understanding. *Artificial Intelligence Surgery*, *4*(3), 109–138.

Doshi-Velez, F., & Kim, B. (2017). Towards a rigorous science of interpretable machine learning. arXiv preprint arXiv:1702.08608.

Edemekong, P. F., Annamaraju, P., & Haydel, M. J. (2018). Health insurance portability and accountability act.

Esteva, A., Kuprel, B., Novoa, R. A., Ko, J., Swetter, S. M., Blau, H. M., & Thrun, S. (2017). Dermatologist-level classification of skin cancer with deep neural networks. *Nature*, *542*(7639), 115–118.

Faiz, M., Sandhu, R., Akbar, M., Shaikh, A. A., Bhasin, C., & Fatima, N. (2023). Machine Learning Techniques in Wireless Sensor Networks: Algorithms Strategies and Applications. *International Journal of Intelligent Systems and Applications in Engineering*, *11*(9s), 685–694.

Garcia-Gonzalez, A., Fuentes-Aguilar, R. Q., Salgado, I., & Chairez, I. (2022). A review on the application of autonomous and intelligent robotic devices in medical rehabilitation. *Journal of the Brazilian Society of Mechanical Sciences and Engineering*, *44*(9), 393.

Ghai, D., Tripathi, S. L., Saxena, S., Chanda, M., & Alazab, M. (Eds.). (2022). *Machine learning algorithms for signal and image processing*. John Wiley & Sons.

Grieves, M. (2014). Digital twin: manufacturing excellence through virtual factory replication. White paper, 1(2014), 1-7.

Haidegger, T., Sándor, J., & Benyó, Z. (2011). Surgery in space: The future of robotic telesurgery. *Surgical Endoscopy*, *25*, 681–690.

Hassani, H., Huang, X., & MacFeely, S. (2022). Impactful digital twin in the healthcare revolution. *Big Data and Cognitive Computing*, *6*(3), 83.

Hastie, T. (2009). The elements of statistical learning: data mining, inference, and prediction.

Henry, K. E., Hager, D. N., Pronovost, P. J., & Saria, S. (2015). A targeted real-time early warning score (TREWScore) for septic shock. Science Translational Medicine, 7(299), 299ra122-299ra122.

Huang, J., Li, Y., & Huang, L. (2020). Spine surgical robotics: Review of the current application and disadvantages for future perspectives. *Journal of Robotic Surgery*, *14*(1), 11–16.

Iroju, O. G., & Olaleke, J. O. (2015). A systematic review of natural language processing in healthcare. *International Journal of Information Technology and Computer Science*, *8*(8), 44–50.

Jobin, A., Ienca, M., & Vayena, E. (2019). The global landscape of AI ethics guidelines. *Nature Machine Intelligence*, *1*(9), 389–399.

Jordan, M. I., & Mitchell, T. M. (2015). Machine learning: Trends, perspectives, and prospects. *Science*, *349*(6245), 255–260.

Kahn, R., & Davidson, M. B. (2014). The reality of type 2 diabetes prevention. *Diabetes Care*, *37*(4), 943–949.

Keramatfar, A., & Amirkhani, H. (2019). Bibliometrics of sentiment analysis literature. *Journal of Information Science*, *45*(1), 3–15.

Koonin, L. M. (2020). Trends in the use of telehealth during the emergence of the COVID-19 pandemic—United States, January–March 2020. *MMWR. Morbidity and Mortality Weekly Report*, 69.

Kourou, K., Exarchos, T. P., Exarchos, K. P., Karamouzis, M. V., & Fotiadis, D. I. (2015). Machine learning applications in cancer prognosis and prediction. *Computational and Structural Biotechnology Journal*, *13*, 8–17.

Lakhani, P. (2017). Deep convolutional neural networks for endotracheal tube position and X-ray image classification: Challenges and opportunities. *Journal of Digital Imaging*, *30*, 460–468.

Lipton, Z. C. (2018). The mythos of model interpretability: In machine learning, the concept of interpretability is both important and slippery. *Queue*, *16*(3), 31–57.

Lundberg, S. M., & Lee, S. I. (2017). A unified approach to interpreting model predictions. *Advances in Neural Information Processing Systems*, 30.

McMahan, B., Moore, E., Ramage, D., Hampson, S., & Arcas, B. A. (2017, April). Communication-efficient learning of deep networks from decentralized data. In *Artificial Intelligence and Statistics* (pp. 1273–1282). PMLR.

Obermeyer, Z., Powers, B., Vogeli, C., & Mullainathan, S. (2019). Dissecting racial bias in an algorithm used to manage the health of populations. *Science, 366*(6464), 447–453.

Patel, V. M., & Misra, S. (2020). Artificial intelligence in healthcare: Past present and future. *Journal of Medical Systems, 44*(8), 1–7.

Petticrew, M., & Roberts, H. (2008). *Systematic reviews in the social sciences: A practical guide*. John Wiley & Sons.

Russell, S. J., & Norvig, P. (2016). *Artificial intelligence: a modern approach*. Pearson.

Sandhu, R., Channi, H. K., Ghai, D., & Kaur, M. (2025). Zero-Trust Approach for Secure Healthcare System. In *Zero-Trust Learning* (pp. 387–409). Apple Academic Press.

Sandhu, R., Ghai, D., Tripathi, S. L., Kaur, R., Rawal, K., & Dhir, K. (2024). Machine learning for cognitive treatment planning in patients with neurodisorder and trauma injuries. In *Computational Intelligence and Deep Learning Methods for Neuro-rehabilitation Applications* (pp. 165–193). Academic Press.

Shortliffe, E. H. (1974, January). A rule-based computer program for advising physicians regarding antimicrobial therapy selection. In *Proceedings of the 1974 Annual ACM Conference-Volume 2* (pp. 739-739).

Singhal, S., & Carlton, S. (2019). The era of exponential improvement in healthcare. McKinsey & Company, 1-16.

Soewu, T., Kaur, H., Sandhu, R., Soni, A., Ghai, D., Dhir, K., & Tripathi, S. L. (2025). Machine learning and deep learning for cancer diagnosis. In *Rehabilitation Robotics and Healthcare Devices* (pp. 83–129). Academic Press.

Sutton, R. S., & Barto, A. G. (1998). *No. 1* (Vol. 1). Reinforcement learning: An introduction. MIT press.

Tomulescu, V. (2009). First year experience of robotic-assisted laparoscopic surgery with 153 cases in a General Surgery Department: Indications technique and results. *Chirurgia*, 2.

Topol, E. (2019). *Deep medicine: how artificial intelligence can make healthcare human again*.

Yala, A., Schuster, T., Miles, R., Barzilay, R., & Lehman, C. (2019). A deep learning model to triage screening mammograms: A simulation study. *Radiology, 293*(1), 38–46.

# Compilation of References


Abbas, A. A., Hansen, B. A., Koesmahargyo, V. A. X., Yadav, V. A., Rosenfield, P. A., Patil, O. A., Dockendorf, M. A., Moyer, M. A., Shipley, L. A., Perez-Rodriguez, M. A., & Galatzer-Levy, I. A. X. (2022). Facial and vocal markers of schizophrenia measured using remote smartphone assessments: Observational study. *JMIR Formative Research*, *6*(1), e26276. Advance online publication. DOI: 10.2196/26276 PMID: 35060906

AbdelAziz, N. M., Fouad, G. A., Al-Saeed, S., & Fawzy, A. M. (2025). Deep Q-Network (DQN) Model for Disease Prediction Using Electronic Health Records (EHRs). *Sci*, *7*(1), 1. Advance online publication. DOI: 10.3390/sci7010014

Abdellatif, A. A., Mhaisen, N., Chkirbene, Z., Mohamed, A., Erbad, A., & Guizani, M. (2021). Reinforcement learning for intelligent healthcare systems: A comprehensive survey. *arXiv preprint arXiv:2108.04087.*

Abell, B., Naicker, S., Rodwell, D., Donovan, T., Tariq, A., Baysari, M., Blythe, R., Parsons, R., & McPhail, S. M. (2023). Identifying barriers and facilitators to successful implementation of computerized clinical decision support systems in hospitals: A NASSS framework-informed scoping review. *Implementation Science : IS*, *18*(1), 32.

Abirami, M. S. (2023, October). AI clinical decision support system (AI-CDSS) for cardiovascular diseases. In *2023 International Conference on Computer Science and Emerging Technologies (CSET)* (pp. 1-7). IEEE.

Adeoye, S., & Adams, R. (2024). Leveraging Artificial Intelligence for Predictive Healthcare: A Data-Driven Approach to Early Diagnosis and Personalized Treatment. *Cogniz. J. Multidiscip. Stud*, *4*, 80–97.

Agamah, F. E., Mazandu, G. K., Hassan, R., Bope, C. D., Thomford, N. E., Ghansah, A., & Chimusa, E. R. (2020). Computational/in silico methods in drug target and lead prediction. *Briefings in Bioinformatics*, *21*(5), 1663–1675. DOI: 10.1093/bib/bbz103 PMID: 31711157

Agatonovic-Kustrin, S., & Beresford, R. (2000). Basic concepts of artificial neural network (ANN) modeling and its application in pharmaceutical research. *Journal of Pharmaceutical and Biomedical Analysis*, *22*(5), 717–727.

Agboklu, M. (2024). The impact of Artificial Intelligence on innovative nanotechnologies for Advanced Medical diagnosis. *Journal of Nanotechnology Research*, *6*, 1–5.

Agboklu, M., Adrah, F. A., & Agbenyo, P. M. (2024). Hope Nyavor. From bits to atoms: Machine learning and nanotechnology for Cancer Therapy. *Journal of Nanotechnology Research*, *6*, 16–26.

Ahmadi, A. (2024). Digital health transformation: Leveraging AI for monitoring and disease management. [IJBLS]. *International Journal of BioLife Sciences*, *3*(1), 10–24.

Ahmed, Z., Mohamed, K., Zeeshan, S., & Dong, X. (2020). Artificial Intelligence with Multi-functional Machine Learning Platform Development for Better Healthcare and Precision Medicine. *Database : The Journal of Biological Databases and Curation*, *2020*, baaa010. PMID: 32185396

Ahsan, M., & Damaševičius, R. (2024, October). AI-Based Decision Support Systems to Improve Diagnostic Accuracy via Medical Imaging. In International Conference on Advanced Research in Technologies, Information, Innovation and Sustainability (pp. 197-208). Cham: Springer Nature Switzerland.

Alabi, M. (2025). *Reinforcement Learning: Applications in Gaming*. Robotics, and Real-World Decision-Making.

Alam, M. A., Nabil, A. R., Uddin, M. M., Sarker, M. T. H., & Mahmud, S. (2024). The Role of Predictive Analytics in Early Disease Detection: A Data-Driven Approach to Preventive Healthcare. *Frontiers in Applied Engineering and Technology*, *1*(01), 105–123.

Al-Dmour, R., Al-Dmour, H., Basheer Amin, E., & Al-Dmour, A. (2025). Impact of AI and big data analytics on healthcare outcomes: An empirical study in Jordanian healthcare institutions. *Digital Health*, *11*, 20552076241311052.

Aldoseri, A., Al-Khalifa, K. N., & Hamouda, A. M. (2023). Re-thinking data strategy and integration for artificial intelligence: Concepts, opportunities, and challenges. *Applied Sciences (Basel, Switzerland)*, *13*(12), 7082.

Ali, O., Abdelbaki, W., Shrestha, A., Elbasi, E., Alryalat, M. A. A., & Dwivedi, Y. K. (2023). A systematic literature review of artificial intelligence in the healthcare sector: Benefits, challenges, methodologies, and functionalities. *Journal of Innovation & Knowledge*, *8*(1), 100333.

Al-Jarrah, O. Y., Yoo, P. D., Muhaidat, S., Karagiannidis, G. K., & Taha, K. (2015). Efficient machine learning for big data: A review. *Big Data Research*, *2*(3), 87–93. DOI: 10.1016/j.bdr.2015.04.001

Almadani, B., Kaisar, H., Thoker, I. R., & Aliyu, F. (2025). A Systematic Survey of Distributed Decision Support Systems in Healthcare. *Systems*, *13*(3), 157.

Amann, J., Blasimme, A., Vayena, E., Frey, D., & Madai, V. I., & Precise4Q consortium. (2020). Explainability for artificial intelligence in healthcare: A multidisciplinary perspective. *BMC Medical Informatics and Decision Making*, *20*(1), 310.

Amarasingham, R., Patzer, R. E., Huesch, M., Nguyen, N. Q., & Xie, B. (2014). Implementing electronic health care predictive analytics: Considerations and challenges. *Health Affairs*, *33*(7), 1148–1154.

Amato, F., López, A., Peña-Méndez, E. M., Vaňhara, P., Hampl, A., & Havel, J. (2013). Artificial neural networks in medical diagnosis. *Journal of Applied Biomedicine*, *11*(2), 47–58. DOI: 10.2478/v10136-012-0031-x

Ambhika, C., Gayathri, S., & Sheena, B. G. (2024, August). Enhancing predictive modeling in high dimensional data using hybrid feature selection. In 2024 5th International Conference on Electronics and Sustainable Communication Systems (ICESC) (pp. 873-879). IEEE.

Amiri, Z. (2024). Leveraging AI-Enabled Information Systems for Healthcare Management. *Journal of Computer Information Systems*, 1–28.

Anagnostou, T., Remzi, M., Lykourinas, M., & Djavan, B. (2003). Artificial neural networks for decision-making in urologic oncology. *European Urology*, *43*(6), 596–603. DOI: 10.1016/S0302-2838(03)00165-5 PMID: 12767358

Anderson, J., & Raine, L. (2018). Artificial intelligence and the future of humans. Pew Research Center. https://www.pewresearch.org/internet/2018/12/10/artificial-intelligence-and-the-future-of-humans/

Annamalai, M., Mittal, T., Sunkara, K. C., Pandey, H., Jadhav, G., & Nemane, V. (2024, December). Revolutionizing Medical Diagnostics with Transparent AI-Driven Decision Support Systems. In 2024 4th International Conference on Mobile Networks and Wireless Communications (ICMNWC) (pp. 1-7). IEEE.

Ansari, A., Kaur, B., Rakhra, M., Singh, A., & Singh, D. (2022, December). Handwritten text recognition using deep learning algorithms. In *2022 4th International Conference on Artificial Intelligence and Speech Technology (AIST)* (pp. 1-6). IEEE.

Antunes, R. S., André da Costa, C., Küderle, A., Yari, I. A., & Eskofier, B. (2022). Federated learning for healthcare: Systematic review and architecture proposal. [TIST]. *ACM Transactions on Intelligent Systems and Technology*, *13*(4), 1–23.

Aouedi, O., Sacco, A., Piamrat, K., & Marchetto, G. (2022). Handling privacy-sensitive medical data with federated learning: Challenges and future directions. *IEEE Journal of Biomedical and Health Informatics*, *27*(2), 790–803.

Armeni, P., & Polat, I., De Rossi Leonardo Maria and Diaferia, L., Meregalli, S., & Gatti, A. (2022). Digital Twins in healthcare: Is it the beginning of a New Era of evidence-based medicine? A critical review. *Journal of Personalized Medicine*, *12*(8), 1255.

Arulkumaran, K., Deisenroth, M. P., Brundage, M., & Bharath, A. A. (2017). Deep reinforcement learning: A brief survey. *IEEE Signal Processing Magazine*, *34*(6), 26–38.

Asan, O., Bayrak, A. E., & Choudhury, A. (2020). Artificial intelligence and human trust in healthcare: Focus on clinicians. *Journal of Medical Internet Research*, *22*(6), e15154.

Ashrafian, H., Darzi, A., & Athanasiou, T. (2015). A review of clinical applications of artificial neural networks. *The Journal of Surgical Research*, *192*(1), 164–170. DOI: 10.1016/j.jss.2014.06.022

Asiri, M. A., Almutairi, A. D., Ozam, T. S., Al Ahmari, R. Y., Alhazmi, S. M., Almoudhi, A. A., & Alqahtani, N. M. (2024). AI-Driven Decision Support Systems: Transforming Hospital Management Strategies. [JICRCR]. *Journal of International Crisis & Risk Communication Research*, *7*(3).

Attiwi, M. H., Almass, J. O., Roukiah, A. S. F., Shakir, K. H., Asaad, L. I., Alabdeli, H., & Hassan, E. (2024, November). Unremarkable AI: Intelligent Decision Support in Critical Clinical Decision-Making. In 2024 International Conference on IoT, Communication and Automation Technology (ICICAT) (pp. 610-616). IEEE.

Autorino, R., Kaouk, J. H., Stolzenburg, J. U., Gill, I. S., Mottrie, A., Tewari, A., & Cadeddu, J. A. (2013). Current status and future directions of robotic single-site surgery: A systematic review. *European Urology*, *63*(2), 266–280.

Avanzo, M., Stancanello, J., Pirrone, G., Drigo, A., & Retico, A. (2024). The evolution of artificial intelligence in medical imaging: From computer science to machine and deep learning. *Cancers (Basel), 16*(21), 3702.

Babu Vimala, B., Srinivasan, S., & Mathivanan, S. K., Mahalakshmi, Jayagopal, P., & Dalu, G. T. (2023). Detection and classification of brain tumor using hybrid deep learning models. *Scientific Reports, 13*(1), 23029. PMID: 38155247

Bajwa, J., Munir, U., Nori, A., & Williams, B. (2021). Artificial intelligence in healthcare: Transforming the practice of medicine. *Future Healthcare Journal, 8*(2), e188–e194. DOI: 10.7861/fhj.2021-0095 PMID: 34286183

Ball, R. A., & Dal Pan, G. (2022). "Artificial intelligence" for pharmacovigilance: Ready for prime time? *Drug Safety, 45*(5), 429–438. DOI: 10.1007/s40264-022-01157-4 PMID: 35579808

Banabilah, S., Aloqaily, M., Alsayed, E., Malik, N., & Jararweh, Y. (2022). Federated learning review: Fundamentals, enabling technologies, and future applications. *Information Processing & Management, 59*(6), 103061.

Bandaru, V. K. R., Gondi, D. S., Gondi, K., & Indugu, V. V. R. (2021). Reinforcement Learning for Optimizing Personalized Treatment Plans in Oncology. *CIT. Journal of Computing and Information Technology, 1*(1).

Bansal, M., Goyal, A., & Choudhary, A. (2022). A comparative analysis of K-nearest neighbor, genetic, support vector machine, decision tree, and long short term memory algorithms in machine learning. *Decision Analytics Journal, 3*, 100071.

Banumathi, K., Venkatesan, L., Benjamin, L. S., Vijayalakshmi, K., Satchi, N. S., & Satchi, N. S.IV. (2025). Reinforcement Learning in Personalized Medicine: A Comprehensive Review of Treatment Optimization Strategies. *Cureus, 17*(4).

Bartschke, A., Börner, Y., & Thun, S. (2021). Accessing the ECG data of the apple watch and accomplishing interoperability through FHIR. In German Medical Data Sciences: Bringing Data to Life (pp. 245-250). IOS Press.

Bashir, A. K., Victor, N., Bhattacharya, S., Huynh-The, T., Chengoden, R., Yenduri, G., & Liyanage, M. (2023). Federated learning for the healthcare metaverse: Concepts, applications, challenges, and future directions. *IEEE Internet of Things Journal, 10*(24), 21873–21891.

Bashshur, R. L., Shannon, G. W., Smith, B. R., Alverson, D. C., Antoniotti, N., Barsan, W. G., & Yellowlees, P. (2014). The empirical foundations of telemedicine interventions for chronic disease management. *Telemedicine Journal and e-Health, 20*(9), 769–800.

Bates, D. W., Cohen, M., Leape, L. L., Overhage, J. M., Shabot, M. M., & Sheridan, T. (2001). Reducing the frequency of errors in medicine using information technology. *Journal of the American Medical Informatics Association : JAMIA*, *8*(4), 299–308.

Battineni, G., Sagaro, G. G., Chinatalapudi, N., Amenta, F., & Tayebati, S. K. (2020). Applications of machine learning predictive models in the chronic disease diagnosis. *Journal of Personalized Medicine*, *10*(2), 21. DOI: 10.3390/jpm10020021 PMID: 32244292

Beam, A. L., & Kohane, I. S. (2018). Big data and machine learning in health care. *Journal of the American Medical Association*, *319*(13), 1317–1318. DOI: 10.1001/jama.2017.18391 PMID: 29532063

Beeler, P. E., Bates, D. W., & Hug, B. L. (2014). Clinical decision support systems. *Swiss Medical Weekly*, *144*, w14073.

Behare, N., Keerthi, V. M., Vasmatkar, A., Waghulkar, S., Behare, S. N., Mohture, A., & Sharma, S. (2025). AI, CI, and Society 5.0: A Historical Overview. *Open AI and Computational Intelligence for Society*, *5*(0), 1–26.

Beniwal, S., Saini, U., Garg, P., & Joon, R. K. (2021). Improving performance during camera surveillance by integration of edge detection in IoT system. [IJEHMC]. *International Journal of E-Health and Medical Communications*, *12*(5), 84–96.

Bergenstal, R. M., Tamborlane, W. V., Ahmann, A., Buse, J. B., Dailey, G., Davis, S. N., & Wood, M. A. (2010). Effectiveness of sensor-augmented insulin-pump therapy in type 1 diabetes. *The New England Journal of Medicine*, *363*(4), 311–320.

Bertl, M., Ross, P., & Draheim, D. (2023). Systematic AI support for decision-making in the healthcare sector: Obstacles and success factors. *Health Policy and Technology*, *12*(3), 100748.

Bhatt, C., Kumar, I., Vijayakumar, V., Singh, K. U., & Kumar, A. (2021). The state of the art of deep learning models in medical science and their challenges. *Multimedia Systems*, *27*(4), 599–613.

Bibault, J. E., Giraud, P., & Burgun, A. (2016). Big data and machine learning in radiation oncology: State of the art and future prospects. *Cancer Letters*, *382*(1), 110–117. DOI: 10.1016/j.canlet.2016.07.036 PMID: 27241666

Binns, R. (2018, January). Fairness in machine learning: Lessons from political philosophy. In *Conference on Fairness, Accountability and Transparency* (pp. 149-159). PMLR.

Bohr, A., & Memarzadeh, K. (2020). The rise of artificial intelligence in healthcare applications. In Bohr, A., & Memarzadeh, K. (Eds.), *Artificial Intelligence in Healthcare* (pp. 25–60). Academic Press., DOI: 10.1016/B978-0-12-818438-7.00002-2

Boopathi, S. (2023). Deep learning techniques applied for automatic sentence generation. In Promoting Diversity, Equity, and Inclusion in Language Learning Environments (pp. 255-273). IGI Global.

Boopathi, S., & Khang, A. (2023). AI-integrated technology for a secure and ethical healthcare ecosystem. In *AI and IoT-Based Technologies for Precision Medicine* (pp. 36–59). IGI Global.

Boppiniti, S. T. (2021). Evolution of Reinforcement Learning: From Q-Learning to Deep. *Available at SSRN* 5061696.

Cadmus-Bertram, L. A., Marcus, B. H., Patterson, R. E., Parker, B. A., & Morey, B. L. (2015). Randomized trial of a Fitbit-based physical activity intervention for women. *American Journal of Preventive Medicine*, *49*(3), 414–418.

Capecchi, A., Probst, D., & Reymond, J.-L. (2020). One molecular fingerprint to rule them all: Drugs, biomolecules, and the metabolome. *Journal of Cheminformatics*, *12*(1), 43. Advance online publication. DOI: 10.1186/s13321-020-00445-4 PMID: 33431010

Cardozo, G. A., Tirloni, S. A., Pereira Moro, A. A., & Marques, J. A. (2022). Use of artificial intelligence in the search for new information through routine laboratory tests: Systematic review. *JMIR Bioinformatics and Biotechnology*, *3*(1), e40473. Advance online publication. DOI: 10.2196/40473 PMID: 36644762

Carta, S., Ferreira, A., Podda, A. S., Recupero, D. R., & Sanna, A. (2021). Multi-DQN: An ensemble of Deep Q-learning agents for stock market forecasting. *Expert Systems with Applications*, *164*, 113820.

Chaddad, A., Peng, J., Xu, J., & Bouridane, A. (2023). Survey of explainable AI techniques in healthcare. *Sensors (Basel)*, *23*(2), 634.

Chan, K. Y., Abu-Salih, B., Qaddoura, R., Al-Zoubi, A. M., Palade, V., Pham, D.-S., Ser, J. D., & Muhammad, K. (2023). Deep neural networks in the cloud: Review, applications, challenges and research directions. *Neurocomputing*, *545*, 126327. DOI: 10.1016/j.neucom.2023.126327

Charow, R., Jeyakumar, T., Younus, S., Dolatabadi, E., & Salhia, M., Al-Mouaswas Dalia and Anderson, M., Balakumar, S., Clare Megan and Dhalla, A., Gillan, C., Haghzare, S., Jackson, E., Lalani, N., Mattson, J., Peteanu, W., Tripp, T., Waldorf, J., Williams, S., Tavares, W., & Wiljer, D. (2021). Artificial intelligence education programs for health care professionals: Scoping review. *JMIR Medical Education*, *7*(4), e31043.

Chauhan, S., Singh, M., &Garg, P. (2021). Rapid forecasting of pandemic outbreak using machine learning. *Enabling Healthcare 4.0 for Pandemics: A Roadmap Using AI, Machine Learning, IoT and Cognitive Technologies*, 59-73.

Chen, H. (2024). Blockchain Targets Integrated IoT for Smart Healthcare Systems - A Bibliometric Analysis. *J. Electr. Syst.*, *20*(6s), 1893–1903.

Chen, H., Mohapatra, S., Michalopoulos, G., He, X., & McKillop, I. (2021). Federated deep learning architecture for personalized healthcare. In *Public Health and Informatics* (pp. 193–197). IOS Press.

Chen, I. Y., Joshi, S., & Ghassemi, M. (2020). Treating health disparities with artificial intelligence. *Nature Medicine*, *26*(1), 16–17. PMID: 31932779

Chen, M., Ma, Y., Li, Y., Wu, D., Zhang, Y., & Youn, C. H. (2017). Wearable 2.0: Enabling human-cloud integration in next generation healthcare systems. *IEEE Communications Magazine*, *55*(1), 54–61. DOI: 10.1109/MCOM.2017.1600278CM

Chen, Z., Liang, N., Zhang, H., Li, H., Yang, Y., Zong, X., & Shi, N. (2023). Harnessing the power of clinical decision support systems: Challenges and opportunities. *Open Heart*, *10*(2), e002432. PMID: 38016787

Choi, E., Schuetz, A., Stewart, W. F., & Sun, J. (2016). Using recurrent neural network models for early detection of heart failure onset. *Journal of the American Medical Informatics Association: JAMIA*, *24*(2), 361–370. DOI: 10.1093/jamia/ocw112 PMID: 27521897

Chowdhury, F., & Link, A. N. (2022a). Public Support for Research in Artificial Intelligence: A descriptive study of U.S. Department of Defense SBIR projects. [van.]. *The Journal of Technology Transfer*, *47*, 762–774.

Chowdhury, F., & Link, A. N. (2022b). The spatial distribution of public support for AI research. [van.]. *Science & Public Policy*, *49*, 573–579.

Churpek, M. M., Adhikari, R., & Edelson, D. P. (2016). The value of vital sign trends for detecting clinical deterioration on the wards. *Resuscitation*, *102*, 1–5.

Collins, F. S., & Varmus, H. (2015). A new initiative on precision medicine. *The New England Journal of Medicine*, *372*(9), 793–795.

Comito, C., Falcone, D., & Forestiero, A. (2022). AI-driven clinical decision support: Enhancing disease diagnosis exploiting patients similarity. *IEEE Access : Practical Innovations, Open Solutions*, *10*, 6878–6888.

Cruz-Roa, A., Basavanhally, A., González, F., Gilmore, H., Feldman, M., Ganesan, S., & Madabhushi, A. (2014, March). Automatic detection of invasive ductal carcinoma in whole slide images with convolutional neural networks. In *Medical Imaging 2014: Digital pathology* (Vol. 9041, p. 904103). SPIE.

Dara, S. A., Dhamercherla, S., Jadav, S. S., Babu, C. M., & Ahsan, M. J. (2022). Machine learning in drug discovery: A review. *Artificial Intelligence Review*, *55*(3), 1947–1999. DOI: 10.1007/s10462-021-10058-4 PMID: 34393317

Darzidehkalani, E., Ghasemi-Rad, M., & van Ooijen, P. (2022). Federated learning in medical imaging: Part II: Methods, challenges, and considerations. *Journal of the American College of Radiology*, *19*, 975–982.

Dash, S., Shakyawar, S. K., Sharma, M., & Kaushik, S. (2019). Big data in healthcare: Management, analysis and future prospects. *Journal of Big Data*, *6*(1), 54. Advance online publication. DOI: 10.1186/s40537-019-0217-0

Davenport, T., & Kalakota, R. (2019). The potential for artificial intelligence in healthcare. *Future Healthcare Journal*, *6*(2), 94–98.

Dayan, I., Roth, H. R., Zhong, A., Harouni, A., Gentili, A., Abidin, A. Z., & Li, Q. (2021). Federated learning for predicting clinical outcomes in patients with COVID-19. *Nature Medicine*, *27*(10), 1735–1743.

Deshmukh, R. (2024). Reinforcement learning in healthcare: Applications for personalized treatment planning and clinical decision support. *Shodh Sagar Journal of Artificial Intelligence and Machine Learning*, *1*(2), 19–24.

Devi, D. H., Duraisamy, K., Armghan, A., Alsharari, M., Aliqab, K., Sorathiya, V., & Rashid, N. (2023). 5G technology in healthcare and wearable devices: A review. *Sensors (Basel)*, *23*(5), 2519.

Devi, R. D. H., Naresh, R., & Kumar, C. V. (2023). Advanced 5G Technology in Healthcare Field. *Resource Management in Advanced Wireless Networks*, *227*, 227.

Dey, N., Ashour, A. S., & Balas, V. E. (2018). *Smart medical data sensing and IoT systems design in healthcare*. Springer., DOI: 10.1007/978-3-319-73960-1

Dhinakaran, D., Kumar, N. J., & Ponnuviji, N. P. (2025). Safeguarding confidentiality and privacy in cloud-enabled healthcare systems with spectrasafe encryption and dynamic k-anonymity algorithm. *Expert Systems with Applications*, *279*, 127584.

Ding, H., Seenivasan, L., Killeen, B. D., Cho, S. M., & Unberath, M. (2024). Digital twins as a unifying framework for surgical data science: The enabling role of geometric scene understanding. *Artificial Intelligence Surgery*, *4*(3), 109–138.

Dlugatch, R., Georgieva, A., & Kerasidou, A. (2024). AI-driven decision support systems and epistemic reliance: A qualitative study on obstetricians' and midwives' perspectives on integrating AI-driven CTG into clinical decision making. *BMC Medical Ethics*, *25*(1), 6. PMID: 38184595

Doshi-Velez, F., & Kim, B. (2017). Towards a rigorous science of interpretable machine learning. arXiv preprint arXiv:1702.08608.

Edemekong, P. F., Annamaraju, P., & Haydel, M. J. (2018). Health insurance portability and accountability act.

Edison, G. (2023). Transforming Medical Decision-Making: A Comprehensive Review of AI's Impact on Diagnostics and Treatment. *BULLET: Jurnal Multidisiplin Ilmu*, *2*(4), 1121–1133.

Ekundayo, F. (2024). Reinforcement learning in treatment pathway optimization: A case study in oncology. *International Journal of Science and Research Archive*, *13*(02), 2187–2205.

Elgin, C. Y., & Elgin, C. (2024). Ethical implications of AI-driven clinical decision support systems on healthcare resource allocation: A qualitative study of healthcare professionals' perspectives. *BMC Medical Ethics*, *25*(1), 148. PMID: 39707327

Elhaddad, M., & Hamam, S. (2024). AI-driven clinical Decision Support Systems: An ongoing pursuit of potential. *Cureus*, *16*(4), e57728.

Elhaddad, M., & Hamam, S. (2024). AI-driven clinical decision support systems: An ongoing pursuit of potential. *Cureus*, *16*(4). PMID: 38711724

Eltawil, F. A., Atalla, M., Boulos, E., Amirabadi, A., & Tyrrell, P. N. (2023). Analyzing barriers and enablers for the acceptance of artificial intelligence innovations into radiology practice: A scoping review. *Tomography : a Journal for Imaging Research*, *9*(4), 1443–1455.

Esteva, A., Kuprel, B., Novoa, R. A., Ko, J., Swetter, S. M., Blau, H. M., &Thrun, S. (2017). Dermatologist-level classification of skin cancer with deep neural networks. *nature, 542*(7639), 115-118.

Esteva, A., Chou, K., Yeung, S., Naik, N., Madani, A., & Mottaghi, A.. (2021). Deep learning-enabled medical computer vision. *NPJ Digital Medicine*, *4*(1), 1–9. PMID: 33420381

Esteva, A., Kuprel, B., Novoa, R. A., Ko, J., Swetter, S. M., Blau, H. M., & Thrun, S. (2017). Dermatologist-level classification of skin cancer with deep neural networks. *Nature*, *542*(7639), 115–118. DOI: 10.1038/nature21056 PMID: 28117445

Esteva, A., Robicquet, A., Ramsundar, B., Kuleshov, V., DePristo, M., Chou, K., Cui, C., Corrado, G., Thrun, S., & Dean, J. (2019). A guide to deep learning in healthcare. *Nature Medicine*, *25*(1), 24–29. DOI: 10.1038/s41591-018-0316-z

Faes, M., & Moens, D. (2020). Recent trends in the modeling and quantification of non-probabilistic uncertainty. *Archives of Computational Methods in Engineering*, *27*, 633–671.

Faheem, F., Haq, M., Derhab, M., Saeed, R., Ahmad, U., & Kalia, J. S. (2025). Integrating Ethical Principles Into the Regulation of AI-Driven Medical Software. *Cureus*, *17*(2), e79506. DOI: 10.7759/cureus.79506

Faiyazuddin, M., Rahman, S. J. Q., Anand, G., Siddiqui, R. K., Mehta, R., Khatib, M. N., & Sah, R. (2025). The Impact of Artificial Intelligence on Healthcare: A Comprehensive Review of Advancements in Diagnostics, Treatment, and Operational Efficiency. *Health Science Reports*, *8*(1), e70312.

Faiz, M., Sandhu, R., Akbar, M., Shaikh, A. A., Bhasin, C., & Fatima, N. (2023). Machine Learning Techniques in Wireless Sensor Networks: Algorithms Strategies and Applications. *International Journal of Intelligent Systems and Applications in Engineering*, *11*(9s), 685–694.

Fatima, S. (2024). Transforming Healthcare with AI and Machine Learning: Revolutionizing Patient Care Through Advanced Analytics. International Journal of Education and Science Research Review, 11.

Financial Times. (2025, January 15). How we can use AI to create a better society. Financial Times. https://www.ft.com/content/33ed8ad0-f8ad-42ed-983a-54d5b9eb2d27

Fisher, S., & Rosella, L. C. (2022). Priorities for successful use of artificial intelligence by public health organizations: A literature review. *BMC Public Health*, *22*(1), 2146. Advance online publication. DOI: 10.1186/s12889-022-14422-z PMID: 36419010

Florescu, L. M., Streba, C. T., erbănescu, M.-S., Mămuleanu, M., Florescu, D. N., Teică, R. V., & Gheonea, I. A. (2022). Federated learning approach with pre-trained deep learning models for COVID-19 detection from unsegmented CT images. *Life (Chicago, Ill.)*, *12*, 958.

Flower, M. A. (2012). *Webb's physics of Medical Imaging*. CRC.

Fogel, D. B. (2018). Factors associated with clinical trials that fail and opportunities for improving the likelihood of success: A review. *Contemporary Clinical Trials Communications*, *11*, 156–164. DOI: 10.1016/j.conctc.2018.08.001 PMID: 30112460

Forczek, E., & Rudzki, E. (2018). Artificial intelligence in healthcare: Opportunities and risks. *European Journal of Medical Research*, *23*(1), 1–5. DOI: 10.1186/s40001-018-0341-0 PMID: 29304843

Fu, C., & Chen, Q. (2025a). The future of pharmaceuticals: Artificial intelligence in drug discovery and development. *Journal of Pharmaceutical Analysis*, *101248*. Advance online publication. DOI: 10.1016/j.jpha.2025.101248

Gandhi, K. I., & Prathyusha, N. S. (2025). Harnessing digital twins and AI integration for enhanced disease prediction in the evolution of healthcare. Digital Healthcare, Digital Transformation and Citizen Empowerment in Asia-Pacific and Europe for a Healthier Society, 361-387.

Garcia-Gonzalez, A., Fuentes-Aguilar, R. Q., Salgado, I., & Chairez, I. (2022). A review on the application of autonomous and intelligent robotic devices in medical rehabilitation. *Journal of the Brazilian Society of Mechanical Sciences and Engineering*, *44*(9), 393.

Garg, P. (2024). Prediction of female pregnancy complication using artificial intelligence. In *Artificial Intelligence and Machine Learning for Women's Health Issues* (pp. 17–35). Academic Press.

Garg, P. (2025). Explainable AI & Model Interpretability in Healthcare: Challenges & Future Directions. *EKSPLORIUM-BULETIN PUSAT TEKNOLOGI BAHAN GALIAN NUKLIR*, *46*(1), 104–133.

Garg, P., Dixit, A., & Sethi, P. (2022). (Forthcoming). Ml-fresh: Novel routing protocol in opportunistic networks using machine learning. *Computer Systems Science and Engineering*.

Garg, P., Srivastava, A. K., Anas, A., Gupta, B., & Mishra, C. (2023). Pneumonia Detection Through X-Ray Images Using Convolution Neural Network. In *Advancements in Bio-Medical Image Processing and Authentication in Telemedicine* (pp. 201–218). IGI Global.

Garralda, E., Dienstmann, R., & Tabernero, J. (2017). Pharmacokinetic/pharmacodynamic modeling for drug development in oncology. *American Society of Clinical Oncology Educational Book*, *37*, 210–215. DOI: 10.1200/EDBK_180460 PMID: 28561730

Gautam, V. K., Gupta, S., & Garg, P. (2024, March). Automatic Irrigation System using IoT. In *2024 International Conference on Automation and Computation (AUTOCOM)* (pp. 100-103). IEEE.

Gawriljuk, V. O., Foil, D. H., Puhl, A. A., Zorn, K. M., Lane, T. R., Riabova, O., Makarov, V., Godoy, A. S., Oliva, G., & Ekins, S. A. (2021). Development of machine learning models and the discovery of a new antiviral compound against yellow fever virus. *Journal of Chemical Information and Modeling*, *61*(8), 3804–3813. DOI: 10.1021/acs.jcim.1c00460 PMID: 34286575

Gerke, S., Minssen, T., & Cohen, G. (2020). Ethical and legal challenges of artificial intelligence-driven healthcare. *Artificial Intelligence in Health*, *295*. Advance online publication. DOI: 10.1016/B978-0-12-818438-7.00012-5

Ghai, D., Tripathi, S. L., Saxena, S., Chanda, M., & Alazab, M. (Eds.). (2022). *Machine learning algorithms for signal and image processing*. John Wiley & Sons.

Ghavidel, A., & Pazos, P., & Del Aguila Suarez Rolando and Atashi, A. (2024). Predicting the need for cardiovascular surgery: A comparative study of Machine Learning models. *J.Electron.Electromedical.Eng.Med.Inform*, *6*(2), 92–106.

Gill, A., Jain, D., Sharma, J., Kumar, A., & Garg, P. (2024, May). Deep learning approach for facial identification for online transactions. In *2024 International Conference on Emerging Innovations and Advanced Computing (INNOCOMP)* (pp. 715-722). IEEE.

Giordano, C., Brennan, M., Mohamed, B., Rashidi, P., Modave, F., & Tighe, P. (2021). Accessing artificial intelligence for clinical decision-making. *Frontiers in Digital Health*, *3*, 645232.

Goodfellow, I., Bengio, Y., & Courville, A. (2016). *Deep learning*. MIT Press.

Gopi, B., Kokila, M. S., Bibin, C. V., Sasikala, D., Howard, E., & Boopathi, S. (2024). Distributed Technologies Using AI/ML Techniques for Healthcare Applications. In Social Innovations in Education, Environment, and Healthcare (pp. 375-396). IGI Global.

Gore, J. C. (2020). Artificial Intelligence in Medical Imaging. *Magnetic Resonance Imaging*, *68*, A1–A4. PMID: 31857130

Gottesman, O., Johansson, F., Komorowski, M., Faisal, A., Sontag, D., Doshi-Velez, F., & Celi, L. A. (2019). Guidelines for reinforcement learning in healthcare. *Nature Medicine*, *25*(1), 16–18. PMID: 30617332

Govindaraj, M., Khan, P., Krishnan, R., Gnanasekaran, C., & Lawrence, J. (2024). Revolutionizing Healthcare: The Transformative Impact of Artificial Intelligence. In Revolutionizing the Healthcare Sector with AI (pp. 54-78). IGI Global Scientific Publishing.

Goyal, N. K., Dandotiya, M., Qurashi, J. A., Kumari, M., & Sharma, S. (2025). AI-Driven Predictive Analytics for Disease Management. In Utilizing AI of Medical Things for Healthcare Security and Sustainability (pp. 231-276). IGI Global Scientific Publishing.

Grieves, M. (2014). Digital twin: manufacturing excellence through virtual factory replication. White paper, 1(2014), 1-7.

Guan, S., & Wang, G. (2024). Drug discovery and development in the era of artificial intelligence: From machine learning to large language models. *Artificial Intelligence Chemistry.*, *2*(1), 100070. DOI: 10.1016/j.aichem.2024.100070

Gulamali, F. F., & Nadkarni, G. N. (2023). Federated learning in risk prediction: A primer and application to COVID-19-associated acute kidney injury. *Nephron*, *147*(1), 52–56.

Gupta, M., Ahmed, S., Kumar, R., & Altrjman, C. (Eds.). (2023). *Computational intelligence in healthcare: Applications, challenges, and management*. CRC Press., https://www.routledge.com/Computational-Intelligence-in-Healthcare-Applications-Challenges-and/Gupta-Ahmed-Kumar-Altrjman/p/book/9781032304939

Haddiya, I., & Ramdani, S. (2024). Artificial intelligence in healthcare: A focus on the best practices. ITM Web of Conferences, 69, 02010. https://doi.org/DOI: 10.1051/itmconf/20246902010

Haidegger, T., Sándor, J., & Benyó, Z. (2011). Surgery in space: The future of robotic telesurgery. *Surgical Endoscopy*, *25*, 681–690.

Haleem, A., Javaid, M., Qadri, M. A., Singh, R. P., & Suman, R. (2022a). Artificial intelligence (AI) applications for marketing: A literature-based study. *International Journal of Intelligent Networks*, *3*, 119–132. DOI: 10.1016/j.ijin.2022.08.005

Haleem, A., Javaid, M., Singh, R. P., & Suman, R. (2022b). Medical 4.0 technologies for healthcare: Features, capabilities, and applications. *Internet of Things and Cyber-Physical Systems*, *2*, 12–30. DOI: 10.1016/j.iotcps.2022.04.001

Hameed, B. Z., Naik, N., Ibrahim, S., Tatkar, N. S., Shah, M. J., Prasad, D., & Somani, B. K. (2023). Breaking barriers: Unveiling factors influencing the adoption of artificial intelligence by healthcare providers. *Big Data and Cognitive Computing*, *7*, 105.

Hameed, B. Z., Shah, M., Naik, N., Singh Khanuja, H., Paul, R., & Somani, B. K. (2021). Application of artificial intelligence-based classifiers to predict the outcome measures and stone-free status following percutaneous nephrolithotomy for staghorn calculi: Cross-validation of data and estimation of accuracy. *European Urology*, *79*, S1375.

Haripriya, R., Khare, N., & Pandey, M. (2025). Privacy-preserving federated learning for collaborative medical data mining in multi-institutional settings. *Scientific Reports*, *15*(1), 12482. DOI: 10.1038/s41598-025-97565-4

Harris, L. A. (2023). Artificial Intelligence: Overview, Recent Advances, and Considerations for the 118th Congress, https://crsreports.congress.gov

Hassani, H., Huang, X., & MacFeely, S. (2022). Impactful digital twin in the healthcare revolution. *Big Data and Cognitive Computing*, *6*(3), 83.

Hastie, T. (2009). The elements of statistical learning: data mining, inference, and prediction.

Hauschild, A. C., Lemanczyk, M., Matschinske, J., Frisch, T., Zolotareva, O., Holzinger, A., & Heider, D. (2022). Federated random forests can improve local performance of predictive models for various healthcare applications. *Bioinformatics (Oxford, England)*, *38*(8), 2278–2286.

Hazarika, I. (2020). Artificial Intelligence: Opportunities and implications for the Health workforce. *International Health*, *12*, 241–245. PMID: 32300794

Helenason, J., & Ekström, C., & Falk Magnus and Papachristou, P. (2024). Exploring the feasibility of an artificial intelligence based clinical decision support system for cutaneous melanoma detection in primary care - a mixed method study. *Scandinavian Journal of Primary Health Care*, *42*(1), 51–60.

Henry, K. E., Hager, D. N., Pronovost, P. J., & Saria, S. (2015). A targeted real-time early warning score (TREWScore) for septic shock. Science Translational Medicine, 7(299), 299ra122-299ra122.

Hider, M. A., Nasiruddin, M., & Al Mukaddim, A. (2024). Early Disease Detection through Advanced Machine Learning Techniques: A Comprehensive Analysis and Implementation in Healthcare Systems. *Revista de Inteligencia Artificial en Medicina*, *15*(1), 1010–1042.

Ho, D., Quake, S. R., McCabe, E. R., Chng, W. J., Chow, E. K., Ding, X., & Zarrinpar, A. (2020). Enabling technologies for personalized and precision medicine. *Trends in Biotechnology*, *38*(5), 497–518.

Holmes, J., Sacchi, L., & Bellazzi, R. (2004). Artificial intelligence in medicine. *Annals of the Royal College of Surgeons of England*, *86*, 334–338. PMID: 15333167

Hossain, M. S., Muhammad, G., & Alhamid, M. F. (2019). Automatic fruit classification using hybrid deep learning model. *IEEE Access : Practical Innovations, Open Solutions*, *7*, 116146–116158. DOI: 10.1109/ACCESS.2019.2933562

Huang, J., Li, Y., & Huang, L. (2020). Spine surgical robotics: Review of the current application and disadvantages for future perspectives. *Journal of Robotic Surgery*, *14*(1), 11–16.

Huang, Y., Kangas, L. J., & Rasco, B. A. (2007). Applications of artificial neural networks (ANNs) in food science. *Critical Reviews in Food Science and Nutrition*, *47*(2), 113–126.

Hudaa, S., Setiyadi, D. B. P., Lydia, E. L., Shankar, K., Nguyen, P. T., Hashim, W., & Maseleno, A. (2019). Natural language processing utilization in healthcare. *International Journal of Engineering and Advanced Technology*, *8*(6), 1117–1120.

Hwang, J., Lee, T., Lee, H., & Byun, S. (2022). A clinical decision support system for sleep staging tasks with explanations from artificial intelligence: User-centered design and evaluation study. *Journal of Medical Internet Research*, *24*(1), e28659.

Iroju, O. G., & Olaleke, J. O. (2015). A systematic review of natural language processing in healthcare. *International Journal of Information Technology and Computer Science*, *8*(8), 44–50.

Islam, M. A., Yeasmin, S., Hosen, A., Vanu, N., Riipa, M. B., Tasnim, A. F., & Nilima, S. I. (2025). Harnessing Predictive Analytics: The Role of Machine Learning in Early Disease Detection and Healthcare Optimization. *Journal of Ecohumanism*, *4*(3), 312–321.

Jabbour, S., Fouhey, D., Shepard, S., Valley, T. S., Kazerooni, E. A., Banovic, N., Wiens, J., & Sjoding, M. W. (2023). Measuring the impact of AI in the diagnosis of hospitalized patients: A randomized clinical vignette survey study. *Journal of the American Medical Association*, *330*(23), 2275–2284.

Jain, S., & Jaidka, P. (2023). Brain Tumor Classification using Deep learning based Novel Hybrid Approach. *2023 2nd International Conference on Edge Computing and Applications (ICECAA)*, 872–876.

Jain, S., & Jain, V. (2022, March). Novel hybrid boosted ensemble learning framework for brain tumor prediction. *2022 9th International Conference on Computing for Sustainable Global Development (INDIACom).*

Jain, S., & Jaidka, P. (2024). Lung cancer classification using deep learning hybrid model. In *Future of AI in Medical Imaging* (pp. 207–223). IGI Global.

Jain, S., & Jain, V. (2023, December). A critical evaluation of deep learning methods for classifying brain tumor: A review. *2023 International Conference on Computational, Networks and Security (ICCINS).*

Jain, S., & Jain, V. (2024). Machine learning and deep learning methods in brain tumor classification: A decade: Systematic literature review. *Intelligent Data Analysis*, 1–32.

Jain, S., Jain, V., & Chatterjee, J. M. (2025). Ensemble based brain tumor classification technique from MRI based on K fold validation approach. *Journal of Integrated Science and Technology, 13*(5), 1114.

Jaladanki, S. K., Vaid, A., Sawant, A. S., Xu, J., Shah, K., Dellepiane, S., & Nadkarni, G. N. (2021). Development of a federated learning approach to predict acute kidney injury in adult hospitalized patients with COVID-19 in New York City. *medRxiv.*

Javaid, M., Haleem, A., Singh, R. P., Suman, R., & Rab, S. (2022). Significance of machine learning in healthcare: Features, pillars and applications. *International Journal of Intelligent Networks, 3*, 58–73. DOI: 10.1016/j.ijin.2022.05.002

Jayachandran, R., Dantapur, B., Antony, A. S., & Nagapadma, R. (2025). Transforming Healthcare Through Smart Health Systems: Harnessing Technology for Enhanced Patient Care. In *Transforming Healthcare Sector through Artificial Intelligence and Environmental Sustainability* (pp. 107–127). Springer Nature Singapore.

Jayaprakasam, B. S. (2025). AI and Big Data-Driven m-Health: Integrating Cloud Computing, Remote Patient Monitoring, Clinical Decision Support Systems, and Self-Supervised Learning with FHIR for Scalable Healthcare Systems. *Indo-American Journal of Life Sciences and Biotechnology, 22*(1), 11–25.

Jayaraman, P., Desman, J., Sabounchi, M., Nadkarni, G. N., & Sakhuja, A. (2024a). A Primer on Reinforcement Learning in Medicine for Clinicians. *NPJ Digital Medicine, 7*(1), 1–10. DOI: 10.1038/s41746-024-01316-0

Jhade, S., & Gangavarapu, S. P., Channabasamma, & Igorevich Rozhdestvenskiy, O. (2024). Smart Medicine: Exploring the landscape of AI-enhanced Clinical Decision Support Systems. *MATEC Web Conf., 392*, 1083.

Jiang, F., Jiang, Y., Zhi, H., Dong, Y., Li, H., Ma, S., & Wang, Y. (2017). Artificial intelligence in healthcare: Past, present and future. *Stroke and Vascular Neurology*, *2*(4), 230–243. DOI: 10.1136/svn-2017-000101 PMID: 29507784

Jiang, M., Wang, S., Zhang, S., Zhou, W., Zhang, Y., & Li, Z. (2022). Sequence-based drug-target affinity prediction using weighted graph neural networks. *BMC Genomics*, *23*(1), 449. Advance online publication. DOI: 10.1186/s12864-022-0868-9 PMID: 35715739

Jobin, A., Ienca, M., & Vayena, E. (2019). The global landscape of AI ethics guidelines. *Nature Machine Intelligence*, *1*(9), 389–399.

Job, S., Tao, X., Li, L., Xie, H., Cai, T., Yong, J., & Li, Q. (2024). Optimal treatment strategies for critical patients with deep reinforcement learning. *ACM Transactions on Intelligent Systems and Technology*, *15*(2), 1–22.

Johnson, K. B., Wei, W.-Q., Weeraratne, D., Frisse, M. E., Misulis, K., Rhee, K., Juan, Z., & Snowdon, J. L. (2021). Precision medicine, AI, and the future of personalized health care. *Clinical and Translational Science*, *14*(1), 86–93.

Jordan, M. I., & Mitchell, T. M. (2015). Machine learning: Trends, perspectives, and prospects. *Science*, *349*(6245), 255–260.

Kahn, R., & Davidson, M. B. (2014). The reality of type 2 diabetes prevention. *Diabetes Care*, *37*(4), 943–949.

Kaissis, G. A.. (2020). Secure, privacy-preserving and federated machine learning in medical imaging. *Nature Machine Intelligence*, *2*(6), 305–311.

Kalusivalingam, A. K., Sharma, A., Patel, N., & Singh, V. (2020). Optimizing Decision-Making with AI-Enhanced Support Systems: Leveraging Reinforcement Learning and Bayesian Networks. *International Journal of AI and ML*, *1*(2).

Kannelønning, M. S. (2024). Navigating uncertainties of introducing Artificial Intelligence (AI) in Healthcare: The role of a Norwegian network of professionals. *Technology in Society*, *76*, 102432.

Kashyap, R., & Piersson, A. D. (2018). Big data challenges and solutions in the medical industries. In *Handbook of Research on Pattern Engineering System Development for Big Data Analytics* (pp. 1–24). IGI Global.

Kathamuthu, N. D., Chinnamuthu, A., Iruthayanathan, N., Ramachandran, M., & Gandomi, A. H. (2022). Deep Q-Learning-Based Neural Network with Privacy Preservation Method for Secure Data Transmission in Internet of Things (IoT) Healthcare Application. *Electronics (Basel), 11*(1), 1. Advance online publication. DOI: 10.3390/electronics11010157

Kaul, A., Ali, S., & Gupta, D. (2020). Evolutionary algorithms in intelligent diagnosis of diseases. *Computers in Biology and Medicine, 124*, 103935. DOI: 10.1016/j.compbiomed.2020.103935

Kaur, J. (2024). Smart Solutions for Health: Computational Intelligence Reshaping the Industry 4.0 Healthcare Paradigm. In Advances in Computational Intelligence for the Healthcare Industry 4.0 (pp. 194-211). IGI Global Scientific Publishing.

Kaur, N., Mittal, A., Kumar, A., & Kumar, R. (2022). Healthcare monitoring through Fog computing: A survey. *ECS Transactions, 107*(1), 7689–7701.

Keerthika, K., Kannan, M., & Saravanan, T. (2024). Clinical Intelligence: Deep Reinforcement Learning for Healthcare and Biomedical Advancements. *Deep Reinforcement Learning and Its Industrial Use Cases: AI for Real-World Applications*, 137-150.

Kendall, J. L., Hoffenberg, S. R., & Smith, R. S. (2007). History of emergency and critical care Ultrasound: The evolution of a New Imaging paradigm. *Critical Care Medicine, 35*, S126–S130. PMID: 17446770

Keramatfar, A., & Amirkhani, H. (2019). Bibliometrics of sentiment analysis literature. *Journal of Information Science, 45*(1), 3–15.

Khalifa, M., Albadawy, M., & Iqbal, U. (2024). Advancing clinical decision support: The role of artificial intelligence across six domains. *Computer Methods and Programs in Biomedicine Update, 5*, 100142.

Khang, A. (Ed.). (2023). *AI and IoT-based technologies for precision medicine*. IGI Global.

Khan, S., Yairi, T., & Torres, J. (2020). A review on machine learning algorithms for the health domain. *Health and Technology, 10*(5), 1087–1109. DOI: 10.1007/s12553-019-00365

Khinvasara, T., Cuthrell, K. M., & Tzenios, N. (2024). Harnessing artificial intelligence in healthcare analytics: From diagnosis to treatment optimization. *Asian Journal of Medicine and Health, 22*(8), 15–31.

Knudsen, J. E., Ghaffar, U., Ma, R., & Hung, A. J. (2024). Clinical applications of artificial intelligence in robotic surgery. *Journal of Robotic Surgery, 18*(1), 102. DOI: 10.1007/s11701-024-01867-0

Kocher, G., & Kumar, G. (2021). Machine learning and deep learning methods for intrusion detection systems: Recent developments and challenges. *Soft Computing, 25*(15), 9731–9763.

Kokila, M. S., Fenil, E., Ponnuviji, N. P., & Nirmala, G. (2024). Securing cloud-based medical data: An optimal dual kernal support vector approach for enhanced EHR management. *International Journal of System Assurance Engineering and Management, 15*(7), 3495–3507.

Komorowski, M., Celi, L. A., Badawi, O., Gordon, A. C., & Faisal, A. A. (2018). The Artificial Intelligence Clinician learns optimal treatment strategies for sepsis in intensive care. *Nature Medicine, 24*(11), 1716–1720. PMID: 30349085

Koonin, L. M. (2020). Trends in the use of telehealth during the emergence of the COVID-19 pandemic—United States, January–March 2020. *MMWR. Morbidity and Mortality Weekly Report*, 69.

Kothinti, R. R. (2024). Artificial intelligence in healthcare: Revolutionizing precision medicine, predictive analytics, and ethical considerations in autonomous diagnostics. *World Journal of Advanced Research and Reviews, 19*(3), 3395–3406.

Kourou, K., Exarchos, T. P., Exarchos, K. P., Karamouzis, M. V., & Fotiadis, D. I. (2015). Machine learning applications in cancer prognosis and prediction. *Computational and Structural Biotechnology Journal, 13*, 8–17.

Kukreti, S., Shrivastava, A., Chandrashekar, R., Rani, K. P., Badhoutiya, A., & Lakhanpal, S. (2025, February). AI-Driven Clinical Decision Support Systems: Revolutionizing Healthcare with Predictive Models. In *2025 International Conference on Computational, Communication and Information Technology (ICCCIT)* (pp. 560-565). IEEE.

Kumar, A., & Sharma, R. (2023). Deep Q-networks in healthcare: A review of applications and challenges. *Journal of Healthcare Informatics Research, 7*(2), 123–138. DOI: 10.1007/s41666-023-001234

Kumar, R., Das, R., Garg, P., & Pandita, N. (2024, April). Duplicate Node Detection Method for Wireless Sensors. In *2024 Sixth International Conference on Computational Intelligence and Communication Technologies (CCICT)* (pp. 512-515). IEEE.

Kumar, V., & Garg, M. L. (2018). Predictive analytics: A review of trends and techniques. *International Journal of Computer Applications, 182*(1), 31–37.

Kuppuswamy, P., Mohan, M., Al Khalidi, S. Q., & Prakash, V. V. (2024). Predictive Analytics Tools and Techniques for Disease Prevention and Early Detection in Healthcare Sector. In *Advancing Healthcare through Data-driven Innovations* (pp. 28–49). CRC Press.

Laal, M. (2013). Innovation process in Medical Imaging. *Procedia: Social and Behavioral Sciences*, *81*, 60–64.

Lake, M. A. (2020). What we know so far: COVID-19 current clinical knowledge and research. *Clinical Medicine*, *20*(2), 124–127.

Lakhani, P. (2017). Deep convolutional neural networks for endotracheal tube position and X-ray image classification: Challenges and opportunities. *Journal of Digital Imaging*, *30*, 460–468.

Lakumarapu, S., Nithyanandhan, R., Bhargavi, V. S., & TP, A. (2024, August). Machine Learning Approaches for Liver Disease Prediction: A Comparative Analysis. In 2024 5th International Conference on Electronics and Sustainable Communication Systems (ICESC) (pp. 159-164). IEEE.

Laroche, R., Trichelair, P., & Des Combes, R. T. (2019, May). Safe policy improvement with baseline bootstrapping. In *International conference on machine learning* (pp. 3652-3661). PMLR.

Lartey, B., Adrah, K., Adrah, F., & Isichei, J. (2023). Application of Machine Learning for Predicting the occurrence of Nephropathy in Diabetic patients. *International Journal of Computer Applications*, *975*, 8887.

Lavanya, M., Ashwini, A., & Balasubramaniam, S. (2025). The Virtual Revolution of Digital Twins in Chronic Healthcare Management. In AI-Powered Digital Twins for Predictive Healthcare: Creating Virtual Replicas of Humans (pp. 169-200). IGI Global Scientific Publishing.

LeCun, Y., Bengio, Y., & Hinton, G. (2015). Deep learning. *Nature*, *521*(7553), 436–444. DOI: 10.1038/nature14539 PMID: 26017442

Lee, H., Park, J., & Kim, S. (2024). Computational intelligence for smart healthcare decision-making: Integrating deep reinforcement learning and clinical data. *Healthcare Analytics*, *5*, 100123. DOI: 10.1016/j.health.2024.100123

Li, T., Sahu, A. K., Zaheer, M., Sanjabi, M., Talwalkar, A., & Smith, V. (2020). Federated optimization in heterogeneous networks. In Proceedings of Machine Learning and Systems, 2, 429–450.

Liang, L., Hu, J., Sun, G., Hong, N., Wu, G., He, Y., Li, Y., Hao, T., Liu, L., & Gong, M. (2022). Artificial intelligence-based pharmacovigilance in the setting of limited resources. *Drug Safety, 45*(5), 511–519. DOI: 10.1007/s40264-022-01170-7 PMID: 35579814

Li, C., Hu, Y., & Deng, Y. (2020). Deep reinforcement learning: Fundamentals, research and applications. *IEEE Access: Practical Innovations, Open Solutions, 8*, 135354–135381. DOI: 10.1109/ACCESS.2020.3011375

Li, L., Xie, N., & Yuan, S. (2022). A federated learning framework for breast cancer histopathological image classification. *Electronics (Basel), 11*, 3767.

Lin, Y. K., Chen, H., Brown, R. A., Li, S. H., & Yang, H. J. (2017). Healthcare predictive analytics for risk profiling in chronic care. *Management Information Systems Quarterly, 41*(2), 473–496.

Lin, Y., Zhang, Y., Wang, D., Yang, B., & Shen, Y. Q. (2022). Computer especially AI-assisted drug virtual screening and design in traditional Chinese medicine. *Phytomedicine, 107*, 154481.

Lipton, Z. C. (2018). The mythos of model interpretability: In machine learning, the concept of interpretability is both important and slippery. *Queue, 16*(3), 31–57.

Liu, S., See, K. C., Ngiam, K. Y., Celi, L. A., Sun, X., & Feng, M. (2020). Reinforcement learning for clinical decision support in critical care: Comprehensive review. *Journal of Medical Internet Research, 22*(7), e18477.

Lopez-Martinez, D., Eschenfeldt, P., Ostvar, S., Ingram, M., Hur, C., & Picard, R. (2019). *Deep Reinforcement Learning for Optimal Critical Care Pain Management with Morphine using Dueling Double-Deep Q Networks* (No. arXiv:1904.11115). arXiv. https://doi.org//arXiv.1904.11115DOI: 10.48550

Lu, M., Shahn, Z., Sow, D., Doshi-Velez, F., & Lehman, L. W. H. (2021, January). Is deep reinforcement learning ready for practical applications in healthcare? A sensitivity analysis of duel-DDQN for hemodynamic management in sepsis patients. *AMIA ... Annual Symposium Proceedings - AMIA Symposium. AMIA Symposium, 2020*, 773.

Lundberg, S. M., & Lee, S. I. (2017). A unified approach to interpreting model predictions. *Advances in Neural Information Processing Systems*, 30.

Madgule, M., Vinayaka, N., Sonkhaskar, Y. M., Patel, D. R., Karthikeyan, R., & Selvakumar, P. (2023). Mechanical properties and microstructure of activated TIG welded similar joints of Inconel alloys by desirability approaches. *Materials Today: Proceedings, 77*, 528–533. DOI: 10.1016/j.matpr.2022.11.251

Maha, C. C., Kolawole, T. O., & Abdul, S. (2024). Harnessing data analytics: A new frontier in predicting and preventing non-communicable diseases in the US and Africa. *Computer Science & IT Research Journal*, *5*(6), 1247–1264.

Maithili, K., Ponmalar, A., Yamini, B., Karthikeyan, M., Anish, T. P., Maheswari, B., & Subramanian, R. S. (2024). Advances in AI and Machine Learning for Healthcare Informatics. In Machine Learning and Generative AI in Smart Healthcare (pp. 1-22). IGI Global.

Makanjee, C. R., Hoffmann, W. A., & Bergh, A. M. (2015). Healthcare provider and patient perspectives on diagnostic imaging investigations. *African Journal of Primary Health Care & Family Medicine*, *7*(1), 1–10.

Malik, A., &Solaiman, B. (2024). AI in hospital administration and management: Ethical and legal implications. *Research handbook on health, AI and the Law*, 20-40.

Malik, A., Nandal, D., Gupta, V., Garg, P., &Nandal, V. INTELLIGENT SYSTEMS AND APPLICATIONS IN ENGINEERING.

Malik, M., Garg, P., & Malik, C. (2024). Artificial intelligence-based prediction of health risks among women during menopause. *Artificial Intelligence and Machine Learning for Women's Health Issues*, 137-150.

Malik, M., Singh, Y., Garg, P., & Gupta, S. (2020). Deep Learning in Healthcare system. *International Journal of Grid and Distributed Computing*, *13*(2), 469–468.

Malik, P., Pathania, M., & Rathaur, V. K. (2019). Overview of artificial intelligence in medicine. *Journal of Family Medicine and Primary Care*, *8*(7), 2328–2331.

Malik, T., Nandal, V., & Garg, P. (2024, May). Deep Learning-Based Classification of Diabetic Retinopathy: Leveraging the Power of VGG-19. In *2024 International Conference on Emerging Innovations and Advanced Computing (INNOCOMP)* (pp. 645-651). IEEE.

Mall, P. K., Singh, P. K., Srivastav, S., Narayan, V., Paprzycki, M., Jaworska, T., & Ganzha, M. (2023). A comprehensive review of deep neural networks for medical image processing: Recent developments and future opportunities. *Healthcare Analytics*, *4*, 100216. DOI: 10.1016/j.health.2023.100216

Malsia, E., & Loku, A. (2024). Generative artificial intelligence in health system management: Transformative insights. *Journal of Service Science and Management*, *17*(02), 107–117.

Mangairkarasi, S., Ramana, T. V., Vaishnavi, R., Agalya, S., Sathya, V., & Subramanian, R. S. (2025). Advancing Healthcare Through Artificial Intelligence: Applications, Challenges, and Future Directions. In Responsible AI for Digital Health and Medical Analytics (pp. 113-134). IGI Global Scientific Publishing.

Manocha, A. K., Jain, S., Singh, M., & Paul, S. (Eds.). (2021). *Computational Intelligence in Healthcare*. Springer.

Manocha, A. K., Singh, M., Jain, S., & Jain, V. (Eds.). (2022). *Smart computational intelligence in biomedical and health informatics*. CRC Press., https://www.routledge.com/Smart-Computational-Intelligence-in-Biomedical-and-Health-Informatics/KumarManocha-Singh-Jain-Jain/p/book/9780367624149

Marey, A., Arjmand, P., Alerab, A. D. S., Eslami, M. J., Saad, A. M., Sanchez, N., & Umair, M. (2024). Explainability, transparency and black box challenges of AI in radiology: Impact on patient care in cardiovascular radiology. *The Egyptian Journal of Radiology and Nuclear Medicine*, *55*(1), 183. DOI: 10.1186/s43055-024-01356-2

Matheus Mr, S., & Barzani Den Mr, V. (2021). An analysis of Artificial Intelligence based clinical decision support systems. *Journal of Biomedical and Sustainable Healthcare Applications*, 9–17.

Mayo, R. C., Sen, L. Q. C., & Leung, J. W. (2020). Financing Artificial Intelligence in Medical Imaging: Show me the money. *Journal of the American College of Radiology*, *17*, 175–177. PMID: 31918877

Ma, Z., Zhang, M., Liu, J., Yang, A., Li, H., Wang, J., & Li, M. (2022). An assisted diagnosis model for cancer patients based on federated learning. *Frontiers in Oncology*, *12*, 860532.

McGinnis, J. M., Stuckhardt, L., Saunders, R., & Smith, M. (2013). *Best care at lower cost: The path to Continuously Learning Health Care in America*. National Academy.

McMahan, B., Moore, E., Ramage, D., Hampson, S., & Arcas, B. A. (2017, April). Communication-efficient learning of deep networks from decentralized data. In *Artificial Intelligence and Statistics* (pp. 1273–1282). PMLR.

McMahan, H. B., Moore, E., Ramage, D., Hampson, S., & Arcas, B. A. (2017). Communication-efficient learning of deep networks from decentralized data. In *Proceedings of the 20th International Conference on Artificial Intelligence and Statistics*, 54, 1273–1282.

Mehmood, Y. (2025). Reinforcement learning in intelligent applications: Algorithms and case studies. *Journal of AI Spectrum*, *2*(1), 12–22.

Melissourgos, D., Gao, H., Ma, C., Chen, S., & Wu, S. S. (2021). On outsourcing artificial neural network learning of privacy-sensitive medical data to the cloud. In *2021 IEEE 33rd International Conference on Tools with Artificial Intelligence (ICTAI)* (pp. 381–385). IEEE.

Mennella, C., Maniscalco, U., De Pietro, G., & Esposito, M. (2024). Ethical and regulatory challenges of AI technologies in healthcare: A narrative review. *Heliyon, 10*(4), e26297. DOI: 10.1016/j.heliyon.2024.e26297

Mhlanga, D. (2025). AI in Hospital Administration: Revolutionizing Healthcare.

Miotto, R., Wang, F., Wang, S., Jiang, X., & Dudley, J. T. (2018). Deep learning for healthcare: Review, opportunities and challenges. *Briefings in Bioinformatics, 19*(6), 1236–1246. PMID: 28481991

Mishra, N., & Silakari, S. (2012). Predictive analytics: A survey, trends, applications, oppurtunities & challenges. *International Journal of Computer Science and Information Technologies, 3*(3), 4434–4438.

Mitra, U., & Rehman, S. U. (2025). Leveraging AI and Machine Learning for Next-Generation Clinical Decision Support Systems (CDSS). In AI-Driven Innovation in Healthcare Data Analytics (pp. 83-112). IGI Global Scientific Publishing.

Mittal, H. K., Dalal, P., Garg, P., & Joon, R. (2024, May). Forecasting Pollution Trends: Comparing Linear, Logistic Regression, and Neural Networks. In *2024 International Conference on Emerging Innovations and Advanced Computing (INNOCOMP)* (pp. 411-419). IEEE.

Mnih, V., Kavukcuoglu, K., Silver, D., Rusu, A. A., Veness, J., & Bellemare, M. G.. (2015). Human-level control through deep reinforcement learning. *Nature, 518*(7540), 529–533. PMID: 25719670

Mohammed, A. S., Neravetla, A. R., Nomula, V. K., Gupta, K., & Dhanasekaran, S. (2024, June). Understanding the Impact of AI-driven Clinical Decision Support Systems. In 2024 15th International Conference on Computing Communication and Networking Technologies (ICCCNT) (pp. 1-6). IEEE.

Mouhni, N., Elkalay, A., Chakraoui, M., Abdali, A., Ammoumou, A., & Amalou, I. (2022). Federated learning for medical imaging: An updated state of the art. *Ingénierie des Systèmes d'Information, 27*, 143–150.

Muhiyaddin, R., Abd-Alrazaq, A. A., Househ, M., Alam, T., & Shah, Z. (2020). The impact of clinical decision support systems (CDSS) on physicians: a scoping review. *The Importance of Health Informatics in Public Health during a Pandemic*, 470-473.

Nag, S., Baidya, A. T. K., Mandal, A., Mathew, A. T., Das, B., Devi, B., & Kumar, R. A. (2022). Deep learning tools for advancing drug discovery and development. *3 Biotech, 12*(5), Article 110. https://doi.org/DOI: 10.1007/s13205-022-03165-8

Najjar, R. (2023). Redefining Radiology: A review of Artificial Intelligence Integration in Medical Imaging. *Diagnostics (Basel), 13*, 2760. PMID: 37685300

Namanja, A. T., Xu, J., Wu, H., Sun, Q., Upadhyay, A. K., Sun, C., Van Doren, S. R., & Petros, A. A. X. (2019). NMR-based fragment screening and lead discovery accelerated by principal component analysis. *Journal of Biomolecular NMR, 73*(12), 675–685. DOI: 10.1007/s10858-019-00279-9 PMID: 31541395

Nanehkaran, Y. A., Licai, Z., Chengyong, J., Chen, J., Anwar, S., Azarafza, M., & Derakhshani, R. (2023). Comparative analysis for slope stability by using machine learning methods. *Applied Sciences (Basel, Switzerland), 13*(3), 1555.

Nascimben, M. (2024). Machine learning approaches for personalized medicine.

Neravetla, A. R., Nomula, V. K., Mohammed, A. S., & Dhanasekaran, S. (2024, June). Implementing AI-driven Diagnostic Decision Support Systems for Smart Healthcare. In 2024 15th International Conference on Computing Communication and Networking Technologies (ICCCNT) (pp. 1-6). IEEE.

Nguyen, D. C., Pham, Q. V., Pathirana, P. N., Ding, M., Seneviratne, A., Lin, Z., & Hwang, W. J. (2022). Federated learning for smart healthcare: A survey. *ACM Computing Surveys, 55*(3), 1–37.

Nguyen, D. S. W., & Odigie, R. (2023). Toward Artificial General Intelligence: Deep Reinforcement Learning Method to AI in Medicine. *Journal of Computer and Communications, 11*(9), 9. Advance online publication. DOI: 10.4236/jcc.2023.119006

Nguyen, T. X., Ran, A. R., Hu, X., Yang, D., Jiang, M., Dou, Q., & Cheung, C. Y. (2022). Federated learning in ocular imaging: Current progress and future direction. *Diagnostics (Basel), 12*, 2835.

Nivedhaa, N. (2024). A comprehensive study of artificial intelligence's contribution to streamlining healthcare workflows and enhancing decision-making practices. [IJITEE]. *International Journal of Information Technology and Electrical Engineering, 13*(5), 1–7.

Noor, A. A., Manzoor, A., Mazhar Qureshi, M. D., Qureshi, M. A., & Rashwan, W. (2025). Unveiling Explainable AI in Healthcare: Current Trends, Challenges, and Future Directions. *Wiley Interdisciplinary Reviews. Data Mining and Knowledge Discovery, 15*(2), e70018. DOI: 10.1002/widm.70018

Obermeyer, Z., Powers, B., Vogeli, C., & Mullainathan, S. (2019). Dissecting racial bias in an algorithm used to manage the health of populations. *Science*, *366*(6464), 447–453. DOI: 10.1126/science.aax2342

OECD. (2023). OECD Employment Outlook 2023. https://www.oecd-ilibrary.org/content/publication/08785bba-en

Olalekan Kehinde, A. (2025). Leveraging Machine Learning for Predictive Models in Healthcare to Enhance Patient Outcome Management. *International Research Journal of Modernization in Engineering Technology and Science*, *7*(1), 1465.

Orji, C., Reghefaoui, M., Saavedra Palacios, M. S., Thota, P., Peresuodei Tariladei, S., Gill, A., & Hamid, P. (2023). Application of artificial intelligence and machine learning in diagnosing scaphoid fractures: A systematic review. *Cureus*, *15*(10), e47732.

Ouanes, K., & Farhah, N. (2024). Effectiveness of Artificial Intelligence (AI) in clinical decision support systems and care delivery. *Journal of Medical Systems*, *48*(1), 74. PMID: 39133332

Pagallo, U., O'Sullivan, S., Nevejans, N., Holzinger, A., Friebe, M., Jeanquartie, F., Jean-Quartier, C., & Miernik, A. (2023). The underuse of AI in the Health Sector: Opportunity costs, success stories, risks and recommendations. *Health and Technology*. Advance online publication. DOI: 10.1007/s12553-023-00806-7 PMID: 38229886

Pakdemirli, E. (2019). New Subspecialty or Close Ally emerging on the Radiology Horizon: Artificial Intelligence. *Acta Radiologica Open*, *8*, 2058460119837498. PMID: 30923633

Panayides, A. S., Amini, A., Filipovic, N. D., Sharma, A., Tsaftaris, S. A., Young, A., Foran, D., Do, N., Golemati, S., & Kurc, T. (2020). AI in Medical Imaging Informatics: Current challenges and future directions. *IEEE Journal of Biomedical and Health Informatics*, *24*, 1837–1857. PMID: 32609615

Pandelu, A. P. (2024, December 28). *Day 62: Reinforcement Learning basics — agent, environment, rewards*. Medium. https://medium.com/@bhatadithya54764118/day-62-reinforcement-learning-basics-agent-environment-rewards-306b8e7e555c

Patel, L., Shukla, T., Huang, X., Ussery, D. A., & Wang, S. A. (2020). Machine learning methods in drug discovery. *Molecules (Basel, Switzerland)*, *25*(22), 5277. Advance online publication. DOI: 10.3390/molecules25225277 PMID: 33198233

Patel, V. M., & Misra, S. (2020). Artificial intelligence in healthcare: Past present and future. *Journal of Medical Systems*, *44*(8), 1–7.

Pathan, R. R., Osei-Asiamah, J., Jadhav, P. N., Saravanan, S., Singh, A. K., & Sahoo, S. K. (2025). Developing Decision Support Systems for Healthcare Administration using AI. *Journal of Neonatal Surgery, 14*(10s).

Patil, S., & Shankar, H. (2023). Transforming healthcare: Harnessing the power of AI in the modern era. *International Journal of Multidisciplinary Sciences and Arts, 2*(2), 60–70.

Peek, N., Capurro, D., Rozova, V., & van der Veer, S. N. (2024). Bridging the gap: Challenges and strategies for the implementation of artificial intelligence-based clinical decision support systems in clinical practice. *Yearbook of Medical Informatics, 33*(1), 103–114.

Petticrew, M., & Roberts, H. (2008). *Systematic reviews in the social sciences: A practical guide*. John Wiley & Sons.

Pohane, L, A., J Dighade, S., S Rithe, E., R Mangwani, R., S Raut, A., & S Bhamburkar, S. (2025). AI-Driven Advancements in Pharmacy: Enhancing Drug Discovery, Optimization and Clinical Decision-Making. *International Journal of Innovative Science and Research Technology, 10*(3), 615–626.

Ponnuviji, N. P., Elangovan, G., Sujatha, K., Jambulingam, U., Ganesan, I., & Lalitha, S. D. (2024). IoT-Enabled Assistive Technologies Approach for Personalized Geriatric Health Monitoring and Safety. In Future of AI in Biomedicine and Biotechnology (pp. 125-146). IGI Global.

Ponnuviji, N. P., Nirmala, G., Kokila, M. S., & Priyadharshini, S. I. (2025). Optimizing Image Retrieval in Cloud Servers with TN-AGW: A Secure and Efficient Approach. Journal of The Institution of Engineers (India): Series B, 106(2), 459-473.

Ponnuviji, N. P., Sumaiya Begum, A., Gnanasekaran, T., Rajendiran, M., & Shenbaga Ezhil, S. (2023, April). Leveraging Random Forest for Intelligent IoT Systems in Industrial Environments. In International Conference on Internet of Things (pp. 46-57). Cham: Springer Nature Switzerland.

Popolo, V., Trunfio, T. A., & Scala, A. A Literature Review on the Application of Reinforcement Learning in Healthcare Management.

Prasad, N., Cheng, L. F., Chivers, C., Draugelis, M., & Engelhardt, B. E. (2020). A reinforcement learning approach to weaning of mechanical ventilation in intensive care units. In *Conference on Uncertainty in Artificial Intelligence* (pp. 818-827). PMLR.

Prayitno, Shyu, C.-R., Putra, K. T., Chen, H.-C., Tsai, Y.-Y., Hossain, K. S. M. T., & Shae, Z.-Y. (2021). A systematic review of federated learning in the healthcare area: From the perspective of data properties and applications. *Applied Sciences (Basel, Switzerland)*, *11*, 11191.

Priyadharshini, S. I., Irene, D. S., Beulah, J. R., & Ponnuviji, N. P. (2025). Enhancing real-time health monitoring with hybrid recurrent long short-term tyrannosaurus search for menstrual cups. *Biomedical Signal Processing and Control*, *100*, 107065.

Puri, N., Saggar, P., Kaur, A., & Garg, P. (2022, July). Application of ensemble Machine Learning models for phishing detection on web networks. In *2022 Fifth International Conference on Computational Intelligence and Communication Technologies (CCICT)* (pp. 296-303). IEEE.

Quazi, F., Mohammed PhD, A. S., & Gorrepati, N. (2024). Transforming treatment and diagnosis in healthcare through AI. *International Journal of Global Innovations and Solutions(IJGIS)*.

Qureshi, F. M., Golan, R., Ghomeshi, A., & Ramasamy, R. (2023). An update on the use of wearable devices in men's health. *The World Journal of Men's Health*, *41*(4), 785–795.

Rácz, A., Bajusz, D., Miranda-Quintana, R. A., & Héberger, K. (2021). Machine learning models for classification tasks related to drug safety. *Molecular Diversity*, *25*(3), 1409–1424. DOI: 10.1007/s11030-021-10239-x PMID: 34110577

Raghu, A., Komorowski, M., Ahmed, I., Celi, L., Szolovits, P., & Ghassemi, M. (2017). Deep reinforcement learning for sepsis treatment. *arXiv preprint arXiv:1711.09602*.

Rahim, M. J., Afroz, A., & Akinola, O. (2025). Predictive Analytics in Healthcare: Big Data, Better Decisions. *International Journal of Scientific Research and Modern Technology*, *4*(1), 1–21.

Rai, A. K., Sharma, M., Saravanan, V., Shalini, N., Kumar, M., & Singh, P. (2023). *Personalized Healthcare Recommendations with Q-Learning Reinforcement Learning*. 1–6. https://doi.org/DOI: 10.1109/ICAIIHI57871.2023.10489223

Rai, A. K., Sharma, M., Saravanan, V., Shalini, N., Kumar, M., & Singh, P. (2023, December). Personalized healthcare recommendations with Q-Learning reinforcement learning. In *2023 International Conference on Artificial Intelligence for Innovations in Healthcare Industries (ICAIIHI)* (Vol. 1, pp. 1-6). IEEE.

Rajendran, S., Obeid, J. S., & Binol, H., DAgostino Jr, R., Foley, K., Zhang, W., & Topaloglu, U. (2021). Cloud-based federated learning implementation across medical centers. *JCO Clinical Cancer Informatics*, *5*, 1–11.

Rajkomar, A., Hardt, M., Howell, M. D., Corrado, G., & Chin, M. H. (2018). Ensuring Fairness in Machine Learning to Advance Health Equity. *Annals of Internal Medicine, 169*(12), 866–872. DOI: 10.7326/M18-1990

Rajkomar, A., Hardt, M., Howell, M. D., Corrado, G., & Chin, M. H. (2018). Ensuring fairness in machine learning to advance health equity. *Annals of Internal Medicine, 169*(12), 866–872. PMID: 30508424

Rajpurkar, P., & Lungren, M. P. (2023). The current and future state of AI interpretation of medical images. *The New England Journal of Medicine, 388*, 1981–1990. PMID: 37224199

Rajput, R., Sukumar, V., Patnaik, P., Garg, P., & Ranjan, M. (2024, March). The Cognitive Analysis for an Approach to Neuroscience. In *2024 International Conference on Automation and Computation (AUTOCOM)* (pp. 524-528). IEEE.

Ramakrishnan, T., Mohan Gift, M. D., Chitradevi, S., Jegan, R., & Subha Hency Jose, P. Nagaraja, Rajneesh Sharma H.N., Selvakumar P., Sintayehu Mekuria Hailegiorgis, (2022). "Study of Numerous Resins Used in Polymer Matrix Composite Materials", Advances in Materials Science and Engineering, vol. 2022, Article ID 1088926, 8 pages, 2022. https://doi.org/DOI: 10.1155/2022/1088926

Ramasamy, L. K., Khan, F., Joghee, S., Dempere, J., & Garg, P. (2024, March). Forecast of Students' Mental Health Combining an Artificial Intelligence Technique and Fuzzy Inference System. In *2024 International Conference on Automation and Computation (AUTOCOM)* (pp. 85-90). IEEE.

Rana, M. S., & Shuford, J. (2024). AI in healthcare: transforming patient care through predictive analytics and decision support systems. Journal of Artificial Intelligence General Science (JAIGS) ISSN: 3006-4023, 1(1).

Rane, N., Choudhary, S., & Rane, J. (2024). Machine learning and deep learning: A comprehensive review on methods, techniques, applications, challenges, and future directions. *Techniques, Applications, Challenges, and Future Directions (May 31, 2024).*

Ratta, R., Sodhi, J., & Saxana, U. (2025). The Relevance of Trust in the Implementation of AI-Driven Clinical Decision Support Systems by Healthcare Professionals: An Extended UTAUT Model. *Electronic Journal of Knowledge Management, 23*(1), 47–66.

Recharla, M., Chakilam, C., Kannan, S., Nuka, S. T., & Suura, S. R. (2025). Harnessing AI and Machine Learning for Precision Medicine: Advancements in Genomic Research, Disease Detection, and Personalized Healthcare. *American Journal of Psychiatric Rehabilitation*, *28*(1), 112–123.

Reddy, S., Rogers, W., Makinen, V.-P., Coiera, E., Brown, P., Wenzel, M., Weicken, E., Ansari, S., Mathur, P., Casey, A., & Kelly, B. (2021). Evaluation framework to guide implementation of AI systems into healthcare settings. *BMJ Health & Care Informatics*, *28*(1), e100444.

Rehan, H. (2024). Enhancing Early Detection and Management of Chronic Diseases with AI-Driven Predictive Analytics on Healthcare Cloud Platforms. *Journal of AI-Assisted Scientific Discovery*, *4*(2), 1–38.

Rehman, A. U., Li, M., Wu, B., Ali, Y., Rasheed, S., Shaheen, S., Liu, X., Luo, R., & Zhang, J. (2025). Role of artificial intelligence in revolutionizing drug discovery. *Fundamental Research (Beijing)*, *5*(3), 1273–1287. DOI: 10.1016/j.fmre.2024.04.021

Reuters. (2024, March 25). Can artificial intelligence extend healthcare to all? Reuters. https://www.reuters.com/sustainability/can-artificial-intelligence-extend-healthcare-all-2024-03-25/

Rieke, N., (2020). The future of digital health with federated learning. *NPJ Digital Medicine*, *3*(119).

Rogers, T. N. (2025, May 27). Robots take on some of the 'busy work' at US hospitals. *Financial Times*. https://www.ft.com/content/aabb7d4b-1e2d-47b9-97f4-c3fc96448aa7

Rosenbacke, R., Melhus, Å., McKee, M., & Stuckler, D. (2024). How Explainable Artificial Intelligence Can Increase or Decrease Clinicians' Trust in AI Applications in Health Care: Systematic Review. *JMIR AI*, *3*, e53207.

Roy, K., Debdas, S., Kundu, S., Chouhan, S., Mohanty, S., & Biswas, B. (2021). Application of natural language processing in healthcare. *Computational Intelligence and Healthcare Informatics*, 393-407.

Roy, P. P., Teju, V., Kandula, S. R., Sowmya, K. V., Stan, A. I., & Stan, O. P. (2024). Secure Healthcare Model Using Multi-Step Deep Q Learning Network in Internet of Things. *Electronics (Basel)*, *13*(3), 3. Advance online publication. DOI: 10.3390/electronics13030669

Roy, P. P., Teju, V., Kandula, S. R., Sowmya, K. V., Stan, A. I., & Stan, O. P. (2024). Secure healthcare model using multi-step deep q learning network in internet of things. *Electronics (Basel)*, *13*(3), 669.

Russell, S. J., & Norvig, P. (2016). *Artificial intelligence: a modern approach*. Pearson.

Sagor, D. H., Chowdhory, U. G., Dey, A., & Sagor, D. H. (2025). *AI and Machine Learning in Healthcare: Advancing Diagnostics, Personalized Treatment, and Predictive Modeling* (No. 2025040007). *Preprints*. https://doi.org/DOI: 10.20944/preprints202504.0007.v1

Saini, P., Nagpal, B., Garg, P., & Kumar, S. (2023). CNN-BI-LSTM-CYP: A deep learning approach for sugarcane yield prediction. *Sustainable Energy Technologies and Assessments*, *57*, 103263.

Salehi, F. (2024). The transformative role of artificial intelligence in the healthcare industry: A comprehensive analysis. *Asian Journal of Research in Medicine and Medical Science*, *6*(1), 62–70.

Sandhu, R., Channi, H. K., Ghai, D., & Kaur, M. (2025). Zero-Trust Approach for Secure Healthcare System. In *Zero-Trust Learning* (pp. 387–409). Apple Academic Press.

Sandhu, R., Ghai, D., Tripathi, S. L., Kaur, R., Rawal, K., & Dhir, K. (2024). Machine learning for cognitive treatment planning in patients with neurodisorder and trauma injuries. In *Computational Intelligence and Deep Learning Methods for Neuro-rehabilitation Applications* (pp. 165–193). Academic Press.

Saraswat, D., Bhattacharya, P., Verma, A., Prasad, V. K., Tanwar, S., Sharma, G., & Sharma, R. (2022). Explainable AI for healthcare 5.0: Opportunities and challenges. *IEEE Access : Practical Innovations, Open Solutions*, *10*, 84486–84517.

Sarker, I. A. (2021). Deep learning: A comprehensive overview on techniques, taxonomy, applications and research directions. *SN Computer Science*, *2*(6), 420. Advance online publication. DOI: 10.1007/s42979-021-00815-1 PMID: 34426802

Schönberger, D. (2019). Artificial intelligence in healthcare: A critical analysis of the legal and ethical implications. *International Journal of Law and Information Technology*, *27*(2), 171–203.

Secinaro, S., Calandra, D., Secinaro, A., Muthurangu, V., & Biancone, P. (2021). The role of artificial intelligence in healthcare: A structured literature review. *BMC Medical Informatics and Decision Making*, *21*(1), 125.

Selvam, D. T., Vinothkumar, J., & Madhubala, S. (2024, November). Two-Phase Deep Q Learning Network for Secure Healthcare Model in the Internet of Things. In *2024 2nd International Conference on Advances in Computation, Communication and Information Technology (ICAICCIT)* (Vol. 1, pp. 365-370). IEEE.

Shah, A. D., Bartlett, J. W., Carpenter, J., Nicholas, O., & Hemingway, H. (2014). Comparison of random forest and parametric imputation models for imputing missing data using MICE: A CALIBER study. *American Journal of Epidemiology, 179*(6), 764–774.

Shah, N., & Chen, H. (2024). Optimizing healthcare delivery: Investigating key areas for AI integration and impact in clinical settings. In *Preprints.*

Shahsavarani, A. M., Azad MarzAbadi, E., HakimiKalkhoran, M., Jafari, S., &Qaranli, S. (2015). Clinical decision support systems (CDSSs): State of the art review of literature. *International Journal of Medical Reviews, 2*(4), 299–308.

Shajari, S., Kuruvinashetti, K., Komeili, A., & Sundararaj, U. (2023). The Emergence of AI-Based Wearable Sensors for Digital Health Technology: A Review. *Sensors (Basel), 23*(23), 9498. DOI: 10.3390/s23239498

Shamshad, F., Khan, S., Zamir, S. W., Khan, M. H., Hayat, M., Khan, F. S., & Fu, H. (2023). Transformers in medical imaging: A survey. *Medical Image Analysis, 88*, 102802. DOI: 10.1016/j.media.2023.102802 PMID: 37315483

Shamszare, H., & Choudhury, A. (2023, August). Clinicians' perceptions of artificial intelligence: focus on workload, risk, trust, clinical decision making, and clinical integration. In Healthcare (Vol. 11, No. 16, p. 2308). MDPI.

Shao, Z. (2024). Analysis of diabetes based on Tree Decision, Logistic Regression and Artificial Neural Network. *Applied and Computational Engineering, 47*(1), 248–256.

Sharma, J., Kumar, D., & Gupta, T. (2024, July). Optimizing Pneumonia Detection: Integrating Quadratic Discriminant Analysis and Deep Q-Networks Through Reinforcement Learning. In *2024 2nd World Conference on Communication & Computing (WCONF)* (pp. 1-5). IEEE.

Sharma, R. Gupta, S. and Garg, P., "Model for Predicting Cardiac Health using Deep Learning Classifier," (2022) Fifth International Conference on Computational Intelligence and Communication Technologies (CCICT), pp. 25-30, doi: DOI: 10.1109/CCiCT56684.2022.00017

Sharma, R., Gupta, S., & Garg, P. (2022, July). Model for predicting cardiac health using deep learning classifier. In *2022 Fifth International Conference on Computational Intelligence and Communication Technologies (CCICT)* (pp. 25-30). IEEE.

Sharma, V., Vashishth, T. K., Kumar, B., Sharma, K. K., Vidyant, S., & Chaudhary, S. (2023, December). Health Interpretation of Covid-19 Patients using Artificial Intelligence. In *2023 International Conference on Artificial Intelligence for Innovations in Healthcare Industries (ICAIIHI)* (Vol. 1, pp. 1-5). IEEE Computer Society.

Sheller, M. J., (2020). Federated learning in medicine. *Scientific Reports, 10*(12598).

Shen, R. (2024). The transformative impact of artificial intelligence in healthcare: Innovations, applications, and future prospects. SHS Web of Conferences, 207, 03018. https://doi.org/DOI: 10.1051/shsconf/202420703018

Shen, Y. T., Chen, L., Yue, W. W., & Xu, H. X. (2021). Artificial intelligence in ultrasound. *European Journal of Radiology, 139*, 109717. PMID: 33962110

Shiny Irene, D., Ponnuviji, N. P., & Kalaivani, A. (2025). EHECA-HSWS: A Holistic Method for Improving Menstrual Health App User Experience. *Journal of the Institution of Electronics and Telecommunication Engineers*, •••, 1–12.

Shortliffe, E. H. (1974, January). A rule-based computer program for advising physicians regarding antimicrobial therapy selection. In *Proceedings of the 1974 Annual ACM Conference-Volume 2* (pp. 739-739).

Shortliffe, E. H. (1976). *Computer-based medical consultations: MYCIN* (Vol. 2). Elsevier.

Shuford, J. (2024). Deep Reinforcement Learning unleashing the power of AI in decision-making. *Journal of Artificial Intelligence General Science (JAIGS) ISSN:3006-4023, 1*(1).

Sikdar, S., & Guha, S. (2020). Advancements of healthcare technologies: Paradigm towards smart healthcare systems. In *Recent trends in image and signal processing in computer vision* (pp. 113–132). Springer Singapore.

Singh, A. P., Saxena, R., Saxena, S., & Maurya, N. K. (2024). Artificial intelligence revolution in healthcare: Transforming diagnosis, treatment, and patient care. *Asian Journal of Advances in Research, 7*(1), 241–263.

Singhal, S., & Carlton, S. (2019). The era of exponential improvement in healthcare. McKinsey & Company, 1-16.

Singh, G., Violi, V., & Fisichella, M. (2023). Federated learning to safeguard patients' data: A medical image retrieval case. *Big Data and Cognitive Computing, 7*, 18.

Singh, M., Garg, P., Srivastava, S., & Saggu, A. K. (2024, April). Revolutionizing Arrhythmia Classification: Unleashing the Power of Machine Learning and Data Amplification for Precision Healthcare. In *2024 Sixth International Conference on Computational Intelligence and Communication Technologies (CCICT)* (pp. 516-522). IEEE.

Singh, R., Arya, P., & Dubey, S. H. (2024). Artificial Intelligence in Pharmaceutics: Revolutionizing Drug Formulation and Optimization. *Journal of Drug Discovery and Health Sciences*, *1*(03), 138–145.

Soewu, T., Kaur, H., Sandhu, R., Soni, A., Ghai, D., Dhir, K., & Tripathi, S. L. (2025). Machine learning and deep learning for cancer diagnosis. In *Rehabilitation Robotics and Healthcare Devices* (pp. 83–129). Academic Press.

Solanki, S. L., Pandrowala, S., Nayak, A., Bhandare, M., Ambulkar, R. P., & Shrikhande, S. V. (2021). Artificial intelligence in perioperative management of major gastrointestinal surgeries. *World Journal of Gastroenterology*, *27*(21), 2758–2770.

Soni, E., Nagpal, A., Garg, P., & Pinheiro, P. R. (2022). Assessment of compressed and decompressed ECG databases for telecardiology applying a convolution neural network. *Electronics (Basel)*, *11*(17), 2708.

Soori, M., Arezoo, B., & Dastres, R. (2023). Artificial intelligence, machine learning and deep learning in advanced robotics, a review. *Cognitive Robotics*, *3*, 54–70. DOI: 10.1016/j.cogr.2023.04.001

Sorte, S. R., Rawekar, A., & Rathod, S. B. (2024). Understanding AI in healthcare: Perspectives of future healthcare professionals. *Cureus*, *16*(8), e66285.

Sreelakshmi, S., Babu, A. A., Lakshmipriya, C., Gracious, L. A., Nalini, M., & Subramanian, R. S. (2024, October). Enhancing Intrusion Detection Systems with Machine Learning. In 2024 2nd International Conference on Self Sustainable Artificial Intelligence Systems (ICSSAS) (pp. 557-564). IEEE.

Sreenivasulu, A., & Manimozhi, T. Satheesh kumar P., Selvakumar P. and Singh P. (2022). "The Model of Smart Sensing Device For Sensitive Nanoclusters Modification in Sensing Properties," 2022 2nd International Conference on Advance Computing and Innovative Technologies in Engineering (ICACITE), Greater Noida, India, 2022, pp. 1043-1047, doi: DOI: 10.1109/ICACITE53722.2022.9823846

Srivastava, A. K., Verma, I., & Garg, P. (2024, May). Improvements in Recommendation Systems Using Graph Neural Networks. In *2024 International Conference on Emerging Innovations and Advanced Computing (INNOCOMP)* (pp. 668-672). IEEE.

Subha, S., Balakrishnan, C., & Anish, T. P. (2024, August). Optimizing Machine Learning Algorithms for Heart Disease Prediction in Healthcare: A Comparative Study. In 2024 5th International Conference on Electronics and Sustainable Communication Systems (ICESC) (pp. 866-872). IEEE.

Sugumaran, K. M. D., Pandiyarajan V., Y. B S, Selvakumar P. and M. S, (2024). "Analysis of Electromyography Signals for Control of Mechanical Prosthesis using Machine Learning Techniques," 2024 2nd International Conference on Intelligent Data Communication Technologies and Internet of Things (IDCIoT), Bengaluru, India, 2024, pp. 1059-1067, doi: DOI: 10.1109/IDCIoT59759.2024.10467707

Sun, Y., Yan, J., Lu, L., Zhang, H., & Shang, Y. (2025). Semantic Fusion-Oriented Bi-Typed Multi-Relational Heterogeneous Graph Neural Network. *IEEE Access : Practical Innovations, Open Solutions.*

Sutton, R. S., & Barto, A. G. (1998). *No. 1* (Vol. 1). Reinforcement learning: An introduction. MIT press.

Sutton, R. S., & Barto, A. G. (2018). *Reinforcement learning: An introduction.* MIT press.

Su, X., Fang, X., Cheng, Z., Gong, Z., & Choi, C. (2024). Deep reinforcement learning based latency-energy minimization in smart healthcare network. *Digital Communications and Networks.* Advance online publication. DOI: 10.1016/j.dcan.2024.06.008

Swayne, M. (2025, March 26). National Quantum Computing Centre's Paper Explores Quantum Computing's Transformative Potential in Healthcare And Pharmaceuticals. *The Quantum Insider.* https://thequantuminsider.com/2025/03/26/national-quantum-computing-centres-paper-explores-quantum-computings-transformative-potential-in-healthcare-and-pharmaceuticals/

Talaat, F. M. (2022). Effective deep Q-networks (EDQN) strategy for resource allocation based on optimized reinforcement learning algorithm. *Multimedia Tools and Applications, 81*(28), 39945–39961.

Tamrakar, P., Pathak, G. R., Lal, M., Goel, A., & Bhende, M. (2024, February). Personalized Healthcare Recommendations with Q-Learning Reinforcement Learning. In *International Conference on Machine Learning Algorithms* (pp. 182-193). Cham: Springer Nature Switzerland.

Tanguay-Sela, M., & Benrimoh, D., Popescu Christina and Perez, T., Rollins, C., Snook, E., Lundrigan, E., Armstrong, C., Perlman, K., Fratila, R., Mehltretter, J., Israel, S., Champagne, M., Williams, J., Simard Jade and Parikh, S. V, Karp, J. F., Heller, K., Linnaranta, O., Cardona, L. G., & Turecki Gustavo and Margolese, H. C. (2022). Evaluating the perceived utility of an artificial intelligence-powered clinical decision support system for depression treatment using a simulation center. *Psychiatry Research*, *308*(114336), 114336.

Tanveer, H., Faheem, M., & Khan, A. H. (2022). Explainable AI in Medical Decision-Making: Challenges and Opportunities. *Iconic Research and Engineering Journals*, *5*(12), 423–435.

Team, D. R. L. (2025, January 14). *The State of Reinforcement Learning in 2025*. DataRoot Labs. https://datarootlabs.com/blog/state-of-reinforcement-learning-2025

Teles, H. R., Ferreira, L. A., Valli, M. A. X., Coelho, F., & Andricopulo, A. A. X. (2022). Hierarchical clustering and target-independent QSAR for antileishmanial oxazole and oxadiazole derivatives. *International Journal of Molecular Sciences*, *23*(16), 8898. Advance online publication. DOI: 10.3390/ijms23168898 PMID: 36012163

Temsah, M.-H., Alhuzaimi, A. N., Almansour, M., Aljamaan, F., Alhasan, K., Batarfi, M. A., Altamimi, I., Alharbi, A., Alsuhaibani, A. A., Alwakeel, L., Alzahrani, A. A., & Alsulaim, K. B., Jamal Amr and Khayat, A., Alghamdi, M. H., Halwani, R., Khan, M. K., Al-Eyadhy, A., & Nazer, R. (2024). Art or artifact: Evaluating the accuracy, appeal, and educational value of AI-Generated Imagery in DALL·E 3 for illustrating congenital heart diseases. *Journal of Medical Systems*, *48*(1), 54.

Thakkar, A., Johansson, S., Jorner, K., Buttar, D., Reymond, J.-L., & Engkvist, O. (2021). Artificial intelligence and automation in computer aided synthesis planning. *Reaction Chemistry & Engineering*, *6*(1), 27–51. DOI: 10.1039/D0RE00340A

Tomulescu, V. (2009). First year experience of robotic-assisted laparoscopic surgery with 153 cases in a General Surgery Department: Indications technique and results. *Chirurgia*, 2.

Topol, E. J. (2019). *Deep Medicine: How Artificial Intelligence Can Make Healthcare Human Again*. Basic Books.Topol, E. J. (2019). *Deep medicine: How artificial intelligence can make healthcare human again*. Basic Books.

Topol, E. (2019). *Deep medicine: how artificial intelligence can make healthcare human again*.

Topol, E. J. (2019). High-performance medicine: The convergence of human and artificial intelligence. *Nature Medicine*, *25*(1), 44–56. PMID: 30617339

Tsai, M. L., Chen, K. F., & Chen, P. C. (2025). Harnessing Electronic Health Records and Artificial Intelligence for Enhanced Cardiovascular Risk Prediction: A Comprehensive Review. *Journal of the American Heart Association*, *14*(6), e036946. PMID: 40079336

Tupe, S., & Kulkarni, N. P. (2015). eca: Evolutionary Computing Algorithm for E-Healthcare Information System. *iPGCON-2015*, 24-25.

University of Pittsburgh & Leidos. (2025, April 18). Pitt, Leidos use AI to fight cancer and health disparities. Axios. https://www.axios.com/local/pittsburgh/2025/04/18/pitt-leidos-use-ai-to-fight-cancer-and-health-disparities

Upadhyay, D., Garg, P., Aldossary, S. M., Shafi, J., & Kumar, S. (2023). A Linear Quadratic Regression-Based Synchronised Health Monitoring System (SHMS) for IoT Applications. *Electronics (Basel)*, *12*(2), 309.

Van Cauwenberge, D., & Van Biesen, W., Decruyenaere Johan and Leune, T., & Sterckx, S. (2022). "Many roads lead to Rome and the Artificial Intelligence only shows me one road": An interview study on physician attitudes regarding the implementation of computerised clinical decision support systems. *BMC Medical Ethics*, *23*(1), 50.

Varadi, M., Anyango, S., Deshpande, M., Nair, S., Natassia, C., Yordanova, G., Yuan, D., Stroe, O., Wood, G., Laydon, A., Žídek, A., Green, T., Tunyasuvunakool, K., Petersen, S., Jumper, J., Clancy, E., Green, R., Vora, A., Lutfi, M., & Velankar, S. (2022). AlphaFold protein structure database: Massively expanding the structural coverage of protein-sequence space with high-accuracy models. *Nucleic Acids Research*, *50*(D1), D439–D444. DOI: 10.1093/nar/gkab1061 PMID: 34791371

Varshney, A., Lamba, S., & Garg, P. (2022, July). A Comprehensive Survey on Event Analysis Using Deep Learning. In *2022 Fifth International Conference on Computational Intelligence and Communication Technologies (CCICT)* (pp. 146-150). IEEE.

Vashishth, T. K., Chaudhary, S., & Sharma, V. (2023). Optimum Utilization of Bed Resources in Hospitals: A Stochastic Approach. In: Manju, Kumar, S., Islam, S.M.N. (eds) Artificial Intelligence-based Healthcare Systems. The Springer Series in Applied Machine Learning. Springer, Cham.

Vashishth, T. K., Sharma, V., Kumar, B., Panwar, R., Sharma, K. K., & Chaudhary, S. (2024). AI-Integrated IoT in Healthcare Ecosystem: Opportunities, Challenges, and Future Directions. AI and IoT Technology and Applications for Smart Healthcare Systems, 37-54.

Vashishth, T. K., Sharma, V., Sharma, K. K., Chaudhary, S., Kumar, B., & Panwar, R. (2024, March). Artificial neural networks & discrete Wavelet transform enabled healthcare model for stress and emotion assessment using speech signal recognition. In AIP Conference Proceedings (Vol. 3072, No. 1). AIP Publishing.

Vashishth, T. K., Sharma, V., Sharma, K. K., Kumar, B., Chaudhary, S., & Panwar, R. (2024). Enhancing biomedical signal processing with machine learning: A comprehensive review. Digital Transformation in Healthcare 5.0: Volume 1: IoT, AI and Digital Twin, 277.

Vashishth, T. K., Sharma, V., Sharma, K. K., Kumar, B., Chaudhary, S., & Panwar, R. (2024). Intrusion Detection and Prevention Techniques in FL Cloud-Based Healthcare 5.0: A Comprehensive Review. Pioneering Smart Healthcare 5.0 with IoT, Federated Learning, and Cloud Security, 152-174.

Vashishth, T. K., Sharma, V., Sharma, M. K., & Sharma, R. (2025). Healthcare and Smart Cities Applications of Secure 6G Infrastructure. In Building Tomorrow's Smart Cities With 6G Infrastructure Technology (pp. 399-432). IGI Global Scientific Publishing.

Vashishth, T. K., Sharma, V., Kumar, S., Verma, N., Vidyant, S., & Kaushik, S. (2025). The Integration of AI in Telemedicine Transforming Healthcare Delivery and Patient Outcomes. In *AI-Driven Personalized Healthcare Solutions* (pp. 71–98). IGI Global Scientific Publishing.

Vashishth, T. K., Sharma, V., Sharma, K. K., & Kumar, B. (2024). Elevating healthcare services: The integration of cloud with fog computing. In *Web 3.0* (pp. 54–75). CRC Press.

Vashishth, T. K., Sharma, V., Sharma, K. K., Kumar, B., Chaudhary, S., & Panwar, R. (2024). Security Challenges in Storing and Exchanging Medical Information. In *Medical Robotics and AI-Assisted Diagnostics for a High-Tech Healthcare Industry* (pp. 378–402). IGI Global.

Vashishth, T. K., Sharma, V., Sharma, K. K., Kumar, B., Chaudhary, S., & Panwar, R. (2025). Data-driven healthcare: Leveraging AoT and metaverse for better diagnosis. In *Leveraging Metaverse and Analytics of Things (AoT) in Medical Systems* (pp. 41–60). Academic Press.

Vashishth, T. K., Sharma, V., Sharma, K. K., Sethi, P., Chaudhary, T., & Bhardwaj, A. (2024). Future Implications of Blockchain for Biomedical and Healthcare. In *Blockchain for Biomedical Research and Healthcare: Concept, Trends, and Future Implications* (pp. 367–404). Springer Nature Singapore.

Vaz, J. M., & Balaji, S. (2021). Convolutional neural networks (CNNs): Concepts and applications in pharmacogenomics. *Molecular Diversity*, *25*(3), 1569–1584. DOI: 10.1007/s11030-021-10225-3 PMID: 34031788

Veiga, R., Both, C. B., Medeiros, I., Rosário, D., & Cerqueira, E. (2023). A federated learning approach for authentication and user identification based on behavioral biometrics. In *Anais do XLI Simpósio Brasileiro de Redes de Computadores e Sistemas Distribuídos* (pp. 15–28).

Verma, J. K., Paul, S., & Johri, P. (Eds.). (2020). *Computational Intelligence and Its Applications in Healthcare*. Academic Press.

Vigneswari, J., & Yamini, B. (2024, November). Smart Health Monitoring System Using IoT Sensors in Cloud Environment. In *2024 International Conference on Smart Technologies for Sustainable Development Goals (ICSTSDG)* (pp. 1-5). IEEE.

Vijayakumar, G. (2024). Muniyandi Rajkumar, Rajiv Chandar N, Selvakumar P and Ramesh Duraisamy, (2024). Environmentally friendly TDS removal from waste water by electrochemical ion exchange batch-type recirculation (EIR) technique. *Environmental Science. Water Research & Technology*, *10*, 826–835. DOI: 10.1039/D3EW00793F

Wable, P. M., Bhargavi, G., Kishore, G. B. V., Sathish, K., & Reuben, G. V. (2024). Leveraging Artificial Intelligence for Predictive Health Diagnostics: Innovations, Applications, and Ethical Considerations in Modern Healthcare. Library of Progress-Library Science, Information Technology & Computer, 44(3).

Wahl, B., Cossy-Gantner, A., Germann, S., & Schwalbe, N. R. (2018). Artificial intelligence (AI) and global health: How can AI contribute to health in resource-poor settings? *BMJ Global Health*, *3*(4), e000798. PMID: 30233828

Wang, D., Wang, L., Zhang, Z., Ding, W., Zhu, H., Gao, Y., Fan, X., & Tian, F. (2021, May). ``brilliant AI doctor'' in rural clinics: Challenges in AI-powered clinical decision support system deployment. *Proceedings of the 2021 CHI Conference on Human Factors in Computing Systems.*

Wang, J., Liu, Q., Liang, H., Joshi, G., & Poor, H. V. (2020). Tackling the objective inconsistency problem in heterogeneous federated optimization. *Advances in Neural Information Processing Systems*, *33*, 7611–7623.

Weissler, E. H., Naumann, T., Andersson, T., Ranganath, R., Elemento, O., Luo, Y., Freitag, D. F., Benoit, J., Hughes, M. C., Khan, F., Slater, P., Shameer, K., Roe, M., Hutchison, E., Kollins, S. H., Broedl, U., Meng, Z., Wong, J. L., Curtis, L., & Ghassemi, M. (2021). The role of machine learning in clinical research: Transforming the future of evidence generation. *Trials*, *22*(1), 537. Advance online publication. DOI: 10.1186/s13063-021-05489-x PMID: 34399832

Wood, E. A., Ange, B. L., & Miller, D. D. (2021). Are we ready to integrate Artificial Intelligence literacy into medical school curriculum: Students and faculty survey. *Journal of Medical Education and Curricular Development*, *8*, 23821205211024080.

World Health Organization. (2021). Ethics and Governance of Artificial Intelligence for Health: WHO Guidance, Geneva.

World Health Organization. (2021). Ethics and governance of artificial intelligence for health: WHO guidance: executive summary. In *Ethics and governance of artificial intelligence for health: WHO guidance: executive summary*.

Wu, Q., Han, J., Yan, Y., Kuo, Y.-H., & Shen, Z.-J. M. (2025). Reinforcement learning for healthcare operations management: Methodological framework, recent developments, and future research directions. *Health Care Management Science*. Advance online publication. DOI: 10.1007/s10729-025-09699-6

Xia, L., Zhen, K., Chen, Z., Liang, R., Zhang, X., Gao, Q., Sheng, M., Bing, L., Xia, J., Si, C., Tian, Y., Jia, L., Xu, Y., Wang, W., Zhong, L., Zuo, X., Wang, D., Xie, W., Wan, J., & Zhai, Z. (2024). Current status of VTE risk assessment and prevention using clinical decision support system: a cross-sectional survey from China. In *Research Square*.

Xia, Q., Zheng, H., Zou, H., Luo, D., Tang, H., Li, L., & Jiang, B. (2025). A comprehensive review of deep learning for medical image segmentation. *Neurocomputing*, *613*, 128740. DOI: 10.1016/j.neucom.2024.128740

Xu, H., & Shuttleworth, K. M. J. (2024). Medical artificial intelligence and the black box problem: A view based on the ethical principle of "do no harm.". *Intelligent Medicine*, *4*(1), 52–57. DOI: 10.1016/j.imed.2023.08.001

Xu, J., Glicksberg, B. S., Su, C., Walker, P., Bian, J., & Wang, F. (2021). Federated learning for healthcare informatics. *Journal of Healthcare Informatics Research*, *5*, 1–19.

Xu, L., Zhu, S., & Wen, N. (2022). Deep reinforcement learning and its applications in medical imaging and radiation therapy: A survey. *Physics in Medicine and Biology*, *67*(22), 22TR02.

Xu, Q., Xie, W., Liao, B., Hu, C., Qin, L., Yang, Z., Xiong, H., Lyu, Y., Zhou, Y., & Luo, A. (2023). Interpretability of clinical decision support systems based on artificial intelligence from technological and medical perspective: A systematic review. *Journal of Healthcare Engineering*, *2023*(1), 9919269.

Yadav, P. S., Khan, S., Singh, Y. V., Garg, P., & Singh, R. S. (2022). A Lightweight Deep Learning-Based Approach for Jazz Music Generation in MIDI Format. *Computational Intelligence and Neuroscience*, *2022*(1), 2140895. PMID: 36035841

Yala, A., Schuster, T., Miles, R., Barzilay, R., & Lehman, C. (2019). A deep learning model to triage screening mammograms: A simulation study. *Radiology*, *293*(1), 38–46.

Yamini, B., Sudha, K., Nalini, M., Kavitha, G., Subramanian, R. S., & Sugumar, R. (2023, June). Predictive modelling for lung cancer detection using machine learning techniques. In 2023 8th International Conference on Communication and Electronics Systems (ICCES) (pp. 1220-1226). IEEE.

Yang, Z., Shi, Y., Li, P., Pan, K., Li, G., Li, X., Yao, S., & Zhang, D. (2022). Application of principal component analysis (PCA) to the evaluation and screening of multiactivity fungi. *Journal of Ocean University of China*, *21*(3), 763–772. DOI: 10.1007/s11802-022-5096-x PMID: 35582545

Yazdani, D., Omidvar, M. N., Yazdani, D., Branke, J., Nguyen, T. T., Gandomi, A. H., & Yao, X. (2023). Robust optimization over time: A critical review. *IEEE Transactions on Evolutionary Computation*.

Yazzourh, S. (2024). *Reinforcement learning and Bayesian outcome-weighted learning for precision medicine: integrating medical knowledge into decision-making algorithms* (Doctoral dissertation, Université de Toulouse).

Yingngam, B., Navabhatra, A., & Sillapapibool, P. (2024). AI-Driven Decision-Making Applications in Pharmaceutical Sciences. In Using Traditional Design Methods to Enhance AI-Driven Decision Making (pp. 1-63). IGI Global Scientific Publishing.

Yu, C., Liu, J., Nemati, S., & Yin, G. (2021). Reinforcement Learning in Healthcare: A Survey. *ACM Comput. Surv.*, *55*(1), 5:1-5:36. https://doi.org/DOI: 10.1145/3477600

Yu, K. H., Beam, A. L., & Kohane, I. S. (2018). Artificial intelligence in healthcare. *Nature Biomedical Engineering*, *2*(10), 719–731. PMID: 31015651

Yu, K. H., Zhang, C., Berry, G. J., Altman, R. B., Re, C., Rubin, D. L., & Snyder, M. (2021). Predicting non-small cell lung cancer prognosis by fully automated microscopic pathology image features. *Nature Communications*, *7*, 12474. PMID: 27527408

Zhang, C., Lu, Y., & Zang, T. A. (2022). CNN-DDI: A learning-based method for predicting drug-drug interactions using convolution neural networks. *BMC Bioinformatics*, *23*(Suppl 3), 88. Advance online publication. DOI: 10.1186/s12859-022-04612-2 PMID: 35255808

Zhang, Q. (2023). Dynamic routing policies for multi-skill call centers using Deep Q Network. *Mathematics*, *11*(22), 4662.

Zhou, B., Yang, G., Shi, Z., & Ma, S. (2022). Natural language processing for smart healthcare. *IEEE Reviews in Biomedical Engineering*, *17*, 4–18.

Zicari, R. V, Ahmed, S., Amann, J., Braun, S. A., Brodersen, J., Bruneault, F., Brusseau, J., Campano, E., Coffee, M., Dengel, A., Düdder, B., Gallucci, A., Gilbert, T. K., Gottfrois, P., Goffi, E., Haase, C. B., Hagendorff, T., Hickman, E., Hildt, E., Wurth, R. (2021). Co-design of a trustworthy AI system in healthcare: Deep learning based skin lesion classifier. *Front. Hum. Dyn., 3*.

# About the Contributors

**Danish Ather** is an accomplished book editor with a robust academic and professional background. Currently as Professor at Amity University in Tashkent, Uzbekistan, Dr. Ather brings over 18 years of experience in teaching, research, and administration. He holds dual Ph.D. degrees in Computer Science and Computer Science & Engineering. His editorial expertise is highlighted through his role as Editor of the proceedings submitted yearly to IEEE USA for the SMART Series conferences. Dr. Ather has authored a book titled "Level up Your Programming with Core Dragon" and published 54 research papers in international journals and conferences, with 15 indexed in Scopus. He is a Senior Member of the IEEE Society and has received numerous awards, including a Certificate of Appreciation from the Ministry of Digital Technologies, Republic of Uzbekistan. His technical proficiency and dedication to advancing knowledge in fields such as IoT, AI, and programming make him a valuable asset in the realm of academic publishing.

**Ng Khai Mun** currently serves as the Acting Deputy Vice Chancellor (Academic & Research) at Infrastructure University Kuala Lumpur, Malaysia. Before becoming Acting Deputy Vice Chancellor, he was the Dean of the Faculty of Engineering, Science & Technology. With over 15 years in academia, Dr. Ng has significantly contributed to engineering education and research. A Chartered Engineer with the Engineering Council UK, and a Professional Technologist with the Malaysia Board of Technologies, he actively engages in academic and industry collaborations. His scholarly work includes multiple journal publications, conference proceedings, and a registered copyright for a solar absorber system. He has been involved in various funded research projects. His research expertise spans renewable energy systems, thermo fluids, and sustainable engineering solutions.He has served as a reviewer for high-impact journals such as Solar Energy and the Journal of Building Engineering, as well as a panel evaluator for research funding proposals.Beyond his academic and research commitments, Dr. Ng is dedicated to fostering innovation and industry-driven research collaborations.

**Sachin Jain** is working as an Associate Professor in the Department of Computer Science and Engineering at Ajay Kumar Garg Engineering College, Ghaziabad. He completed his B.Tech in Computer Science and Engineering in 2007 from UPTU, Lucknow and M.Tech in Computer Science and Engineering in 2010 from GGSIPU, Delhi. He has completed his Ph.D in Computer Science and Engineering from Sharda University Greater Noida in April, 2025. He is a UGC-NET qualified teacher and has total 16 years of teaching experience. His research interests lie in Artificial Intelligence, Deep Learning and Machine Learning. He has published several research papers in Peer-Reviewed Journals and Conference proceedings. Dr. Sachin Jain has filed several patents for his work.

**Vishal Jain** is pursuing Postdoc from Kuala Lumpur University of Science & Technology (KLUST) (formerly known as Infrastructure University Kuala Lumpur (IUKL)), Malaysia. He is presently working as a Professor (CSE) at the Department of Computer Science & Engineering, School of Engineering & Technology, Vivekananda Institute of Professional Studies - Technical Campus, New Delhi. Before that, he worked as Professor at Sharda University, Greater Noida and Associate Professor at Bharati Vidyapeeth's Institute of Computer Applications and Management (BVICAM), New Delhi. He has associated as a member of the Faculty Board, Board of Planning and Management, Executive Council, Academic Council, Curriculum Development and Review Committee and Academic Audit of various higher education Institutions. His research areas include machine learning, information retrieval, semantic web, ontology engineering, data mining, ad hoc networks, sensor networks and network security.

**Vinay Kukreja** currently holds the distinguished position of Professor and Director (Research) at the Office of Research Publications (CURIN), Chitkara University, Punjab. With an illustrious academic career spanning 18 years, he has guided numerous Ph.D. and Master of Engineering students. His scholarly accomplishments are equally impressive, encompassing over 600 articles indexed in Scopus, an h-index of 48, more than 6,000 citations, and upwards of 50 patents, reflecting his significant impact on academia and research. An accomplished author, he has contributed to the academic landscape with three authored books and four edited volumes. Demonstrating his innovative prowess, he secured the prestigious first prize at the 2018 SIH Hackathon, a competition supported by India's Ministry of Housing & Urban Affairs. Prof. Kukreja's research interests are both diverse and cutting-edge, encompassing machine learning, deep learning, agile software development, image processing, data analysis, and structural equation modeling. His achievements underscore his dedication to advancing knowledge and his unwavering commitment to academic and intellectual excellence.

**A. Adaikkammai** is an Assistant Professor in the Department of Computer Science and Business Systems at RMD Engineering College, Chennai. She is committed to academic excellence and student engagement in the evolving field of computing and business integration. Her areas of interest include data analytics, business intelligence, and modern software technologies.

**Satheeshkumar** is working as the assistant professor in the Department of Computer Engineering in Nandha Engineering College, Erode, India

**Mohammad abu Kausar** currently serving as the Associate Professor of the Department of Information Systems and holding the vital role of College Academic Advising Officer and Media Officer, Dr. Mohammad Abu Kausar brings a wealth of experience and dedication to the academic arena. His journey at the University of Nizwa began in 2016 when he joined the Department of Economics, Management, and Information Systems, leaving an indelible mark on the institution. Before assuming his current esteemed position, Dr. Mohammad Abu Kausar demonstrated versatility by working as both an Assistant Professor and a Software Engineer. This dual role showcases his comprehensive understanding of academia and practical applications in the realm of Information Systems. Dr. Mohammad Abu Kausar`s research pursuits delve into the realms of Information Retrieval, Web applications, Programming Languages, and Databases. His scholarly endeavors contribute significantly to the ever-evolving landscape of these domains. Beyond his academic endeavors, Dr. Mohammad Abu Kausar actively participates in numerous professional associations, underscoring his commitment to staying at the forefront of technological advancements. His affiliations include prestigious organizations such as the Computer Society of India (CSI), IEEE, International Association of Engineers (IAENG), The World Association of Technology Teachers (WATT), Computer Science Teachers Association (CSTA), The Institute of Computer Science, Social Informatics and Telecommunication Engineering (ICST), International Society on Multiple Criteria Decision Making (MCDM), and Universal Association of Computer and Electronics Engineers (UACEE).

**Vivek Agarwal** is Assistant Professor in the department of CSE at AKGEC, Ghaziabad, UP, India since August 2024. He received his Bachelor's degree in Computer Science Engineering from UPTU in 2009 and Master degree in Computer Science and Engineering in 2014 from UPTU. He has a vast experience in Academics as well as he has 7 years (from 2017 to 2024) of industry exposure too. The major fields of his interest and research are IoT, Cloud Computing, Machine Learning and & Soft Computing etc.

**Nasser Al Musalhi** is an academic and researcher in Computer Engineering with a PhD and over 5 years of teaching experience. His research focuses on machine learning, artificial intelligence, and cybersecurity, with several peer-reviewed publications. He is also actively involved in editorial roles for East Publications' peer-reviewed journals and contributes to developing smart systems integrating IoT and AI technologies.

**D. Raja** is a faculty member in the Department of Electrical and Electronics Engineering at Thiagarajar College of Engineering, Madurai. He is actively involved in teaching, research, His areas of expertise include power systems, control engineering, and renewable energy technologies.

**Neha Dhule** is a dedicated academician and healthcare management professional currently serving in the Department of MBA (Healthcare Management) at Datta Meghe Institute of Management Studies (DMIMS), Nagpur, Maharashtra. With a strong foundation in healthcare systems and management practices, Dr. Dhule brings a blend of academic expertise and industry insight to her role. She is committed to nurturing future healthcare leaders through innovative teaching methods, research-driven instruction, and a passion for improving healthcare delivery and administration in India.

**Suraj Garg** is currently an Assistant Professor of Forensic Science at the Department of Forensic Sciences, Chandigarh Group of Colleges, Jhanjeri, Mohali, a position he has held since March 27, 2025. He holds an M.Sc. in Forensic Science from Panjab University, Chandigarh, completed between 2020 and 2022. He also earned a B.Sc. in Chemistry from S.V.S.D. College, Bhatoli, affiliated with Himachal Pradesh University, Shimla, from 2017 to 2020. Mr. Garg has significant experience in forensic science, including ten months of training in the Document & Photo Division at the State Forensic Science Laboratory, Dharamshala, and three months of research in Forensic Document Examination at Panjab University, Chandigarh. His research background includes a six-month M.Sc. dissertation on "A Novel approach based on chemometrics coupled to ATR- FTIR Spectroscopy for wood species identification: Application to Wildlife Forensics." He has been awarded the UGC-NET (Forensic Science) twice (June 2024 and Dec. 2024) and the Forensic Aptitude and Caliber Test Plus (FACT) in Forensic Document Examination. He has published work in Forensic Science International: Reports and Microchemical Journal.

**J. Sangeetha** is a faculty member in the Department of Computer Science and Engineering at S.A. Engineering College, Chennai. She is dedicated to teaching and research in core areas of computer science. Her interests include software engineering, data analytics, and emerging technologies in computing.

**Muhabbat Jumaniyozova** is working at Department of Methodology of Primary Education, Urgench state university, Urgench, Uzbekistan.

**Jeyakarthika K** is an Assistant Professor in the Department of Computer Science and Engineering at Ramco Institute of Technology, Rajapalayam, Tamil Nadu. She is dedicated to imparting quality education and fostering innovation among students. Her academic interests include software engineering, artificial intelligence, and data analytics.

**Manpreet Kaur** is currently serving as an Assistant Professor in the Department of Forensic Science at Chandigarh Group of Colleges, Jhanjeri. She is a UGC-NET qualified postgraduate in Forensic Science and Criminology from Panjab University, Chandigarh, and holds a Bachelor's degree in Biotechnology from IK Gujral Punjab Technical University. With a strong academic foundation and passion for research, she has authored multiple publications in the field of forensic science, including studies on the susceptibility of ABO blood groups to COVID-19 and the application of DNA barcoding in plant identification. She is also certified in Cyber Forensics through FACT and FACT-PLUS and has served as a mentor under the Cyber Swachhta Mission 2.0 of Chandigarh Police, promoting cyber awareness. Proficient in forensic software tools like Autopsy and FTK Manager, Manpreet is deeply committed to advancing forensic education and interdisciplinary research, contributing significantly to both academic and practical domains of applied sciences.

**Parminder Kaur** is working as an Professor in the Department of Computer Science, at Guru Nanak Dev University Amritsar, India. She has done her post-graduation in Mathematics as well as System Software and doctorate in the field of Computer Science. She has more than 80 publications in International/National Journals/Conferences. Her research interests include Component-based Software Engineering, Web Engineering, Software Security, Semantic Web, Digital Image Processing, Artificial Intelligence, Requirement Engineering and Service-Oriented Architecture.

**Renu Kumar** is an Assistant Professor in the Department of Computer Science and Engineering at IIMT Engineering College, Meerut. Holding MCA and M.Tech degrees, he brings a blend of academic excellence and dedication to teaching. His passion lies in guiding students through the evolving landscape of computer science and nurturing the next generation of skilled technologists.

**Anto Gracious L. A.** is a faculty member in the Department of Computer Science and Engineering at R.M.K. College of Engineering and Technology, Tiruvallur District, Tamil Nadu. He is actively involved in teaching, student mentoring, and academic development. His interests lie in software engineering, programming, and emerging technologies in computer science.

**Amruta Mahalle** is currently serving as an Assistant Professor at Datta Meghe Institute of Management Studies, Nagpur. With a strong academic foundation and a passion for teaching, she specializes in the areas of Marketing and Human Resource Management.Her academic journey is marked by a commitment to developing industry-relevant knowledge and fostering practical learning among management students. She actively engages in research and scholarly activities, contributing to academic publications and participating in conferences and seminars. Amruta is known for her dynamic teaching approach, blending theoretical insights with real-world applications to enhance student engagement and understanding. Her interests include consumer behavior, digital marketing strategies, financial planning, and investment analysis. She is dedicated to continuous learning and professional development and aims to bridge the gap between academic theory and industry practices. Amruta Mahalle's contributions are instrumental in nurturing future business leaders and promoting academic excellence in the field of management education.

**T.C. Manjunath** was born on 6th February 1967. He did his BE from RV College of Engg. in 1989, ME in Robotics & Automation from LD College of Engg. in 1992 with First Rank and PhD in Systems & Control Engg. from IIT Bombay in the year 2007. He is currently working as the Dean Research R D and as Professor in the Dept. of Computer Science & Engineering with specialization in IoT, Cyber Security & Blockchain Technology in Rajarajeswari College of Engineering, Bengaluru, Karnataka. He has completed B.E. Degree from R.V. College of Engg., M.E. Govt.'s LD College of Engg., Gujarat Univ., Ahmedabad in First Rank and Ph.D. in Systems and Control Engineering from the Indian Institute of Technology Bombay IIT Bombay He has got a teaching academic, research and administrative experience of more than 35+ years 10 years as Principal, 8 years as HoD rest as faculty and has published more than 1200+ research papers in various national & international journals and conferences, with 175+ patents, 25 book-chapters, 25 awards and also published 25 text books in various field of science, engineering and technology, completed projects worth Rs. 9 Crores till date apart from guiding 10

PhD scholars. He is a member of 30 Professional Society Chapters and is a fellow of IE, IETE, AMIEE and a chartered engineer. He got the best research scholar award in 2006 in IIT Bombay amongst all the research scholars of the institute. He has got 10 awards in academics and research activities.

**N. Subhash Chandra** is a Professor at CVR College of Engineering, Hyderabad, Telangana. He is committed to academic excellence and research in the field of engineering and technology. His areas of expertise include computer networks, cybersecurity, and advanced computing systems.

**Mohammad Nasar** is an Assistant Professor and Head of the Department of Computing & Informatics at Mazoon College, Muscat, Oman (Missouri University of Science and Technology, USA). He holds a Ph.D. in Computer Science from Galgotias University, India, and has over 15 years of diverse experience in teaching, research, and industry. His academic interests span software engineering, database systems, and programming languages. Dr. Nasar has authored a book and published over 20 research papers in reputed international journals and conferences. He has participated in several academic events and serves on the editorial boards of seven international journals. He is also a certified Microsoft and Oracle professional and an active member of professional bodies such as IEEE, CSI, IAENG, and IACSIT. His contributions reflect a strong commitment to academic excellence and technological advancement.

**Arpita Nayak** is currently serving as an Assistant Professor, offering courses in management. She completed her Ph.D. in management from the KIIT School of Management. Her MBA and strong interest in Human Resource Management (HRM) led her to pursue further studies in HRM. Her passion for talent management inspired her doctoral research on "A Comparative Study on Talent Management in Private and Public Manufacturing Industries in Odisha." Dr. Nayak has presented research papers at both national and international conferences and has published articles in SCOPUS-listed journals. Over the years, she has taught a variety of subjects, including Human Resource Management, Principles of Management, Business Studies Management, Tribal Entrepreneurship, and Organizational Behaviour. In addition to her academic career, she also has several years of corporate work experience.

**V. N. V. L. S. Swathi** is a committed educator and researcher in the CSE field, blending a decade of teaching experience with active engagement in workshops, and contributions in machine learning and data science. She continues to strengthen CVR's academic and research environment through her roles and scholarly work.

**Aparna P** is a faculty member in the Department of Computer Science and Engineering at RMK College of Engineering and Technology, RSM Nagar, Puduvoyal – 601206. She is dedicated to teaching and guiding students in the field of computer science. Her areas of interest include programming, web technologies, and software development.

**P. Selvakumar** is currently an Associate Professor in the Department of Science and Humanities at Nehru Institute of Technology, Coimbatore, Tamil Nadu, India. Prior to joining Nehru Institute of Technology, he held positions as an Assistant Professor in the Department of Science and Humanities various engineering colleges in Coimbatore, Tamil Nadu, India, spanning from 2011 to 2023. Dr.P. Selvakumar's academic and research interests lie primarily in the field of phytochemistry. He has made significant contributions to his field, with an impressive record that includes 30 journal publications, 12 patents, and 20 conference papers. Additionally, he has organized 5 seminars and conferences, further demonstrating his commitment to academic and scientific exchange. Throughout his career, Dr. P.Selvakumar has been recognized for his dedication and excellence in teaching, having been honored with several awards, including the Best Teacher Awards. He holds a prominent position in the academic community, contributing actively to research.

**Asheesh Pandey** is a seasoned academician with over 20 years of rich experience spanning teaching, research, and the software industry. He holds an MCA, MTech (Computer Science), and a PhD in Computer Science. Currently serving in the Department of Computer Applications at ABES Engineering College, Ghaziabad. He has previously been associated with several reputed institutions under Dr. A.P.J. Abdul Kalam Technical University, Lucknow, and CCS University, Meerut. He also brings two years of industry experience as a software developer at HCL Technologies. A senior member of IEEE, CSI Ghaziabad, CEGR, and ACM, Dr. Pandey specializes in Artificial Intelligence and Machine Learning. He has authored numerous research papers published in prestigious Scopus, SCI, WoS, and UGC CARE journals. His published books cover a wide range of computer science topics including Python for Beginners, Digital Electronics & Computer Organization, Software Engineering, Basics of Artificial Intelligence & Machine Learning, and more.

**R. Anand Babu** is an Associate Professor in the Department of Artificial Intelligence and Machine Learning at Panimalar Engineering College, Chennai. He is passionate about teaching and research in the areas of AI, machine learning, and data science. His work focuses on developing intelligent systems and guiding students in cutting-edge technological advancements.

**R. Asha** is an Assistant Professor in the Department of Computer Science and Engineering at Sathyabama Institute of Science and Technology, Chennai. She is actively involved in teaching, research, and student development. Her areas of interest include artificial intelligence, machine learning, and data science.

**Siva Subramanian R** is an academician at the School of Computing, SRM Institute of Science and Technology, Trichy Campus. He specializes in advanced computing, software development, and artificial intelligence. His research interests include deep learning, data science, and smart systems.

**Ravikumar R. Natarajan** is an experienced academician with over 12+ years of teaching and research expertise across institutions in India, the UAE, and the Maldives. He currently serves as an Assistant Professor at Marwadi University, Rajkot, specializing in Machine Learning, Recommender Systems, and AI-driven applications in healthcare and security. He holds a Ph.D. in Machine Learning and Recommender Systems from Amity University, Jaipur, a Master of Engineering in CSE from VMRF University, Salem, and a Bachelor of Engineering in CSE from Anna University. He also has a MiniMBA from the Swiss eLearning Institute. Dr. Ravikumar has authored more than 8+ multiple SCIE/Scopus-indexed journal articles, 25+ IEEE/Springer conference papers, and co-authored a book on Artificial Intelligence. He has also published 9 patents and contributed 10+ book chapters in emerging domains such as Federated Learning, Blockchain, and Digital Twins for IGI Global, Wiley and Springer publisher. He actively mentors students through initiatives like the Research Activities Club (RAC) and Student Research Internship Training (SRIT), promoting innovation and research culture.

**Aarthi S** is a dedicated Assistant Professor in Computer Science with over six years of teaching experience. She is currently pursuing her Ph.D. at Marwadi University, Gujarat, and holds an M.Phil. and MCA from Bharathiar University, Tamil Nadu. Throughout her academic career, Aarthi has specialized in programming languages such as C++, Java, and C, and contributed to research in recommender systems and AI-related data privacy. She has published journal articles, contributed to book chapters, and actively participated in technical workshops. Known for her student mentorship and engagement in academic events, Aarthi remains committed to fostering innovation and excellence in computer science education.

**S. Sugapriya** is a distinguished academician and an integral pillar of the department and institution. With an M.A. and M.Phil in English, she brings a wealth of knowledge and expertise to her role as an educator. Her administrative and managerial acumen has been instrumental in her responsibilities as the Coordinator for NBA, NAAC, and AU Affiliation, ensuring the institution's adherence to the highest standards of academic excellence. A prolific scholar, Ms. Sugapriya has published seven articles and authored one book, contributing significantly to the field of English education. Her active participation in numerous conferences reflects her commitment to continuous learning and professional development. Beyond her academic and administrative achievements, Ms. Sugapriya is admired for her impeccable dressing sense and her nurturing, motherly affection towards students and colleagues alike. Her dedication, warmth, and leadership make her an invaluable asset to the department and a source of inspiration for all.

**S. Vijayaselvarani** is an Assistant Professor in the Department of Computer Science and Business Systems at Vel Tech Multi Tech Dr. Rangarajan Dr. Sakunthala Engineering College, Avadi, Chennai. She is committed to delivering quality education and mentoring students in the intersection of computer science and business applications. Her academic interests include data analytics, business intelligence, and software development.

**Barkha Samania** is an Assistant Professor at SRM Institute of Science and Technology (SRM IST), Delhi NCR Campus, Ghaziabad. With a strong academic foundation and a deep commitment to teaching, she has contributed significantly to the academic community through her research and scholarly work. Her areas of interest span across emerging technologies and innovative teaching methodologies. Ms. Barkha is known for her dedication to student development and academic excellence.

**Bekhzod Ruzimbaev Saparbaevich** is working at Department Romano-Germanic Philology. Mamun University, Khiva, Uzbekistan

**Narinderjit Singh Sawaran Singh** is an Associate Professor at INTI International University, Malaysia. He graduated from Universiti Teknologi PETRONAS (UTP) in 2016 with Ph.D in Electrical & Electronic Engineering specialized in Probabilistic Methods for Fault Tolerant Computing. Currently, he is appointed as the research cluster head for Computational Mathematics and Technology focuses on the areas like Expert Systems and Artificial Intelligence, Exploratory Data Analysis, Optimization Algorithms, Data Modelling and Computational Intelligence - Swarm Intelligence. He is one of the appointed Editorial Board Members for Journal of Data Science (JoDS) - an international journal indexed by Google Scholar and MyJurnal. He is a very dedicated and committed academician with 20+ years of experience in teaching and more than 10 years of research experience. He is a very resourceful researcher with wide-ranging research interests - Computational, Modeling & Simulation, Mathematical & Statistical Modeling, Fault-tolerant

Computing (reliability - VLSI circuit design), Data Modelling & Computational Intelligence and Healthcare Data Analysis are on the top of the list.

**Mukul Sharma** is a dedicated Lecturer in the Department of Computer Applications at Swami Vivekanand Subharti University, Meerut. With a strong academic foundation and a passion for teaching, he plays a vital role in shaping the technical skills of his students. His primary area of interest lies in Software Engineering, where he focuses on modern development methodologies, software design principles, and emerging technologies. Mr. Sharma is committed to bridging theoretical knowledge with practical applications, inspiring students to innovate and excel in the evolving field of software development.

**Vikas Sharma** is a distinguished researcher affiliated with IIMT University in Meerut, Uttar Pradesh, India. His academic endeavors are centered around the integration of Artificial Intelligence (AI) and Machine Learning (ML) to address complex challenges across various domains. Vikas Sharma's research portfolio includes significant contributions to the field of cybersecurity, particularly in enhancing security protocols within Mobile Ad-Hoc Networks (MANETs). His work emphasizes the development of advanced intrusion detection mechanisms that leverage machine learning algorithms to identify and mitigate potential threats in real-time. International Publications In addition to cybersecurity, Vikas Sharma has explored the application of AI in healthcare, focusing on the interpretation of COVID-19 patient data. His research utilizes deep learning models to analyze respiratory sounds, aiming to improve diagnostic accuracy and patient monitoring during the pandemic.

**Ikvinderpal Singh**, Assistant Professor, P. G. Deptt. Of Computer Science & Applications, Trai Shatabdi GGS Khalsa College, Amritsar. He obtained his MCA with distinction from Guru Nanak Dev University, Amritsar. He has written Thirty Seven books during such a short time span. He has Published Twenty Seven research papers in international/ national journals. He is an editorial board member of 30 international/ national journals. He brought name for himself when he topped the college in B.Sc. His other areas of interest include Soft Computing, Computer Networks and Databases.

**Siva Subramanian R** is an academician at the School of Computing, SRM Institute of Science and Technology, Trichy Campus. He specializes in advanced computing, software development, and artificial intelligence. His research interests include deep learning, data science, and smart systems.

**T. Thilagam** is an Assistant Professor (Senior Grade) in the Department of Computer Science and Engineering at Vel Tech Rangarajan Dr. Sagunthala R&D Institute of Science and Technology, Chennai. She is actively involved in teaching, academic research, and mentoring students. Her areas of interest include artificial intelligence, data structures, and software engineering.

**Shashiraj Teotia** is working as Associate Professor in the Department of Computer Application, Swami Vivekanand Subharti university Meerut. He has total 18 years of experience in teaching and research. He is an active member of IAENG AND IJMRA. He has published about 40 publications in various national and international journals. Four various books.

**Shakhnoza Toshova** is working in the Department of Medical Fundamental Sciences at Termez University of Economics and Service, Termez, Uzbekistan.

**Dipesh Uike** is a distinguished professor at the Dr. Ambedkar Institute of Management Studies and Research, Nagpur, Maharashtra, where he teaches in the MBA program with a specialization in Business Analytics. With a strong command over analytical tools such as SPSS and Power BI, Dr. Uike brings a data-driven approach to business education and research. He has authored numerous research papers published in SCOPUS-indexed journals, contributing significantly to the field of business analytics. In addition to his academic roles, he actively conducts workshops focused on research methodologies and their practical applications in the business world, helping students and professionals bridge the gap between theoretical knowledge and real-world business challenges.

**Tarun Kumar Vashishth** is an active academician and researcher in the field of Computer Science with 22 years of experience. He earned Ph.D. Mathematics degree specialized in Operations Research; served several academic positions such as Dy. Director, HoD, NAAC Coordinator, Academic Coordinator, Member Secretary of Department Research Committee, Assistant Center Superintendent and Head Examiner in University Examinations. He is involved in academic development and scholarly activities. He is member of International Association of Engineers, The Society of Digital Information and Wireless Communications, Global Professors Welfare Association, International Association of Academic plus Corporate (IAAC), Computer Science Teachers Association and Internet Society . His research interest includes Cloud Computing, Artificial Intelligence, Machine Learning and Operations Research; published more than 50 research articles & conference papers with 2 book and 80 book chapters. He is contributing as member of editorial and reviewers boards in conferences and various computer journals and edited books published by

Elsevier, CRC Press, Taylor and Francis, Springer, IGI global, Wiley Publication, IET Publication, De Gruyter, River Publication etc.

**Sanjukta Vidyant** is an Assistant Professor in the Department of Biotechnology at Shobhit University, Meerut, Uttar Pradesh. She holds a Ph.D. from Dr. A.P.J. Abdul Kalam Technical University (AKTU), with her doctoral research focusing on the genetic association of Toll-like receptor (TLR) genes with the risk of HIV-1 infection in the North Indian population. With a robust background in microbiology, Dr. Vidyant has previously served as a Senior Fellow and Research Assistant at the Sanjay Gandhi Postgraduate Institute of Medical Sciences, where she contributed to significant projects, including the WHO-funded Polio Eradication Program and an ICMR-funded study on TLR gene associations in HIV-1 seropositive individuals.

**Atharva Umakant Yewale** is a passionate and ambitious management student pursuing an MBA at Datta Meghe Institute of Management Studies, Nagpur, Maharashtra. With a strong interest in business strategy, leadership, and organizational development, Atharva is committed to gaining comprehensive knowledge and practical skills to excel in the dynamic world of management. He actively participates in academic and co-curricular activities, aiming to become a future leader in the corporate sector.

# Index

## A


Artificial Intelligence 1, 2, 4, 7, 11, 13, 14, 15, 18, 19, 21, 22, 23, 24, 27, 28, 32, 33, 34, 35, 36, 37, 39, 41, 44, 46, 47, 49, 51, 52, 54, 55, 56, 57, 58, 66, 67, 69, 79, 83, 84, 85, 88, 89, 91, 106, 107, 130, 131, 134, 136, 145, 149, 150, 158, 159, 160, 161, 164, 188, 189, 192, 210, 215, 216, 217, 220, 222, 223, 232, 234, 236, 237, 242, 243, 245, 246, 250, 251, 258, 259, 260, 261, 262, 263, 264, 265, 266, 267, 268, 269, 270, 271, 272, 273, 275, 276, 277, 278, 279, 282, 313, 314, 319, 320, 323, 324, 327, 329, 332, 334, 337, 338, 341, 342, 343, 345, 346, 348, 349, 350, 352, 353, 354, 356, 357, 358, 359, 360, 361, 362, 363, 365, 366, 367, 368, 369, 370, 371, 373, 374, 375, 376, 377, 386, 395, 401, 402, 404, 405, 406, 410, 413, 414, 419, 433, 434, 435


## C


Clinical Decision Support Systems 9, 10, 23, 24, 25, 47, 93, 97, 122, 213, 219, 220, 225, 228, 232, 240, 241, 243, 244, 245, 246, 249, 250, 254, 255, 257, 258, 259, 260, 261, 273, 275, 277, 278, 279, 287, 288, 291, 411, 418

Computational Intelligence 1, 3, 4, 5, 11, 14, 19, 22, 23, 24, 25, 27, 28, 29, 30, 32, 34, 39, 40, 41, 42, 43, 44, 47, 49, 50, 51, 52, 55, 56, 84, 85, 87, 88, 89, 91, 92, 93, 97, 98, 99, 100, 101, 102, 105, 108, 109, 281, 282, 286, 287, 309, 311, 315, 319, 435


## D


Data Heterogeneity 92, 115, 163, 165, 169, 172, 177, 186, 288

Decision-Making 1, 2, 7, 8, 9, 18, 19, 27, 28, 29, 30, 31, 32, 33, 34, 35, 36, 37, 38, 39, 40, 41, 44, 45, 48, 49, 50, 51, 52, 53, 54, 56, 89, 100, 101, 102, 106, 107, 108, 127, 128, 138, 146, 147, 149, 150, 155, 161, 170, 192, 195, 197, 198, 199, 202, 203, 204, 209, 210, 213, 214, 219, 220, 222, 225, 228, 229, 240, 241, 243, 244, 245, 246, 248, 249, 250, 252, 253, 254, 269, 270, 272, 273, 276, 278, 318, 319, 326, 330, 332, 333, 335, 337, 340, 344, 350, 357, 359, 362, 365, 367, 369, 371, 376, 380, 418, 425, 426

Deep Q Networks 281, 306, 374

Deep Q-Networks 27, 28, 29, 30, 32, 33, 34, 39, 40, 41, 43, 45, 47, 48, 49, 50, 52, 56, 249, 250, 253, 254, 257, 258, 260, 261, 262, 263, 265, 271, 273, 281, 282, 283, 284, 297, 303, 307, 311, 315, 316, 317, 318, 319, 320, 321, 324, 325, 328, 334, 335, 337, 338, 342, 343, 348, 353, 354, 360, 367, 371, 372, 376

Developing Nations 59, 82

Disease Diagnosis 11, 33, 44, 54, 61, 81, 91, 94, 111, 118, 133, 142, 144, 153, 154, 163, 196, 222, 228, 244, 261, 266, 281, 292, 321, 348

Disease Surveillance 21, 146, 154, 181

Drug Discovery 6, 8, 15, 20, 33, 38, 62, 98, 246, 251, 334, 341, 350, 364, 373, 375, 379, 380, 381, 382, 383, 386, 387, 388, 389, 390, 391, 393, 395, 397, 399, 400, 401, 403

Drug Discovery and Optimization with AI 379


## E


Early Detection 7, 15, 21, 54, 118, 133, 135, 136, 140, 143, 145, 159, 181, 191, 192, 198, 201, 207, 208, 211,

222, 231, 232, 233, 249
Ethical AI 104, 274, 359
Explainable AI 20, 23, 31, 51, 52, 83, 88, 90, 106, 110, 115, 123, 155, 197, 206, 330, 375, 376, 405, 425, 426, 427, 430

# F

Federated Learning 19, 32, 51, 52, 53, 72, 88, 90, 93, 96, 103, 105, 106, 109, 110, 112, 113, 115, 125, 126, 128, 160, 163, 164, 165, 166, 167, 168, 169, 170, 171, 172, 173, 174, 175, 176, 177, 178, 179, 180, 181, 182, 183, 184, 185, 186, 187, 188, 189, 190, 207, 213, 247, 323, 324, 328, 355, 360, 361, 370, 373, 405, 425, 430

# G

Global Health 57, 58, 59, 61, 67, 68, 70, 79, 81, 82, 85, 88, 144, 154, 180, 181, 184, 185, 187, 342

# H

Healthcare 1, 2, 3, 4, 5, 6, 7, 8, 9, 10, 11, 12, 13, 14, 15, 16, 18, 19, 20, 21, 22, 23, 24, 25, 27, 28, 29, 30, 31, 32, 33, 34, 36, 37, 38, 39, 40, 41, 42, 43, 44, 45, 46, 47, 48, 49, 50, 51, 52, 53, 54, 55, 56, 57, 61, 76, 77, 81, 83, 85, 87, 88, 89, 90, 91, 92, 93, 95, 99, 100, 101, 102, 103, 105, 106, 107, 108, 109, 110, 111, 112, 113, 114, 115, 116, 117, 118, 121, 122, 123, 124, 125, 126, 127, 128, 129, 130, 131, 133, 134, 135, 136, 137, 138, 139, 140, 141, 142, 144, 145, 146, 147, 150, 151, 152, 153, 154, 155, 156, 157, 158, 159, 160, 161, 163, 164, 165, 166, 167, 168, 169, 171, 172, 174, 175, 179, 183, 184, 186, 187, 188, 189, 190, 191, 192, 193, 199, 203, 208, 211, 212, 213, 214, 215, 219, 220, 221, 222, 223, 224, 225, 226, 227, 228, 229, 230, 231, 232, 233, 235, 238, 239, 240, 241, 242, 243, 244, 245, 246, 247, 248, 249, 250, 251, 252, 254, 255, 256, 257, 258, 259, 260, 261, 262, 263, 264, 265, 266, 267, 268, 269, 270, 271, 272, 273, 274, 275, 277, 278, 279, 281, 282, 283, 284, 285, 286, 288, 289, 290, 291, 297, 301, 302, 303, 304, 306, 307, 308, 309, 310, 311, 312, 313, 314, 315, 317, 318, 319, 320, 321, 322, 323, 324, 325, 326, 327, 328, 329, 330, 331, 332, 333, 334, 335, 337, 338, 339, 340, 341, 342, 343, 344, 347, 348, 350, 352, 353, 354, 356, 357, 358, 360, 361, 362, 363, 364, 365, 366, 367, 368, 369, 370, 371, 372, 373, 374, 375, 376, 377, 381, 396, 401, 402, 405, 406, 407, 408, 409, 410, 411, 413, 414, 415, 416, 417, 419, 422, 423, 424, 425, 426, 427, 428, 429, 430, 431, 433, 434, 435
Healthcare Data 19, 20, 29, 31, 92, 112, 113, 114, 115, 124, 126, 139, 141, 142, 156, 174, 228, 239, 245, 251, 255, 259, 262, 264, 284, 354, 406
Healthcare Informatics 24, 56, 110, 164, 165, 167, 174, 190
Health Equity 184, 313, 342, 372, 375

# M

Machine Learning 2, 6, 7, 8, 9, 12, 13, 14, 22, 25, 28, 30, 31, 32, 33, 34, 36, 37, 39, 40, 44, 50, 51, 54, 55, 83, 84, 85, 87, 88, 89, 91, 92, 93, 94, 95, 97, 105, 108, 109, 110, 111, 113, 115, 118, 119, 126, 128, 130, 131, 134, 136, 137, 141, 144, 145, 146, 147, 154, 158, 159, 160, 161, 189, 196, 215, 216, 217, 219, 220, 222, 223, 228, 229, 230, 231, 232, 233, 235, 237, 241, 242, 243, 245, 246, 247, 254, 256, 257, 262, 265, 266, 273, 276, 277, 283, 313, 317, 319, 323, 332, 333, 334, 335, 338, 344, 348, 373, 375, 376, 380, 383, 384, 386,

387, 390, 391, 392, 396, 398, 401, 402, 403, 404, 406, 408, 409, 410, 413, 415, 416, 417, 419, 425, 426, 430, 432, 433, 434, 435
Medical Decision-Making 44, 52, 53, 245, 249, 252, 318, 362, 376
Medical Diagnosis 28, 35, 54, 215, 219, 261, 265, 272, 315, 319
Medical Imaging 6, 11, 12, 22, 23, 28, 34, 38, 47, 87, 93, 111, 112, 114, 134, 137, 140, 141, 169, 172, 175, 188, 189, 191, 192, 193, 194, 195, 197, 199, 201, 204, 208, 210, 211, 212, 213, 214, 215, 216, 217, 224, 228, 231, 233, 244, 249, 251, 261, 265, 276, 284, 288, 293, 295, 317, 319, 322, 335, 346, 350, 371, 412, 417, 432
Medical Imaging Analysis 6, 93, 193, 194

## P

Personalized Medicine 6, 14, 38, 41, 46, 51, 52, 54, 87, 97, 99, 102, 107, 192, 203, 214, 233, 235, 236, 242, 275, 318, 324, 325, 326, 327, 332, 333, 396, 397, 406, 407, 413, 416, 417
Personalized Treatment Strategies 27, 193, 204, 212
Predictive Analytics 2, 12, 13, 14, 16, 21, 23, 24, 27, 28, 30, 31, 37, 41, 52, 111, 112, 113, 114, 115, 118, 119, 120, 121, 124, 125, 127, 128, 129, 131, 133, 134, 135, 136, 137, 138, 139, 140, 144, 145, 146, 147, 149, 150, 151, 152, 153, 154, 155, 156, 157, 158, 159, 219, 220, 233, 237, 243, 261, 262, 274, 281, 292, 294, 311, 320, 338, 379, 380, 407, 408, 415, 416, 430
Privacy-Preserving AI 19, 105, 163, 166, 213

## R

Real-Time Decision Support 34, 49, 147, 149, 304, 305
Reinforcement Learning 9, 27, 28, 29, 31, 32, 33, 34, 35, 36, 38, 40, 41, 43, 44, 50, 51, 52, 56, 91, 108, 229, 249, 250, 253, 254, 256, 257, 258, 261, 262, 263, 264, 265, 271, 272, 273, 278, 281, 282, 283, 284, 285, 287, 288, 289, 290, 291, 292, 294, 295, 299, 300, 301, 302, 303, 304, 305, 307, 308, 309, 310, 311, 312, 313, 314, 315, 316, 317, 318, 320, 321, 322, 324, 325, 326, 327, 328, 329, 330, 332, 333, 334, 335, 337, 338, 339, 343, 348, 350, 352, 354, 361, 364, 367, 373, 374, 375, 376, 377, 383, 391, 398, 408, 409, 435
Risk Assessment 12, 13, 14, 94, 101, 111, 114, 120, 121, 133, 134, 154, 230, 279, 294, 417, 427

## S

Smart Healthcare 6, 25, 33, 36, 38, 39, 40, 51, 56, 87, 88, 89, 90, 91, 92, 93, 100, 102, 105, 107, 108, 110, 160, 245, 247, 275, 302, 303, 319, 321, 328, 337, 342, 343, 348, 353, 354, 360, 376, 405, 406, 407, 415
Smart Healthcare Systems 36, 38, 51, 90, 93, 105, 108, 110, 160, 247, 275, 319

## T

Telemedicine 6, 21, 29, 38, 40, 43, 46, 48, 61, 63, 66, 81, 83, 90, 156, 160, 247, 337, 352, 353, 423, 424, 432

www.ingramcontent.com/pod-product-compliance
Lightning Source LLC
LaVergne TN
LVHW062335300926
849161LV00007B/1704